Donald School
Atlas of
Fetal Anomalies

Donald School
Atlas of
Fetal Anomalies

2nd Edition

Editors

Asim Kurjak MD PhD
Professor, Department of Obstetrics and Gynecology
Medical School University of Zagreb
Zagreb, Croatia
Professor Emeritus
University Sarajevo School of Science and Technology
Sarajevo, Bosnia and Herzegovina

Ritsuko K Pooh MD MSc PhD LLB
President
Fetal Diagnostic Center
Fetal Brain Center
CRIFM Prenatal Medical Clinic
Osaka, Japan

Frank A Chervenak MD MMM
Chair, Obstetrics and Gynecology
Lenox Hill Hospital
Chair, Obstetrics and Gynecology
Associate Dean for International Medicine
Zucker School of Medicine at Hofstra/Northwell
New York, New York, USA

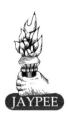

JAYPEE BROTHERS MEDICAL PUBLISHERS
The Health Sciences Publisher
New Delhi | London

Jaypee Brothers Medical Publishers (P) Ltd

Headquarters

Jaypee Brothers Medical Publishers (P) Ltd
EMCA House, 23/23-B
Ansari Road, Daryaganj
New Delhi 110 002, India
Landline: +91-11-23272143, +91-11-23272703
+91-11-23282021, +91-11-23245672
Email: jaypee@jaypeebrothers.com

Corporate Office

Jaypee Brothers Medical Publishers (P) Ltd
4838/24, Ansari Road, Daryaganj
New Delhi 110 002, India
Phone: +91-11-43574357
Fax: +91-11-43574314
Email: jaypee@jaypeebrothers.com

Overseas Office

JP Medical Ltd
83 Victoria Street, London
SW1H 0HW (UK)
Phone: +44 20 3170 8910
Fax: +44 (0)20 3008 6180
Email: info@jpmedpub.com

Website: www.jaypeebrothers.com
Website: www.jaypeedigital.com

Donald School Atlas of Fetal Anomalies

First Edition: 2007

Second Edition: **2023**

ISBN: 978-93-5465-851-8

Printed at: Replika Press Pvt. Ltd.

Dedication

Our book is dedicated to two giants who are no longer with us but have left their imprint for generations to come by enhancing the care of maternal, fetal and neonatal patients throughout the world:

Ian Donald, *Founder of Modern Obstetric and Gynecologic Ultrasound*

Erich Saling, *Father of Perinatal Medicine*

Contributors

Badreldeen Ahmed FRCOG MD
Professor of Obstetrics
Weill Cornell Medical College
Doha, Qatar
Professor of Obstetrics
Qatar University, Doha
Professor of Obstetrics and Gynecology
University Sarajevo School of
Science and Technology
Sarajevo, Bosnia and Herzegovina
Director of Feto-Maternal Centre
Doha, Qatar

Apostolos Athanasiadis MD PhD
Professor of Obstetrics and Gynecology –
Maternal Fetal Medicine
3rd Department of Obstetrics and
Gynecology
Aristotle University of Thessaloniki
Thessaloniki, Greece

Guillermo Azumendi Pérez MD PhD
Professor
Centro Gutenberg, Malaga, Spain

M Lisa Bartholomew MD
Associate Professor
Department of Obstetrics and
Gynecology and Women's Health
John A Burns School of Medicine
University of Hawaii
Honolulu, Hawaii, USA

Alin Basgül Yigiter MD PhD
Former Professor
Department of Obstetrics and Gynecology
Marmara University School of Medicine
Istanbul, Turkey

Fernando Bonilla-Musoles MD PhD
Professor and Doctor Honoris Causa
Department of Obstetrics and
Gynecology
Valencia School of Medicine
Valencia, Spain

Tatjana Božanović MD PhD
Professor
Institute for Obstetrics and Gynecology
Clinical Center of Serbia
School of Medicine University of Belgrade
Belgrade, Serbia

Jacek Brązert MD PhD
Professor
Department of Obstetrics and
Female Health
Chair of Gynecology, Obstetrics and
Gynecological Oncology
Poznan University of Medical Sciences
Poznan, Poland

Jose Maria Carrera MD PhD
Professor
Matres Mundi, Barcelona, Spain

Frank A Chervenak MD MMM
Chair, Obstetrics and Gynecology
Lenox Hill Hospital
Chair, Obstetrics and Gynecology
Associate Dean for International Medicine
Zucker School of Medicine at Hofstra/
Northwell
New York, New York, USA

Dušan Damnjanović MD PhD
Assistant Professor
Ars Medica, School of Medicine
University of Belgrade, Belgrade, Serbia

Milica Đurđić MD
Head
Department of Radiology
Biocell Hospital, Vincula Biotech Group
Belgrade, Serbia

Pamela Grant MD
Assistant Professor
Department of Obstetrics and Gynecology
and Women's Health
John A Burns School of Medicine
University of Hawaii
Honolulu, Hawaii, USA

Toshiyuki Hata MD PhD
Special Adviser
Department of Obstetrics and
Gynecology, Miyake Clinic
Okayama-shi, Okayama, Japan
Professor Emeritus
Department of Perinatology and
Gynecology
Kagawa University
Graduate School of Medicine
Miki, Kagawa, Japan

Rafał Iciek MD PhD
Department of Obstetrics and
Female Health
Chair of Gynecology, Obstetrics and
Gynecological Oncology
Poznan University of Medical Sciences
Poznan, Poland

Ida Jovanović MD PhD
Professor and Head
Department of Pediatrics
Biocell Hospital, Vincula Biotech Group
Belgrade, Serbia

Kenji Kanenishi MD PhD
Professor and Chairman
Department of Perinatology and
Gynecology, Kagawa University
Graduate School of Medicine
Miki, Kagawa, Japan

Aya Koyanagi RMS
Sonographer
Department of Obstetrics and Gynecology
Miyake Clinic
Okayama-shi, Okayama, Japan

Asim Kurjak MD PhD
Professor
Department of Obstetrics and
Gynecology
Medical School University of Zagreb
Zagreb, Croatia
Professor Emeritus
University Sarajevo School of
Science and Technology
Sarajevo, Bosnia and Herzegovina

Alexandra Shera Lieb
Student
American University of Antigua
College of Medicine
Osbourn, Antigua and Barbuda

Aleksandar Ljubić MD PhD
Professor
Department of Obstetrics and Gynecology
Chairman of the Supervisory Board and
Co-Owner
Biocell Hospital, Vincula Biotech Group
Belgrade, Serbia

Luiz Eduardo Machado MD PhD
Professor
Department of Obstetrics and Gynecology
Salvador School of Medicine
Salvador, Brazil

Themistoklis Mikos MD PhD
Associate Professor
1st Department of Obstetrics and
Gynecology
Aristotle University of Thessaloniki
Thessaloniki, Greece

Takahito Miyake MD PhD
President
Department of Obstetrics and
Gynecology, Miyake Clinic
Okayama-shi, Okayama, Japan
Clinical Professor
Department of Perinatology and
Gynecology, Kagawa University
Graduate School of Medicine
Miki, Kagawa, Japan

Zehra Nese Kavak MD PhD
Professor
Department of Obstetrics, Gynecology
and Perinatology
Academic Hospital
Istanbul, Turkey

Ertan Ozen MD
Department of Obstetrics and
Gynecology
Academic Hospital
Istanbul, Turkey

Sonal Panchal MD
Consultant
Dr Nagori's Institute for Infertility and IVF
Ahmedabad, Gujarat, India

Panayiota Papasozomenou MD PhD
Obstetrician-Gynecologist
Fetal Medicine Specialist
International Hellenic University
Thessaloniki, Greece

Andjela Perović MD
Department of Obstetrics and Gynecology
Biocell Hospital, Vincula Biotech Group
Belgrade, Serbia

Dušica Petrović MSc
Clinical Embryologist
IVF Laboratory
Biocell Hospital, Vincula Biotech Group
Belgrade, Serbia

Marek Pietryga MD PhD
Professor
Department of Obstetrics and
Female Health
Chair of Gynecology, Obstetrics and
Gynecological Oncology
Poznan University of Medical Sciences
Poznan, Poland
Prenatal Diagnostic Center
Gynecology and Obstetrics Hospital
Poznan University of Medical Sciences
Poznan, Poland

Ritsuko K Pooh MD MSc PhD LLB
President
Fetal Diagnostic Center
Fetal Brain Center
CRIFM Prenatal Medical Clinic
Osaka, Japan

Bernat Serra Zantop MD PhD
Consultant
Department of Obstetrics and Gynecology
University Hospital Quirón Dexeus
Barcelona, Spain

Milena Srbinović MD
Department of Obstetrics and Gynecology
Medigroup, Belgrade, Serbia

Milan Stanojević MD PhD
Professor
Neonatal Unit, Department of Obstetrics
and Gynecology
Medical School University of Zagreb
Sveti Duh Hospital
Zagreb, Croatia

Riko Takayoshi MD
Consultant
Department of Obstetrics and Gynecology
Miyake Clinic
Okayama-shi, Okayama, Japan
Research Student
Department of Perinatology and
Gynecology
Kagawa University Graduate School of
Medicine, Miki, Kagawa, Japan

Kinga Toboła-Wróbel MD PhD
Department of Obstetrics and
Female Health
Chair of Gynecology, Obstetrics and
Gynecological Oncology
Poznan University of Medical Sciences
Poznan, Poland

Alina Veduta MD PhD
Senior Consultant
Department of Obstetrics and Gynecology
Filantropia Hospital
Bucharest, Romania

Radu Vladareanu MD PhD
Professor and Chairman
Department of Obstetrics and Gynecology
Carol Davila University of
Medicine and Pharmacy
Elias University Hospital
Bucharest, Romania

Simona Vladareanu MD PhD
Professor and Chairman
Department of Neonatology
Carol Davila University of
Medicine and Pharmacy
Elias University Hospital
Bucharest, Romania

Kenneth Ward MD
Professor and Chairman
Department of Obstetrics and Gynecology
and Women's Health
John A Burns School of Medicine
University of Hawaii
Honolulu, Hawaii, USA

Menelaos Zafrakas MD PhD
Professor
Department of Obstetrics and Gynecology
International Hellenic University
Thessaloniki, Greece

Ivica Zalud MD PhD
Professor and Chair
Kosasa Endowed Chair
Department of Obstetrics and Gynecology
and Women's Health
John A Burns School of Medicine
University of Hawaii
Honolulu, Hawaii, USA

Preface

It could be argued that during the past more than 60 years, the three greatest breakthroughs in obstetrics have been ultrasound, ultrasound, and ultrasound. The analysis of fetal growth, fetal gestational age, fetal well-being, fetal behavior, fetal number, even the presence of fetal life itself are now easily performed in clinical obstetrics—whereby they were not prior to the development of ultrasound.

Probably, the greatest impact ultrasound has made on the clinical practice of obstetrics, has been in the diagnosis of fetal anomalies. Prior to the availability of ultrasound, fetal anomalies were diagnosed after delivery as an unwelcome surprise. Many women and their families suffered by the tragic news that their long awaited child would die because of a serious defect. For others, the tragedy was worse in that an anomaly was present which would have benefited by delivery in a tertiary center where morbidity and mortality would be minimized. The genius of Ian Donald, the pioneer of obstetric ultrasound has changed this dramatically. Fetal diagnosis of most anomalies is now possible in second and often the first trimester of pregnancy. This enables the pregnant woman to be informed and have the options of optimal perinatal care and termination of pregnancy available.

This textbook describes all aspects of the ultrasound diagnosis of fetal anomalies. The latest ultrasound technologies, including 4D ultrasound and color Doppler ultrasound are utilized to define the spectrum of ultrasound manifestations of fetal defects. System by system is analyzed in a methodical manner to make the text clinically useful for beginner in the use of ultrasound as well as seasoned veterans.

We are grateful to the contributors to this volume who represent the world' leaders in the field. Most are directors of the Ian Donald Inter-university School of Ultrasound. Since the birth of obstetric ultrasound, it has been truly global in its innovation and clinical application. We believe that we can best honor the spirit of Ian Donald by emphasizing worldwide cooperation in education and research in the ultrasound diagnosis of fetal anomalies.

Asim Kurjak
Ritsuko K Pooh
Frank A Chervenak

Acknowledgments

Our book would not have been possible without the international brotherhood and sisterhood of the Ian Donald School of Ultrasound and the tireless and selfless work of the authors who have contributed to this book and have taught throughout the world.

Contents

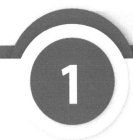

Ultrasound and Fetal Anomalies

Frank A Chervenak, Asim Kurjak, Jose Maria Carrera

■ INTRODUCTION

Antenatal ultrasound scanning at about 18–20 weeks of gestation permits the detection of most major fetal structural anomalies.[1-7] It is important to appreciate, however, that even a thorough ultrasound evaluation during the second trimester will not detect all structural malformations. Such anomalies as hydrocephalus, duodenal atresia, microcephaly, achondroplasia, and polycystic kidneys may not manifest until the third trimester, when the degree of anatomic distortion is sufficient to be sonographically detectable. A useful classification of fetal anomalies is based on the nature of the dysmorphology that permits sonographic detection.

We will review here normal anatomy, diagnosis of fetal anomalies, and management of fetal anomaly. To illustrate diagnostic possibilities few ultrasonograms were used from other chapters in this book with the permission of authors (R Pooh, Z Nese Kavak, A Basgul, G Azumendi).

SONOGRAPHIC EVALUATION OF FETAL ANATOMY

Evaluation of fetal anatomy is an integral part of ultrasound examinations during the second and third trimesters. Ultrasound examinations that document fetal life, fetal number, fetal presentation, gestational age, and growth assessment, amniotic fluid volume assessment, and placental localization without an evaluation of fetal anatomy, therefore, should be considered incomplete. The following is meant to represent the examination of fetal anatomy that should be part of the basic examination. Sonographic examination of fetal anatomy is often more detailed when it is targeted to look for a certain anomaly.[8-19]

The fetal skull should be elliptical with the cranium ossified and intact. The ventricular system should be evaluated by assessment of the width of the atrium and the cerebellum should be visualized **(Fig. 1)** and nuchal thickness measured **(Fig. 2)**. An attempt should be made to visualize the face, especially to rule out a facial cleft **(Figs. 3A and B)**. The spine is easier to evaluate in its entirety in the second trimester than in the third. A sagittal sonogram should be complemented by a series of transverse sonograms to identify normal anterior and normal posterior ossification elements **(Figs. 4A to C)**. A four-chambered view of the heart should be obtained. Ventricles and atria of equal and appropriate sizes and an intact ventricular septum should be observed **(Fig. 5)**. Evaluation of the outflow tracts should be attempted **(Fig. 6)**. The abdominal wall should be intact. The fetal kidneys, bladder, and stomach **(Figs. 7A to F)** should be visualized. The long bones of at least the lower extremities should be visualized **(Fig. 8)**. Although fetal gender often may be identified in the second and third trimesters, this should not be considered an integral part of the examination[8-19] **(Figs. 9A to D)**.

■ TRANSVAGINAL ULTRASOUND

Transvaginal ultrasound with its ability to use higher frequency transducers can result in better visualization of the early pregnancy. The gestational sac, yolk sac, and embryo can be seen earlier and with more detail than transabdominal ultrasound. Extrauterine pathology, such as an ectopic pregnancy or an ovarian mass, can be better evaluated.[20-23] This enhanced visualization with vaginal ultrasound is especially important in the obese patient and when there is a retroverted or myomatous uterus.

A gestational sac can be seen with transvaginal ultrasound as early as 4.5 menstrual weeks.[24,25] This sac is surrounded by an echogenic ring which represents trophoblastic tissue. The normal gestational sac is located in the upper uterine body and has a smooth contour and a round shape. Once seen, the gestational sac grows at a fairly constant rate of 1 mm in mean diameter per day.[26]

The yolk sac is visualized when the gestational sac is >10 mm. Visualization of a yolk sac documents that an

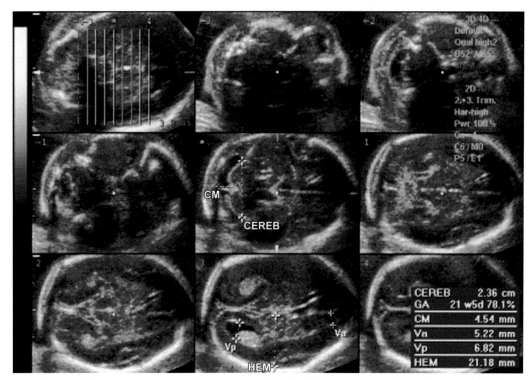

Fig. 1: Measurement of the cerebellum, cysterna magna, hemisphere, and both of the ventricles can be performed easily using multislice imaging.

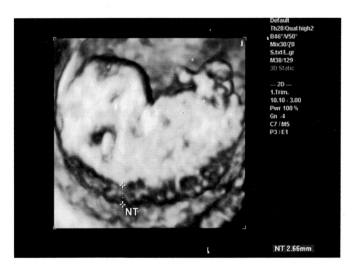

Fig. 2: Visualization of increased nuchal thickness in fetus complicated by Turner syndrome.

anechoic area in the uterus represents a true gestational sac and not the pseudogestational sac seen in ectopic pregnancy. Between the seventh and the thirteenth menstrual week the yolk sac gradually increases in diameter from about 3 to 6 mm[27,28] **(Figs. 10 to 13)**.

The amnion develops about the same time as the yolk sac but, because it is thinner, the amnion is more difficult to visualize. It surrounds the embryo and is opposite to the yolk sac. The amnion grows rapidly during the early pregnancy and fusion with the chorion is usually complete by the 16th week. At that time, the extraembryonic celom is obliterated.

Cardiac activity is usually the first manifestation of the embryo at about six menstrual weeks. Once the embryo is 5 mm, cardiac activity should be present; its absence is indicative of early demise.[29,30] When cardiac activity is not present and the embryo is >5 mm, the findings are not conclusive. The normal heart rate can be as low as 90 BPM at six menstrual weeks and increases during the first trimester.[31] Embryonic movements can be seen between seven and eight menstrual weeks.

Although the gestational sac can be used to date an early pregnancy, the most accurate sonographic method is the crown-rump length.[32] During the first trimester, this method is accurate to within 4–5 days. As this is the best tool to assess gestational age during the whole pregnancy, it should be considered in patients at risk for growth retardation and other prenatal complications.

The embryonic pole, a flat, echogenic structure, can be visualized when it is 2–4 mm during the seventh menstrual week. During the eighth week a large head with a posterior cystic space, representing the rhombencephalon, can be visualized, together with the spinal column and the lower and upper extremities. By the ninth week, the falx cerebri and the choroid plexus can be visualized and, by the 11th week, the echogenic choroid plexus fills the prominent ventricles. The cerebellum may not be visualized until after 12 weeks.[20-24]

Between the 8th and the 12th weeks there is a normal midgut herniation[33] **(Fig. 13)** This should not be confused with an omphalocele, which can be diagnosed with certainty after that time. The liver can be seen at 9–10 weeks; the stomach, at 10–12 weeks; the bladder, at 11–13 weeks; and the four chambers, at about 12 weeks.[20-24]

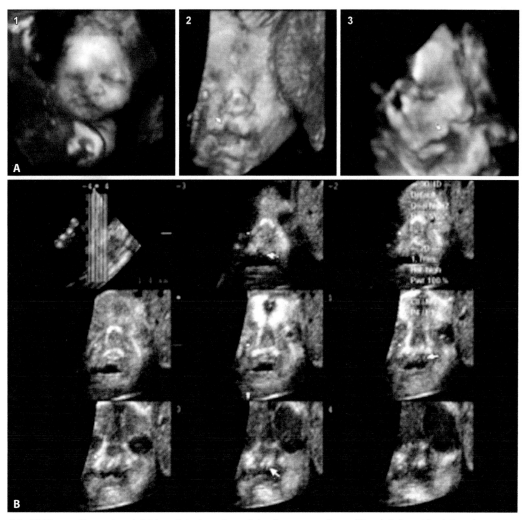

Figs. 3A and B: (A) Three-dimensional (3D) surface imaging of the fetus complicated by cleft lip with cleft palate; (B) Tomographic ultrasound imaging demonstrated slice-by-slice facial anatomy in this anomaly.

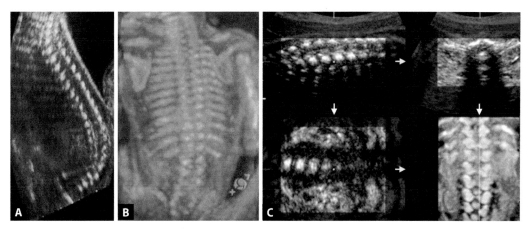

Figs. 4A to C: (A) Two-dimensional (2D) sonogram of normal vertebral structure obtained from the sagittal axis; (B and C) Three-dimensional (3D) maximum mode can be used to assess the whole length of vertebral structure.

Many of the fetal anomalies described above during 18–20 weeks transabdominal anatomic survey can be diagnosed earlier with transvaginal ultrasound. The anomalies with the most serious disruptions of anatomy, such as anencephaly, holoprosencephaly, cystic hygroma, and conjoined twins, could be detected[20-24] **(Figs. 14A to H)**. However, at this time, first trimester vaginal ultrasound is not as accurate in detecting anomalies. This is because some structures, such as the brain, are not as well developed and other structures, such as the heart, are too small, to be adequately evaluated.

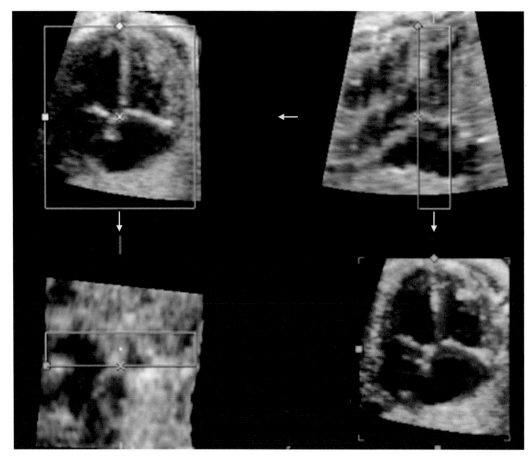

Fig. 5: Spatiotemporal image correlation (STIC) can easily be used to obtain four-chamber view of the heart.

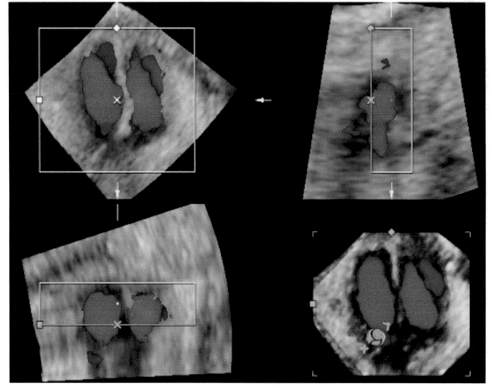

Fig. 6: Visualization of outflow tract can be depicted using spatiotemporal image correlation (STIC) method.

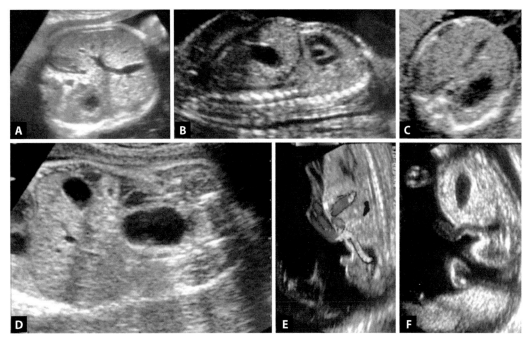

Figs. 7A to F: Normal visualization of abdominal structure by two-dimensional (2D) sonography. (A) Abdominal structure obtained in the transverse plane; (B) Normal appearance of the abdominal organs from the longitudinal axis; (C) Intact abdominal wall structure from the transverse plane; (D) Visualization of fetal bladder from coronal plane; (E and F) Insertion of the umbilical cord can be easily depicted by 2D sonography.

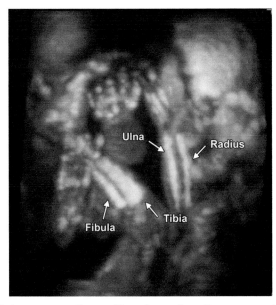

Fig. 8: Appearance of normal long bones from the upper and lower extremities. Three-dimensional (3D) maximum mode can depict the bones structure.

Therefore, first trimester ultrasound should not be used as a substitute for a second trimester evaluation of anatomy.[34]

An important aspect of first trimester vaginal ultrasound is the evaluation of nuchal thickness to predict chromosomal aberrations. Nicolaides has shown that a nuchal translucency >3 mm **(Fig. 15)** at 10–13 weeks of gestation occurs in 86% of trisomic and 4.5% of chromosomally normal fetuses.

In addition, the observed number of trisomies when the nuchal translucency was <3 mm was five times less than the number expected on the basis of maternal age.[35] This simple sonographic sign can therefore discriminate between high-risk and low-risk groups for trisomy and may be of great value to patients in deciding either for or against invasive testing to determine the fetal karyotype.[36]

Although the main value of vaginal ultrasound is in early pregnancy, it may be of clinical use later in gestation. Vaginal ultrasound permits direct visualization of the internal cervical os and therefore permits accurate assessment of the location of the placenta and its distance from the internal os. The diagnosis or exclusion of placenta previa is therefore facilitated.[37] In addition, because the cervix can be accurately visualized, vaginal ultrasound may identify early signs of preterm labor or incompetent cervix, such as funneling or shortening of the cervical length[18] and thereby directly aid in patient care. Lastly, vaginal ultrasound can improve visualization of intracranial anatomy when the head is engaged and permits enhanced views of cranial structures in coronal and sagittal planes.[38]

ABSENCE OF A NORMALLY PRESENT STRUCTURE

A dramatic example of the absence of a structure normally detected by ultrasound is anencephaly, the absence of calvaria and forebrain. Ultrasound clearly reveals the absence of echogenic skull bones and the presence of

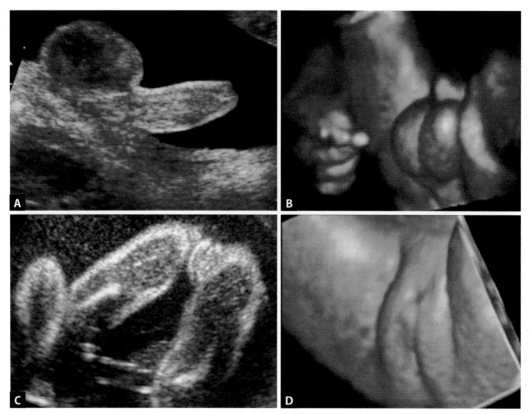

Figs. 9A to D: Normal appearance of male (A and B) and female (C and D) fetal genital using two different methods.

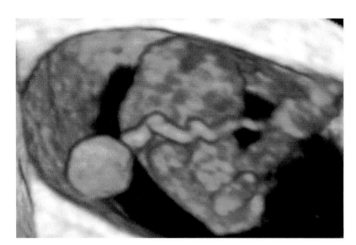

Fig. 10: Three-dimensional (3D) sonogram demonstrating crown-rump length (between crosses) of 8 weeks fetus. Yolk sac is in the near field.

a heterogeneous mass of cystic tissue, called the area cerebrovasculosa, which replaces well-defined cerebral structures. In 1972, anencephaly was the first fetal anomaly to be diagnosed with sufficient certainty to support a decision to terminate a pregnancy[39] **(Figs. 16A to C).**

Alobar holoprosencephaly is the absence of midline cerebral structures, resulting from incomplete cleavage of the primitive forebrain. The "midline echo" of the fetal head, normally generated by acoustic interfaces in the area of the interhemispheric fissure, is absent. However, absence of a midline echo is not specific to alobar holoprosencephaly; an additional sonographic sign should be sought to confirm a diagnosis, which may include hypotelorism, nasal anomalies, and facial clefts. The detection of the facial aberration helps to confirm the diagnosis of alobar holoprosencephaly[40] **(Figs. 17A to C).**

The kidneys are normally visualized as bilateral, ovoid, paraspinal masses with echospared renal pelvises. When not visualized, the diagnosis of renal agenesis should be suspected. Severe oligohydramnios and the inability to visualize the bladder support the diagnosis of renal agenesis. Although antenatal diagnosis of renal agenesis is possible, false-positive and false-negative diagnoses occur from inadequate visualization due to the presence of oligohydramnios and simulation of the sonographic appearance of kidneys by the ovoid-shaped adrenal glands.[41]

■ PRESENCE OF AN ADDITIONAL STRUCTURE

Masses that distort normal fetal anatomy can be readily identified with ultrasound. Fetal teratomas are the most common neoplasms of fetuses. They are derived from pluripotent cells and are composed of a diversity of tissue foreign to the anatomic site from which they arise. They may be visualized as distortions of fetal contour, often in the sacrococcygeal area or along the fetal midline.

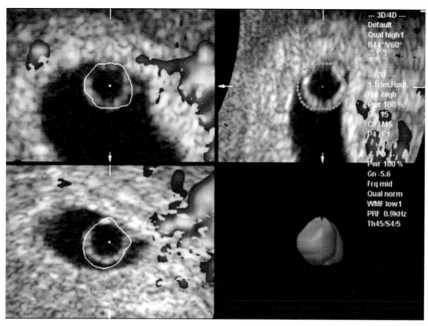

Fig. 11: Volumetric calculation of the yolk sac during 6 weeks of gestation can be performed using VOCAL™ software.

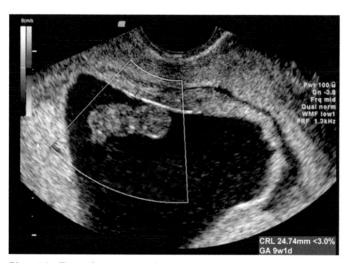

Fig. 12: Two-dimensional (2D) color Doppler sonogram demonstrating embryonic demise in 9 weeks embryo. No heart activity was present.

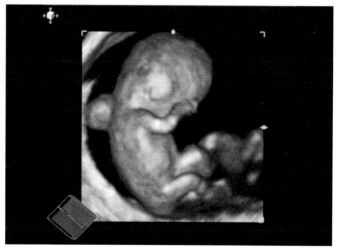

Fig. 13: Crosses outline normal midgut herniation in 10 weeks fetus.

The internal sonographic appearance, characterized by irregular cystic and solid areas and occasional calcifications, helps to identify the lesion[42] **(Figs. 18A to E)**.

Fetal cystic hygromas are fluid-filled masses of the fetal neck which arise from abnormal lymphatic development. They are generally anechoic, with scattered septations and the presence of a midline septum arising from the nuchal ligament. If the lymphatic disorder causing the hygromas is widespread, it may produce fetal hydrops and intrauterine death[43,44] **(Figs. 19A to C)**.

Fetal hydrops or fetal anasarca may be identified by the distortion of the normal fetal surface by skin edema.

Ascites, pleural effusions, and pericardial effusions also may be identified. The etiologies of fetal hydrops are many and varied[45-47] **(Figs. 20A to C)**.

HERNIATION THROUGH STRUCTURAL DEFECTS

A common theme in the development of the fetus is the formation of compartments containing vital structures by folding and midline fusion. Incomplete fusion in a variety of locations can lead to defects and herniations of contained structures.[48]

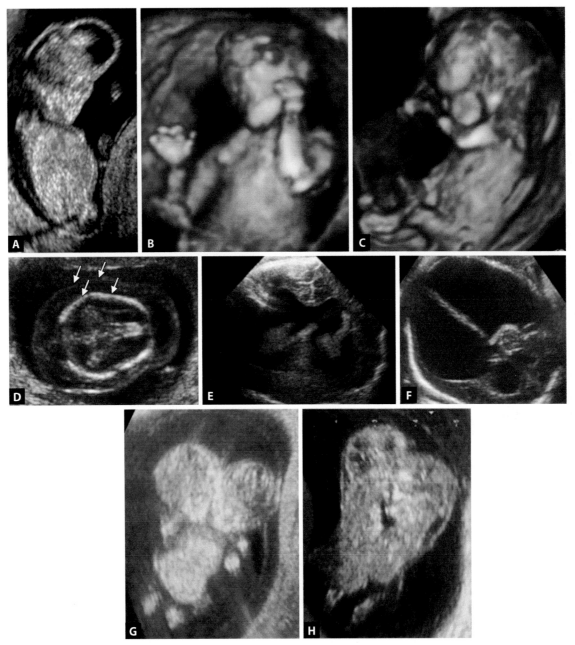

Figs. 14A to H: (A) Two-dimensional (2D) sonogram of acrania fetus at 12 weeks of gestation; (B) Three-dimensional (3D) sonogram of anencephalic fetus at 14 weeks of gestation; (C) 3D surface rendering of fetus complicated by Turner syndrome demonstrated increase nuchal thickness; (D) Early fetal hydrops during the first trimester demonstrated by 2D sonography; (E and F) 2D sonogram of fetus complicated by holoprosencephaly and hydrocephalus; (G and H) Sonograms of conjoined twins.

The neural tube and overlying mesoderm begin their closure in the region of the fourth somite, with fusion extending both rostrally and caudally during the fourth week of fetal life.[17] Incomplete closure at the rostral end produces cephaloceles, with herniations of meninges and, frequently, of brain substance through a defect in the cranium[49] **(Figs. 21A and B)**. Failed fusion at the caudal end produces spina bifida with protruding meningoceles and meningomyeloceles **(Figs. 22A to C)**. Sonographic diagnosis of each of these anomalies depends on the demonstration of

a defect in the normal structure of the cranium or spine and of a protruding sac, often containing tissue.[50,51]

The Arnold–Chiari malformation is an anomaly of the hindbrain that has two components. The first is a variable displacement of a tongue of spinal canal. The second is a similar caudal dislocation of the medulla and fourth ventricle. Most, if not all, cases of spina bifida are complicated by the Arnold–Chiari malformation.[52] The Arnold–Chiari malformation can serve, therefore, as an important marker for spina bifida. Two characteristic sonographic signs

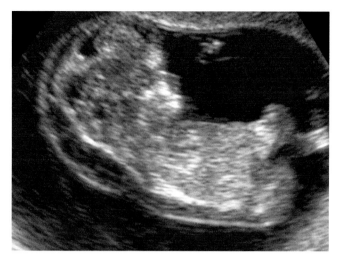

Fig. 15: Sonogram demonstrating nuchal translucency >3 mm in 10 weeks embryo.

(the "lemon" and the "banana") of the Arnold–Chiari malformation have been described. A scalloping of the frontal bones can give a lemon-like configuration, in axial section, to the skull of an affected fetus during the second trimester. The caudal displacement of the cranial contents within a pliable skull is thought to produce this scalloping effect. Similarly, as the cerebellar hemispheres are displaced into the cervical canal, they are flattened rostrocaudally and the cisterna magna is obliterated, thus producing a flattened, centrally curved, banana-like sonographic appearance. In extreme instances, the cerebellar hemispheres may be absent from view during fetal head scanning. These characteristic cranial signs are valuable adjuncts to the sonographer in the search for spina bifida[53] **(Figs. 23A to D)**.

Omphaloceles result from failure of the intestines to retract from their temporary location in the umbilical cord and the subsequent herniation of other abdominal

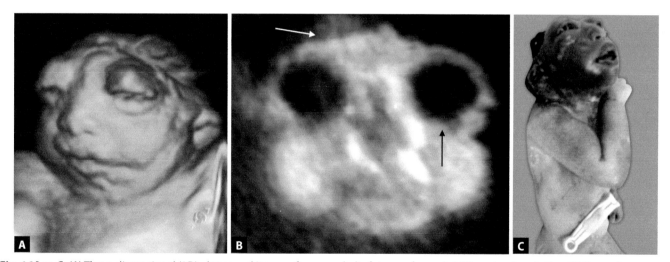

Fig. 16A to C: (A) Three-dimensional (3D) ultrasound image of anencephalic fetus performed at 30 weeks of gestation; (B) Coronal sonogram of fetal head demonstrating anencephaly. Black arrow points to orbits. White arrow points to area cerebrovasculosa; (C) Postmortem photograph of infant with anencephaly demonstrating prominent area cerebrovasculosa.

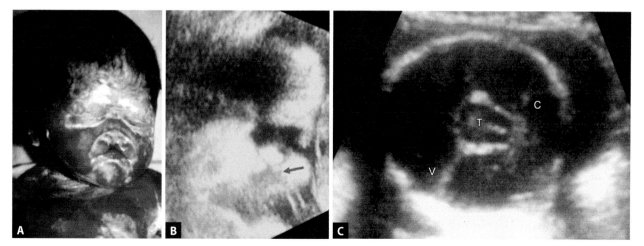

Figs. 17A to C: (A) Postmortem photograph of holoprosencephaly; (B) Ultrasound sonogram of midline facial defects in the same case; (C) Cranial sonogram demonstrating alobar holoprosencephaly. (V: common ventricle, T: prominent fused thalamus; C: compressed cerebral cortex).

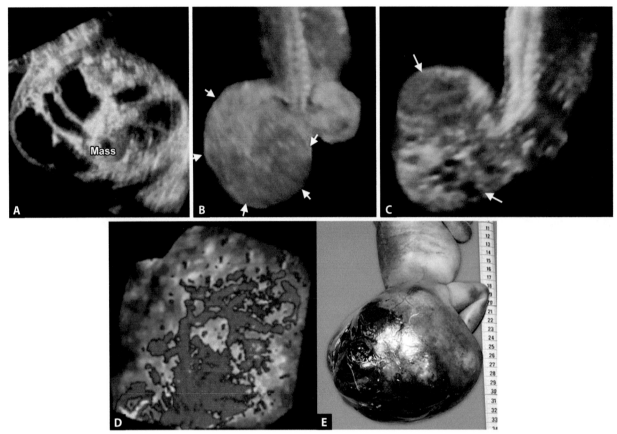

Figs. 18A to E: Sonogram of sacrococcygeal teratoma outlined by protruding beneath fetal spine. (A) Visualization of teratoma mass by two-dimensional (2D) sonography; (B and C) Three-dimensional (3D) surface rendering and maximum mode in visualization of the tumor; and (D) 3D power Doppler of the tumor vascularization; (E) Neonate with sacrococcygeal teratoma.

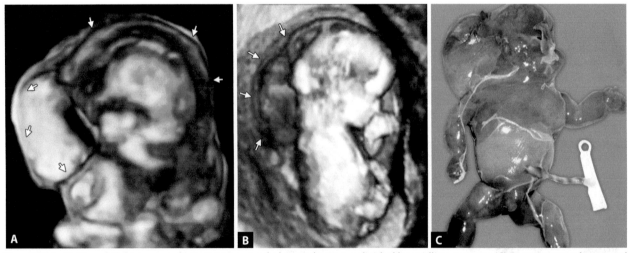

Figs. 19A to C: (A and B) Sonogram demonstrating nuchal cystic hygroma divided by midline septum; (C) Postmortem photograph demonstrating fetus with cystic hygroma protruding from posterolateral neck.

contents, including both hollow and solid structures contained within a peritoneal sac. Insertion of the umbilical cord into the sac helps to differentiate an omphalocele from gastroschisis, which has no covering membrane. Nonetheless, distinguishing these two entities may be difficult[54] **(Figs. 24 and 25).**

The diaphragm forms from four separate structures that fuse to separate the pleural and peritoneal cavities. When a diaphragmatic hernia is present, abdominal contents may be visualized within the chest on transverse sonographic scanning. A disruption in this development of the diaphragm may be seen in the sagittal plane.[55,56]

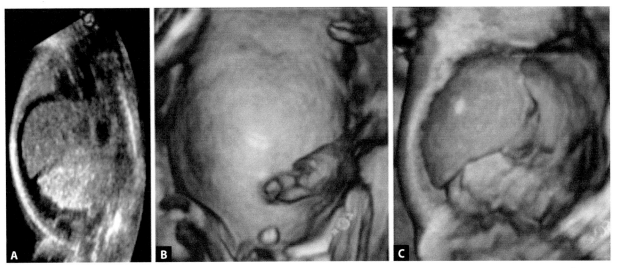

Figs. 20A to C: (A) Visualization of fetal hydrops by two-dimensional (2D) sonography; (B and C) Three-dimensional (3D) surface rendering through fetal abdomen demonstrating fetal hydrops.

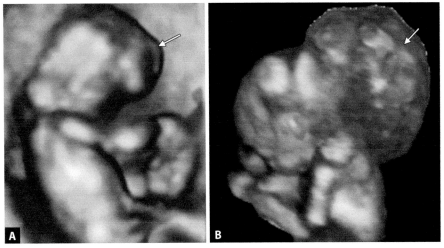

Figs. 21A and B: (A) Three-dimensional (3D) surface rendering of frontal encephalocele; (B) Large encephalocele with resultant microcephaly.

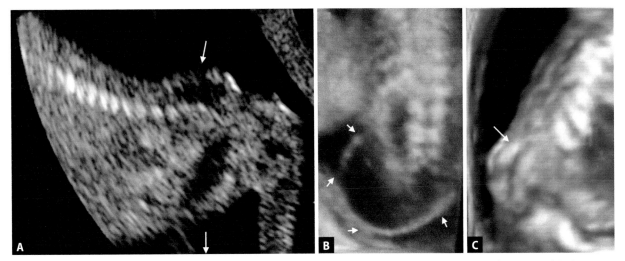

Figs. 22A to C: (A) Two-dimensional (2D) sonogram demonstrated meningomyelocele; (B and C) Three-dimensional (3D) sonogram of fetal spine with arrows pointing to meningomyelocele.

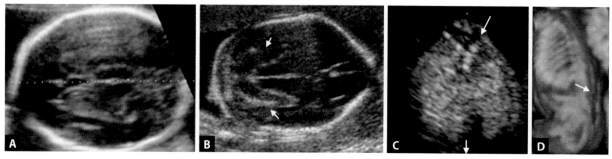

Figs. 23A to D: (A) Transverse section of normal fetal head in an 18-week fetus at level of cavum septi pellucidi; (B and C) Transverse section of fetal head at level of cavum septi pellucidi in an 18-week fetus with open spina bifida showing "lemon" and "banana" sign; (D) Three-dimensional (3D) surface rendering of fetus with spina bifida.

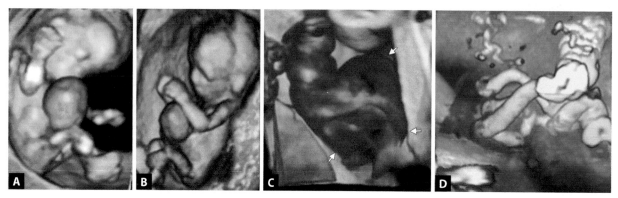

Figs. 24A to D: (A and B) Three-dimensional (3D) surface rendering of fetus with omphalocele at 12 weeks of gestation; (C) 3D sonogram of fetus with omphalocele at 28 weeks of gestation; (D) 3D power Doppler of vascularization inside the omphalocele structure.

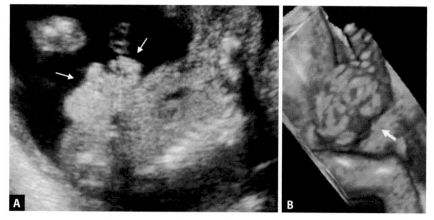

Figs. 25A and B: (A) Two-dimensional (2D) sonogram of fetus with gastroschisis at 20 weeks of gestation; (B) Visualization of gastroschisis by three-dimensional (3D) surface rendering.

■ DILATATION BEHIND AN OBSTRUCTION

In this class of anomalies, the structural defect itself is rarely seen. Rather, what is observed is the distention of structures behind a defect. Such dilatation is caused by obstruction to the normal flow of cerebrospinal fluid, urine, or swallowed amniotic fluid.

Hydrocephalus is characterized by a relative enlargement of the cerebroventricular system with an accompanying increase of pressure of the cerebrospinal fluid within the fetal head. Hydrocephalus is suggested by a lateral ventricular

atrial width >1 cm,[57-59] a dangling choroid plexus,[60] and an asymmetric appearance of the choroid plexus.[59,60] The location of the obstruction may be determined by observing which portions of the ventricular system are enlarged **(Figs. 26A to C)**. There is a frequent association of fetal hydrocephalus with other anomalies, especially spina bifida.[61]

Fetal small bowel obstruction may cause dilatation proximal to the area of obstruction. Duodenal atresia has been observed to produce its characteristic "double

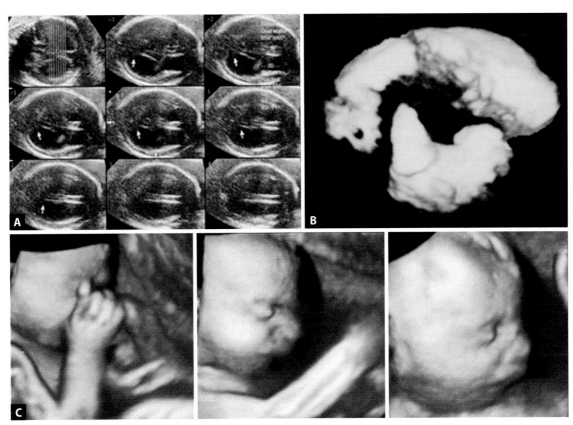

Figs. 26A to C: (A) Tomographic ultrasound imaging of fetal hydrocephalus (arrows); (B) Visualization of entire cerebrospinal fluid in hydrocephalus using three-dimensional (3D) inverse mode; (C) Changing of facial expression of hydrocephalic fetus can be observed using four-dimensional (4D) sonographic technique.

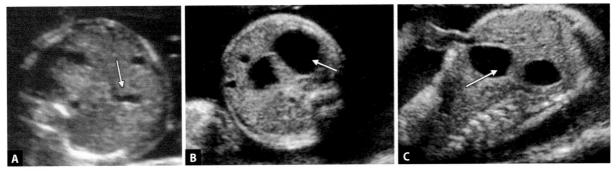

Figs. 27A to C: (A) Sonogram demonstrating normal duodenum (arrow); (B and C) Sonogram illustrating classic "double bubble" sign. The two echofree areas (arrows) represent the stomach and proximal duodenum.

bubble" sign, consisting of enlarged duodenum and stomach with narrowing at the pylorus and duodenum, is commonly associated with Down syndrome[62,63] **(Figs. 27A to C)**. Obstruction in the lower gastrointestinal tract (e.g., imperforate anus) is generally not detected on antenatal ultrasound unless there is an associated lesion.

Obstructions to urinary flow with proximal dilatation have occurred at the uteropelvic and uterovesicular junctions **(Figs. 28A to C)**. These are commonly unilateral defects, whereas obstruction at the urethra from posterior urethral valves characteristically produces bilateral dilatation of the ureters and renal pelves.[64,65] When a posterior urethral valve produces a complete obstruction, renal dysplasia and pulmonary hypoplasia may result.

ABNORMAL FETAL BIOMETRY

Several fetal anomalies are best diagnosed not by observing alterations in shape or consistency, but by determining abnormalities in size. The science of fetal biometry has generated many nomograms defining normal values for parts of the fetal anatomy at various gestational ages.[66]

Fetal microcephaly is usually the result of an underdeveloped brain. Although commonly associated with cerebral structural malformations, microcephaly may be produced by a brain that is normal in configuration but merely small. The accurate diagnosis of microcephaly has proved challenging because compressive forces within the uterus may distort the shape of the fetal head. The best correlation between microcephaly diagnosed in utero and neonatal microcephaly is made when multiple parameters are measured and suggest a small head.[67-69]

A variety of skeletal dysplasias may affect the growth of long bones. Measurement may suggest a particular skeletal dysplasia, depending on which bones are foreshortened. The shape of these bones, their density, the presence of fractures, or the absence of specific bones may aid in differentiating the various bony abnormalities.[70]

When interorbital distances are inconsistent with gestational age, hypotelorism or hypertelorism may be suggested. Abnormal distance between the orbits may serve as a clue to several malformation syndromes (e.g., alobar holoprosencephaly[40] and median cleft face syndrome[71]) **(Figs. 29A to D).**

The internal architecture of the kidneys may be difficult to assess in the presence of oligohydramnios. The diagnosis of polycystic kidneys thus is aided by renal measurement.

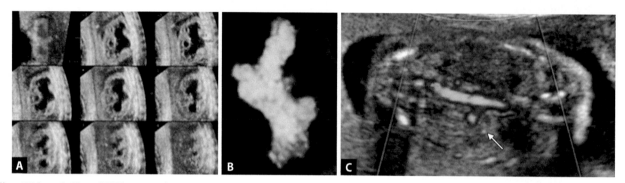

Figs. 28A to C: (A and B) Tomographic sonogram demonstrating hydronephrosis with dilated renal pelvis and calyces; (C) Sonogram demonstrating dysplastic right kidney (arrow) and normal left kidney.

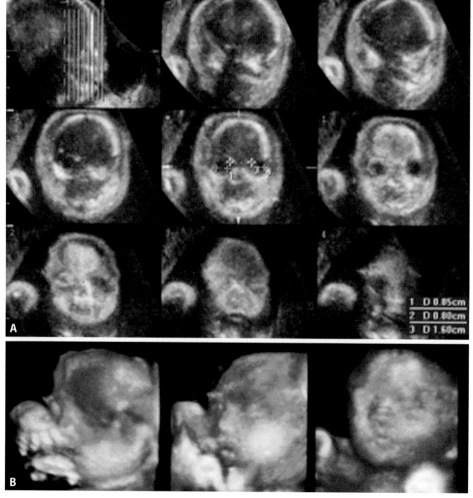

Figs. 29A and B

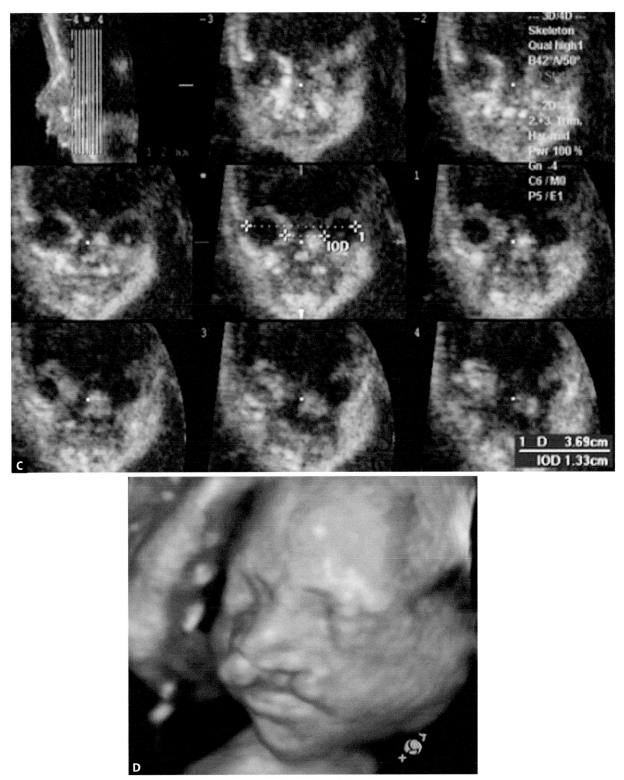

Figs. 29C and D

Figs. 29A to D: (A) Coronal scan through orbits of fetus demonstrates hypertelorism. Inner orbital distance (IOD) and outer orbital distance (OOD) are increased for gestational age of 31 weeks. Tomographic ultrasound imaging demonstrated slice-by-slice facial anatomy and level of the hypertelorism in trisomy 18; (B) Visualization of rounded face and hypertelorism in trisomy 18 by 3D US; (C) Coronal scan through orbits of normal fetus at 37 weeks of gestation demonstrates normal IOD and OOD; (D) Fetus with median cleft face syndrome demonstrated by three-dimensional (3D) surface rendering.

In addition to being echogenic, polycystic kidneys usually are enlarged and display an abnormally increased kidney-circumference/abdominal-circumference ratio.[72,73]

■ ABSENT OR ABNORMAL FETAL MOTION

Abnormalities in fetal motion may suggest a malformation that cannot itself be seen. Although the fetus normally can assume contorted positions in utero, the persistence of such an unusual posture over time may suggest an orthopedic or neurologic anomaly such as clubfoot[74] **(Figs. 30A to C)** or arthrogryposis.[75]

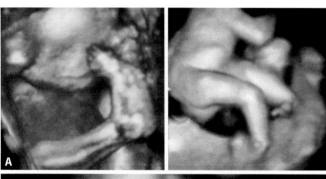
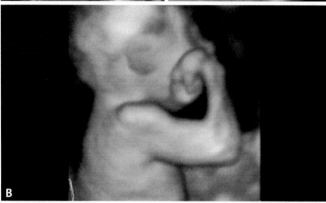
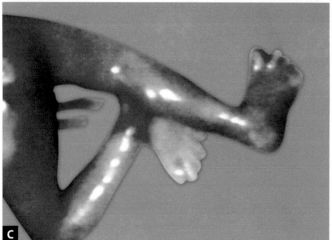

Figs. 30A to C: (A and B) Visualization of club foot by Three-dimensional (3D) surface imaging in the fetus complicated by arthrogryposis multiplex congenital; (C) Postmortem photograph demonstrating clubfoot.

The fetal heart is the most conspicuously dynamic part of the fetus. Real-time ultrasound is invaluable in diagnosing most fetal cardiac anomalies **(Figs. 31A to C)**. A four-chamber view of the heart should be obtained in obstetrical ultrasound examination in which fetal anatomy is surveyed. Examination of the fetal outflow tracts increases the detection of heart anomalies. In cases of a suspected fetal arrhythmia, atrial, and ventricular rates can be determined.[76-81]

■ ULTRASOUND DETECTION OF CHROMOSOMAL ABNORMALITIES

Ultrasound examination can suggest a chromosomal aberration. Sonographic markers for the most serious karyotype abnormalities are often present. Holoprosencephaly, facial clefts, hypotelorism, omphalocele, polydactyly, and heart defects are associated with trisomy 13, while growth retardation, micrognathus, overlapping fingers, omphalocele, horseshoe kidney, and heart defects are associated with trisomy 18. Early onset severe growth retardation, large head, syndactyly, and heart defects suggest triploidy. Turner syndrome (45X) is classically associated with nuchal cystic hygroma but this ultrasound finding can occur in a wide variety of genetic disorders.[31,36,82,83]

Major structural malformations, including hydrops, duodenal atresia, and heart defects are associated with trisomy 21 but are detected sonographically in only about 30% of cases.[84,85] Nuchal skin thickness, defined as >6 mm is a useful screening tool for trisomy 21 and other chromosomal malformations[84,86,87] **(Figs. 32A to D)**. Other sonographers used to screen for Down syndrome, including short femur, short humerus, pyelectasis, mild cerebral ventriculomegaly, clinodactyly with hypoplastic middle phalanx of the fifth digit, widely spaced first and second toe, low set ears, echogenic bowel, and a single palmar crease.[84,85,88]

Choroid plexus cysts can occur in about 1% of fetuses and are most closely associated with trisomy 18 but can be associated with other chromosomal abnormalities[89,90] **(Fig. 33)**. The necessity for karyotype determination is controversial because trisomy 18 usually has other sonographic markers.[91,92] Benaceraff has calculated that the performance of amniocentesis for choroid plexus cysts would result in more fetal loss than detection of unsuspected chromosomal aberrations.[92] In the authors' view, when a choroid plexus cyst is identified with ultrasound, it should be disclosed to the pregnant woman and amniocentesis offered, but not recommended.

In summary, if a major structural malformation is detected with ultrasound, karyotype determination should be considered by the pregnant woman. At the present time, nuchal thickness is a most clinically useful ultrasound marker for trisomy with the relative value of other ultrasound markers under investigation.

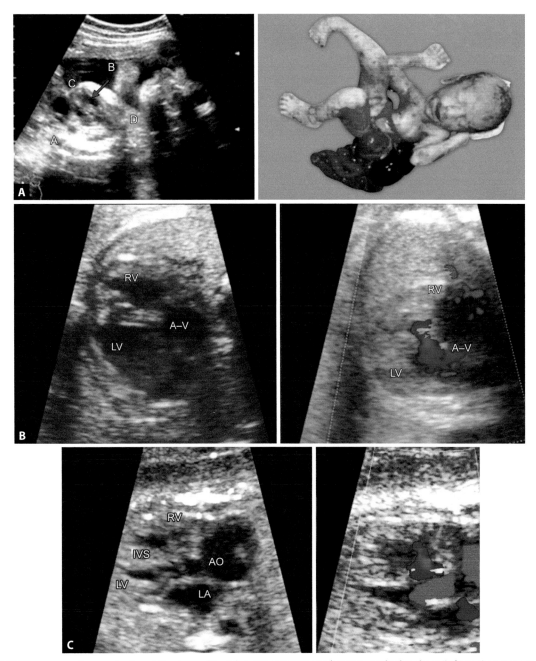

Figs. 31A to C: (A) Sonogram demonstrating ectopic cordis with arrow pointing to heart outside the chest (left) and postmortem photograph of the fetus with body stalk anomaly showing ectopic cordis (right); (B) Sonogram demonstrating A-V canal in fetus with Down syndrome; (C) Sonogram of fetus with tetralogy of Fallot demonstrating enlarged aortic outflow tract (AO). Its anterior wall overrides the interventricular septum (IVS).
(RV: right ventricle; LV: left ventricle: LA: left atrium).

MANAGEMENT OF A PREGNANCY COMPLICATED BY AN ULTRASONICALLY DIAGNOSED FETAL ANOMALY

If a fetal anomaly is diagnosed by obstetric ultrasound, the fetus should be carefully evaluated for other anomalies before management options can be considered. Echocardiography and karyotype determination usually should be part of this evaluation. Copel et al. have shown that 23% of fetuses referred for echocardiography because of an extracardiac anomaly had congenital heart disease.[93] Approximately one-third of fetuses with structural anomalies has a chromosomal disorder.[94-96] This additional information is invaluable to define fetal prognosis. For example, the prognosis for isolated hydrocephalus is substantially better than that for hydrocephalus associated with alobar holoprosencephaly and trisomy 13. Amniocentesis is the most widely utilized technique for determination of fetal karyotype when an ultrasonically diagnosed anomaly is detected, but fetal

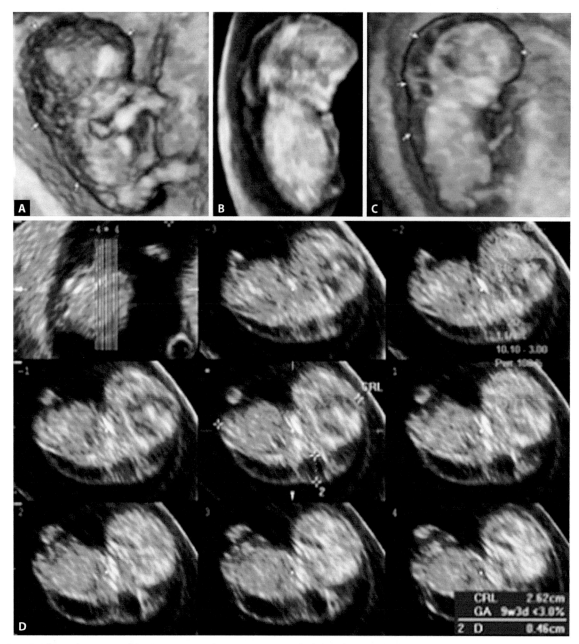

Figs. 32A to D: Three-dimensional (3D) sonogram demonstrating nuchal skin thickness >3 mm (A to C) and Tomographic ultrasound imaging of fetus with increased nuchal thickness (D).

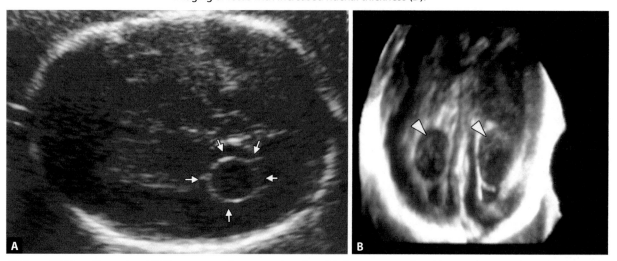

Figs. 33A and B: Two-dimensional (2D) sonogram demonstrating choroid plexus cyst outlined by arrows (A) and visualization of the choroid plexus cyst by three-dimensional (3D) surface imaging (B).

blood sampling or placental biopsy may be necessary if a rapid result is required.

After the fetal evaluation is completed, the certainties and uncertainties of fetal prognosis should be explained to the pregnant woman. The disclosure requirements of the informed consent process require the physician to present information about the range of available management options: aggressive management, termination of pregnancy, nonaggressive management, and cephalocentesis.[97] These disclosure requirements obligate the physician to be objective when presenting this information. That is, the physician is not justified in withholding information about available management options to which he or she might object for reasons of personal conscience.[98]

Aggressive Management

In order to optimize fetal outcome, there should be an interdisciplinary approach, including specialists in maternal-fetal medicine, neonatology, genetics, pediatric surgery, and pediatric cardiology.[99-101] Social work services may provide important support to the family before as well as after birth. Such a team approach is best equipped to address the important questions of where, when, and how the infant should be delivered, as well as the role of invasive fetal therapy.

Most infants with anomalies are best delivered in a referral center with a neonatal intensive care unit experienced in caring for such infants. In such a setting, there is immediate access to diagnostic and therapeutic medical and surgical interventions.

Delivery at term is optimal for most fetal anomalies. For some anomalies, however, such as hydrocephalus, delivery as soon as fetal lung maturation has occurred may be advisable in order to expedite corrective neonatal surgery.[102] Rarely, because of the risk of imminent fetal death, an anomaly such as progressive fetal hydrops may necessitate delivery prior to fetal lung maturity.[100]

Most fetuses with anomalies can be delivered vaginally. Cesarean delivery may necessary to avoid dystocia if certain conditions are present, such as a sacrococcygeal teratoma or conjoined twins. For other anomalies, such as spina bifida, cesarean delivery may be recommended in order to minimize trauma to fetal tissues.[103]

Rarely, an invasive approach during the antenatal period may be considered to optimize outcome when there is a sonographically diagnosed anomaly. This should only be considered when the natural history of the anomaly diagnosed is dismal and a relatively simple intrauterine correction is possible. The sonographic and karyotypic evaluation described above is especially important before an invasive approach can be considered. The disclosure requirements of the informed consent process necessitate that the experimental nature of invasive fetal therapy at

this time and potential harms to the fetus and the mother be carefully explained. In addition, it is generally agreed that such an approach after 32 weeks of gestation offers no clear advantage over delivery and neonatal treatment. Given the risk of inflicted premature delivery as well as the experimental nature of these procedures, a normal coincident twin is considered to be a contraindication to such an approach.[99,100,104]

The most common form of invasive fetal therapy has been intrauterine shunt placement. The purpose of such a shunt is to drain fluid under high pressure in a fetal organ to the lower pressure of the amniotic fluid. Such a shunt may have a role in the treatment of a complete bladder outlet obstruction which would be expected to eventually result in renal failure and pulmonary failure.[104-106] Analysis of fetal urine after bladder aspiration may help to define which fetuses are candidates for this vesiculoamniotic shunt.[106,107] Intrauterine aspiration or shunt placement may also be of value in cases of isolated pleural effusions[108-110] **(Figs. 34A to D)**. In fetal hydrocephalus, however, current experience does not demonstrate a clear benefit to ventriculoamniotic shunt placement which should be avoided.[104,111-113]

The San Francisco group has pioneered open fetal surgery to manage such conditions as congenital diaphragmatic hernia and complete bladder obstruction. In such cases, there is hysterotomy and exteriorization of the fetus then repair, replacement, and continuation of the pregnancy.[99,103] At this time, it is not possible to make a final judgment concerning the place of this fascinating modality in fetal therapy because more clinical experience is needed to better define the benefits to the fetus and the harms to the mother.

Termination of Pregnancy

Prior to fetal viability abortion of any pregnancy is a woman's right as established by Roe versus Wade in the United States.[114] The option of abortion prior to fetal viability is, therefore, available to a pregnant woman when any fetal anomaly is diagnosed by ultrasound. Ethically, this option is supported by an approach that holds that all of obstetric ethics is essentially a function of the pregnant woman's autonomy[115,116] as well as an approach which holds that autonomous-based obligations to the pregnant woman should be balanced against beneficence-based obligations to her and the fetus that she is carrying.[108]

After fetal viability there is limited legal access in the United States to termination of pregnancy because of a fetal anomaly. Ethically, the option of terminating third trimester pregnancies complicated by fetal anomalies has been defended when there is (1) certainty of diagnosis and (2) either (a) certainty of death as an outcome of the anomaly diagnosed or, (b) in some cases of short-term survival, certainty of the absence of cognitive developmental capacity as a result of the anomaly diagnosed. Anencephaly is a clear

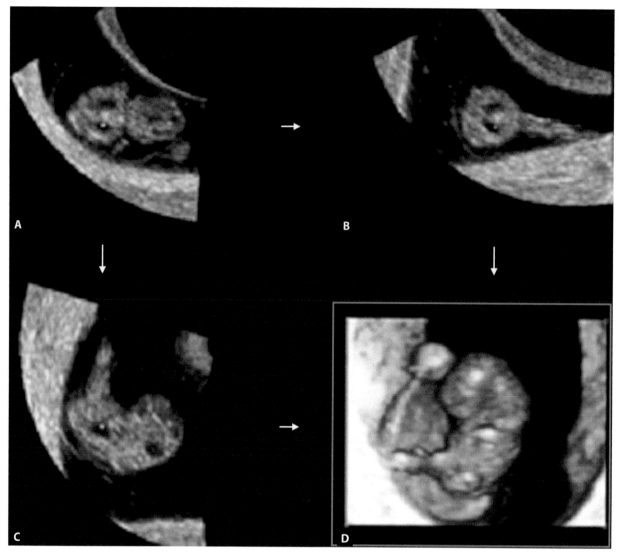

Figs. 34A to D: Pleural effusion at 9 weeks of gestation. Three orthogonal views (A to C) and three-dimensional (3D) surface image (D). Bilateral pleural effusion is clearly demonstrated.

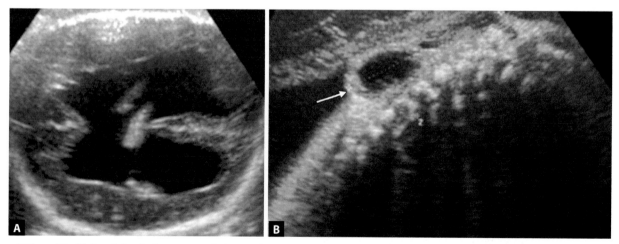

Figs. 35A and B: (A) Semilobar holoprosencephaly visualized by two-dimensional (2D) sonography; (B) The same fetus demonstrated myelomeningocele in the lumbar region.

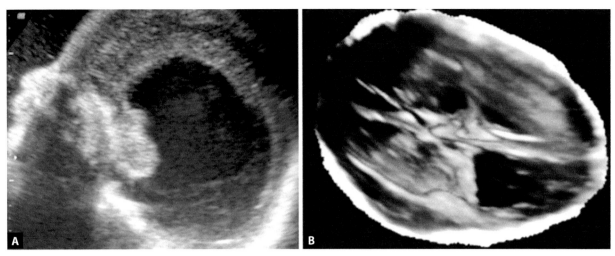

Figs. 36A and B: (A) Fetus at 30 weeks of gestation complicated by hydrocephalus; (B) Three-dimensional (3D) sonogram of the same fetus.

example of a sonographically diagnosed anomaly that meets these criteria.[117] Trisomy 21 is a clear example of an anomaly that does not meet these criteria.[118]

Nonaggressive Management

The abovementioned criteria for termination of pregnancy for fetal anomalies during the third trimester are quite restrictive. In addition, even if ethical criteria for third trimester termination of pregnancy were met, it may not be possible to perform termination in some situations because of legal concerns. Nonaggressive management is the noninclusion of obstetric interventions to benefit the fetus, such as fetal surveillance, tocolysis, cesarean delivery, or delivery in a referral center. Ethically, the option of nonaggressive management for third trimester pregnancies complicated by fetal anomalies has been defended when there is (1) a very high probability of a correct diagnosis and (2) either (a) a very high probability of death as an outcome of the anomaly diagnosed or (b) a very high probability of severe irreversible deficit of cognitive developmental capacity as a result of the anomaly diagnosed.[119]

Cephalocentesis

When a pregnancy is complicated be fetal hydrocephalus with macrocephaly there may be a role for cephalocentesis, which is the transabdominal or transvaginal aspiration of cerebrospinal fluid to avoid cesarean delivery. Ethical justification for this procedure can be based on an analysis of beneficence-based and autonomy-based obligations to the pregnant woman and the fetus she is carrying. Such an analysis needs to respect the heterogeneity of fetal hydrocephalus: isolated fetal hydrocephalus, hydrocephalus with severe associated anomalies (such as holoprosencephaly), and hydrocephalus with other associated anomalies (such as arachnoid cyst)[120,121] **(Figs. 35 and 36)**.

■ REFERENCES

1. Sabbagha R (Ed). Diagnostic Ultrasound Applied to Obstetrics and Gynecology. Philadelphia: JB Lippincott; 1994.
2. Chervenak FA, Isaacson G, Campbell S (Eds). Ultrasound in Obstetrics and Gynecology. Philadelphia: Little, Brown, 1993.
3. Manning FA. The anomalous fetus. In: Manning FA (Ed). Fetal Medicine: Principles and Practice. Norwalk: Appleton and Lange; 1995.
4. McGahan JP, Porto M (Eds). Diagnostic Ultrasound. Philadelphia: JB Lippincott; 1994.
5. Callen P (Ed). Ultrasonography in Obstetrics and Gynecology, 3rd edition. Philadelphia: WB Saunders; 1994.
6. Romero R, Pilu G, Jeanty P, Ghidini A, Hobbins JC (Eds). Prenatal Diagnosis of Congenital Anomalies. Norwalk: Appleton and Lange; 1988.
7. Nyberg DA, Mahony BS, Pretorius DH (Eds). Diagnostic Ultrasound of Fetal Anomalies: Text and Atlas. Chicago: Year Book; 1990.
8. Nyberg DA, Mahony, BS, Pretorius DH. Diagnostic Ultrasound and Fetal Anomalies: Text and Atlas. Chicago: Year Book; 1990.
9. Romero R, Pilu G, Jeanty P, Ghidini A, Hobbins JC (Eds). Prenatal Diagnosis of Congenital Anomalies. Norwalk: Appleton and Lange; 1988.
10. Seeds JS, Azizkhan RG. Congenital Malformations: Antenatal Diagnosis, Perinatal Management, and Counseling. Rockville: Aspen; 1990.
11. Chervenak FA, Isaacson G, Lorber J. Anomalies of the Fetal Head, Neck, and Spine: Ultrasound Diagnosis and Management. Philadelphia: WB Saunders; 1988.
12. Ultrasound in Pregnancy. ACOG Technical Bulletin 116. Washington, DC: American College of Obstetricians and Gynecologists; 1988.
13. Leopold GR. Antepartum obstetrical ultrasound examination guidelines. J Ultrasound Med. 1986;5:241-2.
14. Filly RA. Level 1, level 2, level 3 obstetric sonography: I'll see your level and raise you one. Radiology. 1989;172:312.
15. Callen PN. Ultrasonography in Obstetrics and Gynecology. Philadelphia: WB Saunders; 1994. p. 1.
16. Sabbagha RE, Kamel EM. Standard Ultrasound Obstetric Examination in Diagnostic Ultrasound Applied to Obstetrics and Gynecology. Philadelphia: JB Lippincott; 1994. p. 59.

17. Campbell S. The obstetric ultrasound examination. In: Chervenak FA, Isaacson G, Campbell S (Eds). Ultrasound in Obstetrics and Gynecology. Philadelphia: Little, Brown; 1993. p. 187.

18. Azumendi G, Arenas JB, Andonotopo W. Three dimensional sonoembryology. In: Kurjak A (Ed). Textbook of Transvaginal Sonography. London: Taylor and Francis; 2005. pp. 396-407.

19. Andonotopo W, Kurjak A, Azumendi G. Early normal pregnancy. In: Carrera JM, Kurjak A (Eds). Atlas of Clinical Application of Ultrasound in Obstetrics and Gynecology. New Delhi: Jaypee Brothers Medical Publishers Pvt Ltd.; 2006. pp. 25-50.

20. Timor-Tritsch IE, Rottem S (Eds). Transvaginal Sonography, 2nd edition. New York; Elsevier Science; 1991.

21. Fleischer AC, Kepple DM. Transvaginal Sonography: A Clinical Atlas. Philadelphia: JB Lippincott; 1992.

22. Nyber DA, Hill LM, Bohm-Veley M, Mendelson EB. Transvaginal Ultrasound. Saint Louis: Mosby Year Book; 1992.

23. Dodson MG. Transvaginal Ultrasound. New York: Churchill Livingstone; 1991.

24. Timor-Tritsch IE, Rottem S. Normal and abnormal fetal anatomy in the first fifteen weeks. In: Sabbagha RE (Ed). Diagnostic Ultrasound Applied to Obstetrics and Gynecology, 3rd edition. Philadelphia: JB Lippincott; 1994. p. 353.

25. Fossum GT, Davagan V, Kletzky DA. Early detection of pregnancy with transvaginal ultrasound. Fertil Steril. 1988;49:788-91.

26. Nyberg DA, Mack LA, Laing FC, Palten RM. Distinguishing normal from abnormal gestational sac growth in early pregnancy. J Ultrasound Med. 1987;6:23-7.

27. Reece EA, Scioscia AL, Pinter E, Hobbins JC, Green J, Mahoney MJ, et al. Prognostic significance of the human yolk sac assessed by ultrasonography. Am J Obstet Gynecol. 1988;159:1191-4.

28. Lindsay DJ, Lovett IS, Lyons EA, Levi CS, Zheng XH, Holt SC, et al. Yolk sac diameter and shape at endovaginal US: predictors of pregnancy outcome in the first trimester. Radiology. 1992;183:115-8.

29. Levi CS, Lyons EA, Zheng XH, Lindsay DJ, Holt SC. Endovaginal US: demonstration of cardiac activity in embryos of less than 5.0 mm in crown-rump length. Radiology. 1990;176:71-4.

30. Brown DL, Emerson DS, Felker RE, Cartier MS, Smith WC. Diagnosis of early embryonic demise by endovaginal sonography. J Ultrasound Med. 1990;9:631-6.

31. Howe RS, Isaacson HJ, Albert JL, Contiforis CB. Embryonic heart rate in human pregnancy. J Ultrasound Med. 1991;10:367-71.

32. Robinson HP, Fleming JE. A critical evaluation of sonar crown-rump length measurement. Brit J Obstet Gynæcol. 1975;82:702-10.

33. Timor-Tritsch IE, Warner WB, Peisner DB, Pirrone E. First trimester midgut herniation: a high-frequency transvaginal sonographic study. Am J Obstet Gynecol. 1989;161:831-3.

34. Philips J. Sensitivity and specificity in ultrasonographic screening. In: Simpson Jl, Elias S (Eds). Essentials of Prenatal Diagnosis. New York: Churchill Livingstone; 1993. p. 141.

35. Nicolaides KM. Fetal nuchal translucency: ultrasound screening for fetal trisomy in the first trimester of pregnancy. Brit J Obstet Gynæcol. 1994;101:782-6.

36. Gome ZR, Galasso M, Romero R, Mazor M, Sorokin Y, Gonçalves L, et al. Ultrasonographic examination of the uterine cervix is better than cervical digital examination as a predictor of the likelihood of premature delivery in patients with preterm labor and intact membranes. Am J Obstet Gynecol. 1994;171:956-64.

37. Farine D, FOX HE, Timor-Tritsch IE. Vaginal approach to the ultrasound diagnosis of placenta previa. In: Chervenak FA, Isaacson G, Campbell S (Eds). Ultrasound in Obstetrics and Gynecology. Philadelphia: Little, Brown; 1993. p. 1503.

38. Monteagudo A, Reuss ML, Timor-Tritsch IE. Imaging the fetal brain in the second trimester using transvaginal sonography. Obstet Gynecol. 1991;77:27-32.

39. Campbell S, Johnstone FD, Hold EM, May P. Anencephaly: early ultrasonic diagnosis and active management. Lancet. 1972;2:1226-7.

40. Chervenak FA, Isaacson G, Mahoney MJ, Tortora M, Mesologites T, Hobbins JC, et al. The obstetric significance of holoprosencephaly. Obstet Gynecol. 1984;63:115-21.

41. Romero R, Cullen M, Grannum P, Jeanty P, Reece EA, Venus I, et al. Antenatal diagnosis of renal anomalies with ultrasound. III. Bilateral renal agenesis. Am J Obstet Gynecol. 1985;151:38-43.

42. Chervenak FA, Isaacson G, Touloukian R, Tortora M, Berkowitz RL, Hobbins JC. The diagnosis and management of fetal teratomas. Obstet Gynecol. 1985;66(5):666-71.

43. Chervenak FA, Isaacson G, Blakemore KJ, Breg WR, Hobbins JC, Berkowitz RL, et al. Fetal cystic hygroma: cause and natural history. N Engl J Med. 1984;309:822-5.

44. Johnson MP, Johnson A, Holzgreve W, Isada NB, Wapner RJ, Treadwell MC, et al. First trimester cystic hygromas: cause and outcome. Am J Obstet Gynecol. 1993;168:156-61.

45. Holzgreve W, Curry CJR, Golbus MS. Investigation of nonimmune hydrops fetalis. Am J Obstet Gynecol. 1984; 150:805-12.

46. Machin GA. Hydrops revisited: literature review of 1,414 cases published in the 1980s. Am J Med Genetics. 1989;34:366-90.

47. Santolaya J, Alley D, Jaffe R, Warsof SL. Antenatal classification of hydrops fetalis. Obstet Gynecol. 1992;79:256-9.

48. Arey LB. Developmental Anatomy. Philadelphia: WB Saunders; 1974. pp. 245-262 & 465-499.

49. Chervenak FA, Isaacson G, Mahoney MJ, Berkowitz RL, Tortora M, Hobbins JC. The diagnosis and management of fetal cephalocele. Obstet Gynecol. 1984;64:86-91.

50. Hobbins JC, Venus I, Tortora M, Mayden K, Mahoney MJ. Stage II ultrasound examination for the diagnosis of fetal abnormalities with an elevated amniotic fluid alpha-fetoprotein concentration. Am J Obstet Gynecol. 1982;142:1026-9.

51. Platt LD, Feuchtbaum L, Filly R, Lustig L, Simon M, Cunningham GC. The California maternal serum alpha-fetoprotein screening program: the role of ultrasonography in the detection of spina bifida. Obstet Gynecol. 1992;166:1328-9.

52. McIntosh R. The incidence of congenital malformations: A study of 5,964 pregnancies. Pediatrics. 1954;14:505-22.

53. Nicolaides KH, Campbell S, Gabbe SG, Guidetti R. Ultrasound screening for spina bifida: cranial and cerebellar signs. Lancet. 1986;2(8498):72-4.

54. Nakayama DK, Harrison RM, Gross BH, Callen PW, Filly RA, Golbus MS, et al. Management of the fetus with an abdominal wall defect. J Pediatr Surg. 1984;19:408-13.

55. Marwood RP, Davison OW. Antenatal diagnosis of diaphragmatic hernia. Br J Obstet Gynecol. 1981;88:71-2.

56. Sharlane GK, Lockhart SM, Heward AJ, Allan P. Prognosis in fetal diaphragmatic hernia. Am J Obstet Gynecol. 1992;166:9.

57. Cardoza JD, Goldstein RB, Filly RA. Exclusion of fetal ventriculomegaly with a single measurement: the width of the lateral ventricular atrium. Radiology. 1988;169:711-4.

58. Cardoza JD, Filly RA, Podarsky AE. The dangling choroid plexus: a sonographic observation of value in excluding ventriculomegaly. AJR Am J Roentgenol. 1988;151:767-70.

59. Benaceraff BR, Birnholz JC. The diagnosis of fetal hydrocephalus prior to 22 weeks. J Clin Ultrasound. 1987;15:531-6.

60. Benaceraff BR. Fetal hydrocephalus: diagnosis and significance. Radiology. 1988;169:858-9.

61. Chervenak FA, Duncan C, Ment LR, Hobbins JC, McClure M, Scott D, et al. The outcome of fetal ventriculomegaly. Lancet. 1984;2(8396):179-81.

62. Lees RF, Alford BA, Brenbridge NAG, Buschi AJ, Williamson BR. Sonographic appearance of duodenal atresia in utero. Am J Roentgenol. 1978;131:701-2.

63. Romero R, Ghidini A, Costigan K, Touloukian R, Hobbins JC. The prenatal diagnosis of duodenal atresia: does it make any difference? Obstet Gynecol. 1988;71:739-41.

64. Hobbins JC, Romero R, Grannum P, Berkowitz RL, Cullen M, Mahoney M. Antenatal diagnosis of renal anomalies with ultrasound. I. Obstructive uropathy. Am J Obstet Gynecol. 1984;148:868-77.

65. Corteville JE, Gray DL, Crane JP. Congenital hydronephrosis: correlation of fetal ultrasonographic findings with infant outcome. Am J Obstet Gynecol. 1991;165:384-8.

66. Mandell J, Blyth B, Peters CA, Retik AB, Estroff JA, Benacerraf BR. Structural genitourinary defects detected in utero. Radiology. 1991;178:193-6.

67. Deter RL, Harrist RB, Birnholz JC, Hadlock FP. Quantitative Obstetrical Ultrasonography. New York: Churchill Livingstone; 1986.

68. Chervenak FA, Jeanty P, Cantraine F, Chitkara U, Venus I, Berkowitz RL, et al. The diagnosis of fetal microcephaly. Am J Obstet Gynecol. 1984;149:512-7.

69. Chervenak FA, Rosenberg J, Brigthman RC, Chitkara U, Jeanty P. A prospective study of the accuracy of ultrasound in predicting fetal microcephaly. Obstet Gynecol. 1987;69:908-10.

70. Romero R, Pilu G. Jeanty P, Ghidini A, Hobbins JC. Prenatal Diagnosis of Congenital Anomalies. Norwalk: Appleton and Lange; 1988. p. 311.

71. Chervenak FA, Tortora M, Mayden K, Mesologites T, Isaacson G, Mahoney MJ, et al. Antenatal diagnosis of median cleft face syndrome: sonographic demonstration of cleft lip and hypotelorism. Am J Obstet Gynecol. 1984;149:94-7.

72. Grannum P, Bracken M, Silverman R, Hobbins JC. Assessment of fetal kidney size in normal gestation by comparison of ratio of kidney circumference to abdominal circumference. Am J Obstet Gynecol. 1980;136:249-54.

73. Romero R, Cullen M, Jeanty P, Grannum P, Reece EA, Venus I, et al. The diagnosis of congenital renal anomalies with ultrasound. II. Infantile polycystic kidney disease. Am J Obstet Gynecol. 1984;150:259-62.

74. Chervenak FA, Tortora MN, Hobbins JC. Antenatal sonographic diagnosis of clubfoot. J Ultrasound Med. 1985; 4:49-50.

75. Goldberg JD, Chervenak FA, Lipman RA, Berkowitz RL. Antenatal sonographic diagnosis of arthrogryposis multiplex congenita. Prenat Diagn. 1986;6:45-9.

76. Allan LD, Crawford DC, Anderson RH, Tynan MH. Echocardiographic and anatomical correlations in fetal congenital heart disease. Br Heart J. 1984;52:542-8.

77. Copel JA, Pilu G, Green J, Hobbins JC, Kleinman CS. Fetal echocardiographic screening for congenital heart disease: the importance of the four-chamber view. Am J Obstet Gynecol. 1987;157:648-55.

78. Gertgesell HP (Ed). Symposium of fetal echocardiography. J Clin Ultrasound. 1985;13:227.

79. Devore G. Fetal echocardiography. In: Chervenak FA, Isaacson G, Campbell S (Eds). Ultrasound in Obstetrics and Gynecology. Boston: Little, Brown; 1994. p. 199.

80. Reed KL, Anderson CF, Shenker L. Fetal Echocardiography: An Atlas. New York: Alan R. Liss; 1988.

81. Kleinman CS, Copel JA. Fetal cardiac dysrhythmias: diagnosis and therapy. In: Chervenak FA, Isaacson G, Campbell S (Eds). Ultrasound in Obstetrics and Gynecology. Boston: Little, Brown, 1993. p. 195.

82. Hill LM. Chromosomal abnormalities. In: McGahan JP, Porto M (Eds). Diagnostic Ultrasound. Philadelphia: JB Lippincott, 1994. p. 449.

83. Kalousek DK, Fitch N, Paradice BA. Pathology of the Human Embryo and Previable Fetus: An Atlas. New York: Springer-Verlag; 1990. p. 188.

84. Benaceraff BR, Gelman R, Frigoletto FD. Sonographic identification of second-trimester fetuses with Down syndrome. N Engl J Med. 1987;317:1371-6.

85. Nyberg DA, Resta RG, Luthy DA, Hickok DE, Mahony BS, Hirsch JH. Prenatal sonographic findings of Down syndrome: review of 94 cases. Obstet Gynecol. 1990;76:370-7.

86. Crome JP, Gray DL. Sonographically measured nuchal skinfold as a screening tool for Down syndrome: results of a prospective clinical trial. Obstet Gynecol. 1991;77:533-6.

87. Benaceraff BR, Neuberg D, Bromley B, Frigoletto FD. Sonographic scoring index for prenatal detection of chromosomal abnormalities. J Ultrasound Med. 1992;11: 449-58.

88. Hill LM, Gurzevich D, Belfar ML, Hixson J, Rivello D, Rusnak J. The current role of sonography in the detection of Down syndrome. Obstet Gynecol. 1989;74:620-3.

89. Gabrielli S, Reece AE, Pilu G, Perolo A, Rizzo N, Bovicelli L, et al. The clinical significance of prenatally diagnosed choroid plexus cysts. Am J Obstet Gynecol. 1989;160:1207-10.

90. Rotmensch S, Luo JS, Nores JA, Dimaio MS, Hobbins JC. Bilateral choroid plexus cysts in trisomy 21. Am J Obstet Gynecol. 1992;166:591-2.

91. Platt LD, Carlson DE, Medearis AL, Walla CA. Fetal choroid plexus cysts in the second trimester of pregnancy. A cause for concern. Am J Obstet Gynecol. 1991;64:1652-5; discussion 1655-6.

92. Benacerraf BR, Hanlon B, Frigoletto F. Are choroid plexus cysts an indication for second-trimester amniocentesis? Am J Obstet Gynecol. 1990;162:1001-6.

93. Copel JA, Pilu G, Kleinmann CS. Congenital heart disease and extracardiac anomalies: Associations and indications for fetal echocardiography. Am J Obstet Gynecol. 1986; 154:1121-32.

94. Palmer CG, Miles JH, Howard-Peebles PN, Magenis RE, Patil S, Friedman JM. Fetal karyotype following ascertainment of fetal anomalies by ultrasound. Prenat Diagn. 1987;7: 551-5.

95. Platt LD, DeVore GR, Lopez E, Herbert W, Falk R, Alfi O. Role of amniocentesis in ultrasound-detected fetal malformations. Obstet Gynecol. 1986;68:153-5.

96. Williamson RA, Weiner CP, Patil S, Benda J, Varner MW, Abu-Yousef MM. Abnormal pregnancy sonogram: selective indication for fetal karyotype. Obstet Gynecol. 1987;69:15-20.

97. Chervenak FA, McCullough LB. An ethically justified, clinically comprehensive management strategy for third-trimester pregnancies complicated by fetal anomalies. Obstet Gynecol. 1990;75:311-6.

98. Chervenak FA, McCullough LB. Does obstetric ethics have any role in the obstetrician's response to the abortion controversy? Am J Obstet Gynecol. 1990;163:1425-9.

99. Harrison M, Golbus M, Filly R. The Unborn Patient. 2nd edition. New York; Grune and Stratton; 1991.

100. Seeds JW, Azizkhan RG. Congenital Malformations. Antenatal Diagnosis, Perinatal Management, and Counseling. Rockville: Aspen Publishers; 1990.

101. Romero R, Oyarzun E, Sirtori M, Hobbins JC. Detection and management of anatomic congenital anomalies. Obstet Gynecol Clin N Amer. 1988;15:215-36.

102. Chervenak FA, Berkowitz RL, Tortora M, Hobbins JC. The management of fetal hydrocephalus. Am J Obstet Gynecol. 1985;151:933-42.

103. Luthy DA, Wardinsky T, Shurtleff DB, Hollenbach KA, Hickok DE, Nyberg DA, et al. Cesarean section before the onset of labor and subsequent motor function in infants with open spina bifida. N Engl J Med. 1991;162:662-6.

104. Manning FA, Harrison MR, Rodeck C, Members of the International Fetal Medicine and Surgery Society. Catheter shunts for fetal hydronephrosis and hydrocephalus. Special Report. N Engl J Med. 1986;315:336-40.

105. Manning FA. The anomalous fetus. In: Manning FA (Ed). Fetal Medicine: Principles and Practice. Norwalk: Appleton and Lange; 1995. p. 451.

106. Albar H, Manning FA, Harman CR. Treatment of urinary tract and CNS obstruction. In: Harman CR (Ed). Invasive Fetal Testing and Treatment. Cambridge: Blackwell Scientific; 1995. p. 259.

107. Anderson RL, Golbus MS. Bladder aspiration. In: Chervenak FA, Isaacson G, Campbell S (Eds). Textbook of Ultrasound in Obstetrics and Gynecology. Boston: Little, Brown; 1993.

108. Rodeck CH, Fisk NM, Fraser DI, Nicolini U. Long-term in utero drainage of fetal hydrothorax. N Engl J Med. 1988;319:1135-8.

109. Nicolaides KH, Azar G. Thoracoamniotic shunting. In: Chervenak FA, Isaacson G, Campbell S, (Eds). Textbook of Ultrasound in Obstetrics and Gynecology. Boston: Little, Brown; 1993. p. 1289.

110. Vaughn JI, Fisk NM, Rodeck CM. Fetal pleural effusions. In: Harman CR (Ed). Fetal Testing and Treatment. Cambridge: Blackwell Scientific; 1995. p. 219.

111. Clewell WH, Johnson ML, Meier PR, Newkirk JB, Zide SL, Hendee RW, et al. A surgical approach to the treatment of fetal hydrocephalus. N Engl J Med. 1982;306:1320-5.

112. Clewell W. Current status of ventriculo-amniotic shunt placement. In: Kurjak A, Comstock C, Chervenak FA (Eds). Ultrasound and the Fetal Brain. Carnforth: Parthenon; 1996.

113. Harrison MR, Adzick NS, Longaker MT, Goldberg JD, Rosen MA, Filly RA, et al. Successful repair in utero of a fetal diaphragmatic hernia after removal of herniated viscera from the left thorax. N Engl J Med. 1990;322:1582-4.

114. Supreme Court of the United States. Roe v. Wade. U.S. Reports: Roe v. Wade, 410 U.S. 113. 1973.

115. Elias S, Annas GJ. Reproductive Genetics and the Law. Chicago: Year Book Medical Publishers; 1987.

116. Annas GJ. Protecting the liberty of pregnant patients. N Engl J Med. 1987;316:1213-4.

117. Chervenak FA, Farley MA, Walters L, Hobbins JC, Mahoney MJ. When is termination of pregnancy during the third trimester morally justifiable? N Engl J Med. 1984;310:501-4.

118. Chervenak FA, McCullough LB, Campbell S. Is third trimester abortion justified? Br J Obstet Gynæcol. 1995;102:434-5.

119. Chervenak FA, McCullough LB. Nonaggressive obstetric management. An option for some fetal anomalies during the third trimester. JAMA. 1989;261:3439-40.

120. Chervenak FA, McCullough LB. Ethical challenges in perinatal medicine: the intrapartum management of pregnancy complicated by fetal hydrocephalus with macrocephaly. Semin Perinatol. 1987;11:232-9.

121. Chervenak FA, McCullough LB. Fetal destructive procedures in operative obstetrics. In: O'Grady JP, Gimovsky ML, McIlhargie LJ (Eds). Operative Obstetrics. Baltimore: Williams and Wilkins; 1995. p. 354.

Three-dimensional Sonography in the Evaluation of Normal and Abnormal Fetal Face

Asim Kurjak, Guillermo Azumendi Pérez

■ INTRODUCTION

The face is the anatomical structure that clearly demonstrates the utility and advantages of three-dimensional (3D) and four-dimensional (4D) ultrasound. It is difficult to find a book about ultrasound published during the last few years that does not include a 3D picture about the fetal face on its cover. Even in a text dedicated to gynecological ultrasound, it is usual to find a 3D picture of a fetal face helping illustrate the potential of such a new technology.

Practically, all the pioneering studies on 3D ultrasound provide an example of 3D fetal face reconstruction.[1-29] We have all taken our first steps in 3D ultrasound by exploring the fetal face and our main aim has always been to obtain good pictures of this anatomic structure. It is, therefore, a good opportunity to elaborate on the role of 3D and 4D ultrasound of the fetal face **(Figs. 1 to 118)**.

▌ADVANTAGES AND LIMITATIONS OF 3D ULTRASOUND

The study of the fetal face is of great importance in prenatal medicine because some facial and encephalic structures share the same embryologic origin. This is why every malformation detected at the facial level must necessitate the corresponding study at encephalic level.[30,31] We all recognize the thought of De Meyer and colleagues, who said, "The face predicts the brain".[31,32] In the ever-increasing body of knowledge on this topic, there are papers that demonstrate some advantages of 3D ultrasound compared with the use of two-dimensional (2D) ultrasound in perinatal medicine, mainly in the study of the fetal face.[18,19,32,33] Three-dimensional ultrasound shows perspectives that cannot be obtained with 2D ultrasound and depicts the anatomy in the most appropriate and comprehensive position.[34] This standardized display of images helps us to obtain a better understanding of the fetal anatomy for both the parents and less-experienced doctors. Because of its curvature and small anatomical details, the fetal face can be visualized and analyzed only to a limited extent with 2D sonography.[35,36] The entire face cannot be seen on a single image. Three-dimensional ultrasound provides a spatial reconstruction of the fetal face and simultaneous visualization of all facial structures such as the fetal nose, eyebrows, mouth, jaws, dental germs, and eyelids **(Figs. 11 and 12)**.[28,33-37]

Advantages

Improved Maternal-fetal Bonding

Ji EK and colleagues have stated that, for many parents, the image taken by 2D ultrasound is abstract, while with 3D ultrasound the features of the baby are instantly recognized, regardless of whether they are normal or not, which allows parental bonding with the baby.[38] This is one of the unquestionable benefits of 3D ultrasound over 2D.[18,22,39,40] In a few papers in which no other real benefits are found with the use of 3D, the reinforcement of the affective bonding is unchallengeable.[40] Three-dimensional images give the mother more security and a deeper vision of the psychological aspects of ongoing pregnancy.[41] It has also been noted that these positive and close affective bonds between the mother and the fetus can help her to stop smoking or end any other potentially harmful habits.[42]

Improvement in Identifying Anomalies

The improvement in the identification of anomalies by the performance of images in perspectives and planes that cannot be obtained with 2D ultrasound has proved vital. It is precisely stated that most fetal face deformations have been diagnosed with 3D ultrasound while they had gone unnoticed with 2D ultrasound. Ultrasound cases of micrognathia, cleft lip **(Figs. 88 to 93)**, midfacial hypoplasia, orbitary hypoplasia, facial dysmorphea, defects in the cranium ossification and auricular dysplasia have been picked up.[18,22,31,32] Some of these abnormalities have been diagnosed in the 3D presentations and some others in the planes not available with conventional 2D ultrasound. By allowing evaluation of the volume millimeter by millimeter and in three perspectives, it is possible to study the upper lip in coronal and axial images and the palate in the axial plane. Three-dimensional ultrasound assists by visualizing the facial profile in the correct axis, which is not always obtainable on a 2D image.[43] Merz E and colleagues analyzed the effect of 3D facial profile reconstruction on 125 fetuses.[22] They found that 30.4% of the profiles were turned 3–20° from the real one. Therefore, in only 69.6% of the cases was the true profile obtained with 2D ultrasound. The magnitude of this discovery cannot be disputed, since previously those anomalies could not be detected or were overdiagnosed. Several papers state the clear superiority of 3D ultrasound for the study of the fetal face in both normal and abnormal conditions,[1-7,9-15,17-20,22-29,44,45] although some authors do not find these differences so significant.[40]

Improved Assessment of Extent and Location of Fetal Anomalies

Assessment of the extent and location of fetal anomalies can be improved by using 3D ultrasound **(Figs. 81 to 97)**.[18,28,32,46] A cleft lip and/or a cleft palate are often difficult to diagnose with 2D ultrasound, or at least it has been difficult to precisely evaluate their extent, especially if the operator has little experience or lacks anatomic references with the appropriate image plane. In the RADIUS study, 7,685 low-risk fetuses were studied and only three of nine cleft lips were prenatally identified.[47] Using 3D ultrasound, the operator can evaluate the front alveolar ledge or the primary palate in the appropriate axial plane, using the correct reconstruction or the sagittal planar image as a reference, and can then move on to the parallel axial images. This possibility for studying axial or frontal parallel planes of the fetal face' is not obtained with 2D ultrasound. It is extremely useful to show the anomaly to both relatives and trainee doctors in order to assist their decision regarding future diagnostic and therapeutic options.[18,22,23,28,33,48]

Four-dimensional Ultrasound

Four-dimensional ultrasound has some additional advantages such as the ability to study fetal activity in the surface-rendered mode, and is particularly superior for fast fetal movements.[49] With 2D ultrasound, fetal movements such as yawning, swallowing, and eyelid movements cannot be displayed simultaneously, while, with 4D sonography, the simultaneous facial movements can be clearly depicted.[50] There are several types of jaw movement patterns, such as isolated jaw movement, sucking and swallowing, which can be observed by 2D ultrasound.[51] The variable amplitudes of jaw opening and speed characterize isolated jaw movements **(Fig. 3)**. Yawning can be observed as a movement pattern identical to that seen in infants, children, and adults: slow opening, prolonged wide opening of the jaws followed by quick closure, with simultaneous retroflexion of the head. With 4D ultrasound, it is now feasible to study a full range of facial expressions including smiling, crying, scowling, and eyelid movement.[50,52]

The observation of the facial expression may be of scientific and diagnostic value and this scientific approach opens an entirely new field. There are many unanswered questions. When do facial expressions start? Which expression dominates and at what gestational age do they occur? An important diagnostic aim of the observation of facial expression is prenatal diagnosis of facial paresis. The criterion for the diagnosis is asymmetrical facial movement and detection of the movements limited to only one side of the face. Unfortunately during the relaxed phase, it is not possible to evaluate the status of the facial nerve.

Therefore, during the active phase, the fetus should be scanned by 4D ultrasound. Since the origin of the facial expression can be external, the sonographer should be aware of this pitfall. For example, force of the fetal hand can alter the facial expression on one side of the face, causing asymmetry **(Fig. 80)**. This kind of asymmetry, however, should be differentiated from pathological features such as unilateral facial paresis **(Fig. 6)**. We believe that the largest challenges for 4D ultrasound are in the unexplored areas of parental and fetal behavior.[53-55] Two-dimensional real-time ultrasound and 4D sonography are complementary methods used for evaluation of fetal movements. It is clear that the quality of each fetal movement can be visualized and evaluated more reliably by 4D ultrasound. It appears that there are still not enough prospective studies that may clarify or prove real benefits of 3D ultrasound in daily practice and there is an urgent need for randomized control studies.[40] Our group have been evaluating fetal behavioral patterns in the third trimester between 30th and 33rd week of gestation in 10 gravidas.[56] The continuity between fetal and neonatal behavior have been published recently from Zagreb, Barcelona, and Malaga groups.[57]

Limitations

As with any new technique, there are some limitations. Failure rates are reported in obtaining high-quality images in surface mode under certain circumstances such as oligohydramnios or the shadowing by hands, feet, umbilical cord, or placenta **(Fig. 34)**. Under these circumstances, it is advisable to re-examine the reconstructions together with the planar data of the same volume, in order to evaluate the direction of the ultrasound beam that is more visible on planar images than on those reconstructed. One report described how a totally normal fetal face appeared to have a cleft lip due to the shadow of the umbilical cord adjacent to the upper lip on the multiplanar images.[46] Sometimes, we have difficulties in identifying other surface features such as fingers and toes because they are frequently opposed to the wall of the uterus. An additional limitation of 4D ultrasound, at least for the moment, is the inability to display fetal movements that are too quick (within 1 to 2 sec) and subtle fetal movements such as those of breathing. However, many of these limitations may disappear in the near future as more powerful equipment is developed and appears on the market.

■ ASSESSMENT OF FETAL FACIAL EXPRESSION

We had classified several facial expressions at least to eight different activities.

Classification of Facial Patterns

1. *Yawning:* This movement is similar to the yawn observed after birth. An involuntary wide opening of the mouth, with maximal widening of the jaws followed by quick closure often with retroflexion of the head and sometimes elevation of the arms. This movement pattern is nonrepetitive **(Figs. 54 and 55)**.
2. *Swallowing:* Indicating that the fetus is drinking amniotic fluid. Swallowing consists of displacements of tongue and/or larynx. Swallowing activity develops earlier than sucking in the course of fetal development **(Fig. 115)**.
3. *Sucking:* Rhythmical bursts of regular jaw opening, and closing at a rate of about one per second. Placing the finger or thumb on the roof of the mouth behind the teeth and sucking with lips closed. Thumb sucking is a very frequent fetal behavioral pattern **(Fig. 52)**.
4. *Smiling:* A facial expression characterized by turning up the corners of the mouth **(Fig. 50)**.
5. *Tongue expulsion:* A facial expression characterized by expulsion of the tongue **(Fig. 33)**.
6. *Grimacing:* The wrinkling of the brows or face in frowning to express of displeasure **(Figs. 103 and 104)**.
7. *Mouthing:* A facial expression characterized by mouth manipulation to investigate an object. Mouthing is most common in fetus and it may develop into a persistent, stereotyped behavior pattern **(Fig. 112)**.
8. *Isolated eye blinking:* A reflex that closes and opens the eyes rapidly. Brief closing of the eyelids by involuntary normal periodic closing, as a protective measure, or by voluntary action **(Figs. 1, 16, and 110)**.

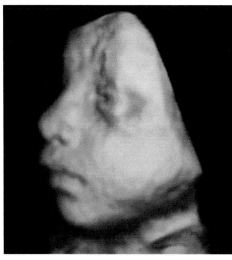

Fig. 2: Three-dimensional (3D) scan of a fetal semiprofile showing facial contours of the facial muscle.

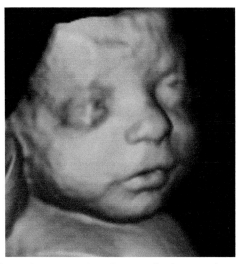

Fig. 3: Three-dimensional (3D) scan of a fetus with semiprofile position showing contours of both eyelids and surrounding soft tissue structures such as nose and cheeks.

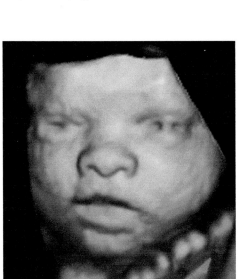

Fig. 1: Three-dimensional (3D) scan of a fetus showing complete face profile at 33rd week of gestation. Eyelids are opened and surface of facial features are discernible.

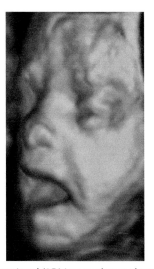

Fig. 4: Three-dimensional (3D) image shows alteration of the facial expression of the fetus. The fetus seems to be glumness.

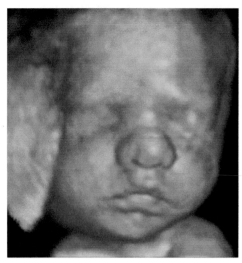

Fig. 5: This image shows alteration of the facial expression. The movements of the facial musculature caused the fetus seems to be sleeping.

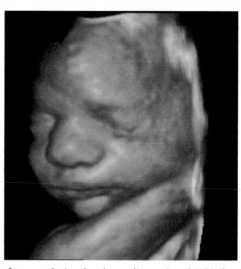

Fig. 8: Surface rendering by three-dimensional (3D) demonstrates the facial contours of the lips and nose. The fetus seems to be sleeping.

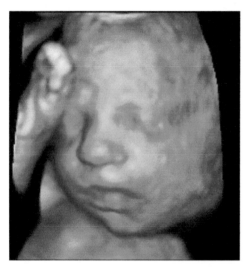

Fig. 6: Sleeping expression of the fetus is clearly visible.

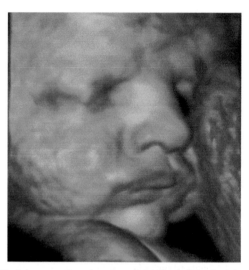

Fig. 9: Facial expression showing distortion of the facial muscles. The fetus seems to be angry.

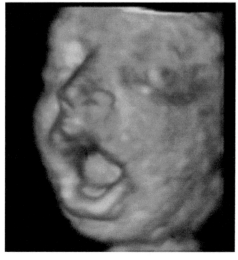

Fig. 7: Other facial expression of the fetus showing mouth opening.

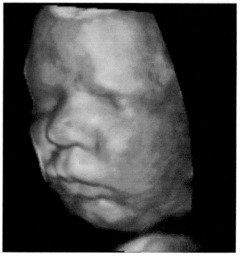

Fig. 10: Semiprofile expression of the facial contour.

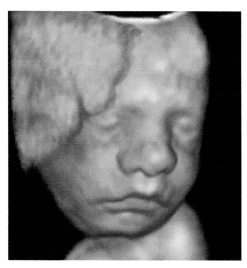

Fig. 11: Semiprofile surface rendering showing the contours of the fetal face, eyelids, and nose.

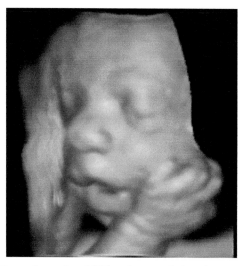

Fig. 14: Three-dimensional (3D) surface rendering showing opening of the mouth and movements of eyebrows.

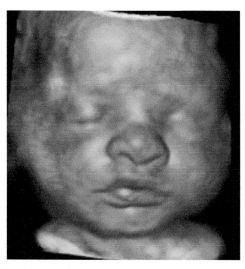

Fig. 12: Complete profile of surface rendering showing movements of the bilateral part of eyebrows is clearly visible.

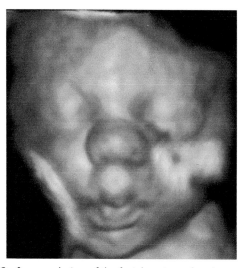

Fig. 15: Surface rendering of the facial contour showing expression of the sleeping fetus.

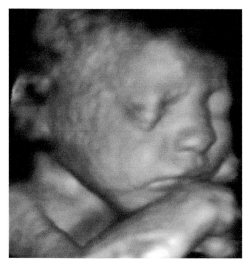

Fig. 13: The entire face is discernible, with clear visualization of nostrils, right ear, and eyelids. The fetal hand is positioned in front of the mouth.

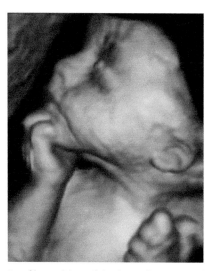

Fig. 16: Semiprofile position of the fetus showing eyelids opening and all facial features.

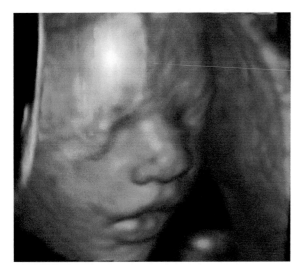

Fig. 17: Semiprofile position showing facial contour of the fetal lips which cause the change in facial expression.

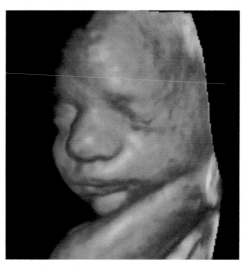

Fig. 20: Semiprofile surface rendering showing sleeping expression of the fetus.

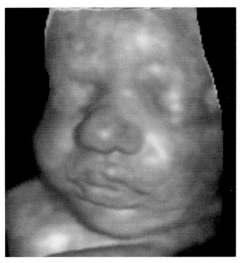

Fig. 18: Surface rendering demonstrates clear visualization of facial anatomical structures.

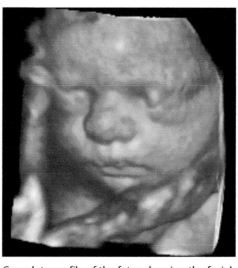

Fig. 21: Complete profile of the fetus showing the facial contour. Even the umbilical cord is observable surrounded by the fetal neck.

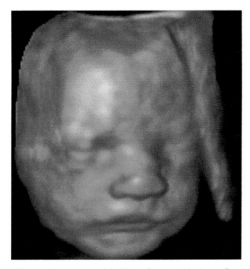

Fig. 19: Three-dimensional (3D) surface rendering of complete profile showing discernible contour of facial musculatures.

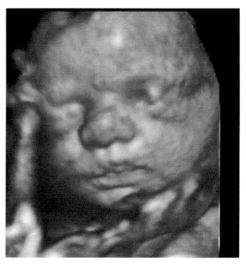

Fig. 22: Three-dimensional (3D) surface rendering shows sleeping expression of the fetus. Note the nuchal cord around the neck is clearly visible.

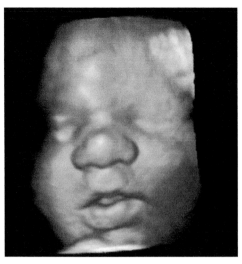

Fig. 23: Asymmetry of the facial expression caused by changing in lateral parts of the cheek.

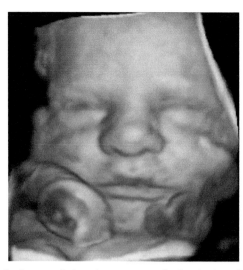

Fig. 26: Surface rendering demonstrates the beginning of opening of the right fetal eyelids.

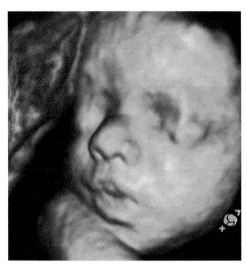

Fig. 24: Changing of the facial expression due to the movements of the bilateral parts of eyebrows.

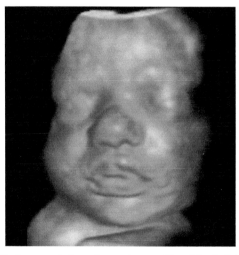

Fig. 27: Surface rendering of complete profile of the facial contour.

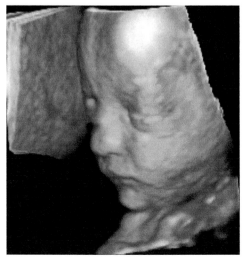

Fig. 25: Fetal profile by three-dimensional (3D) surface rendering showing the facial texture.

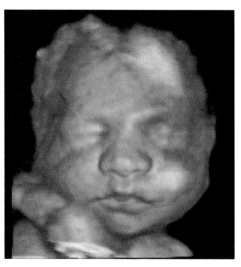

Fig. 28: Sleeping expression is clearly visible on this image.

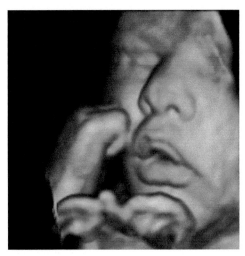

Fig. 29: Three-dimensional (3D) scan of the fetus in complete profile showing opening of the mouth. Note clear demonstration of the fetal lips.

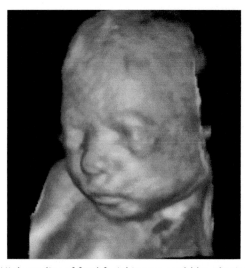

Fig. 32: High quality of fetal facial image could be obtained in the surface rendering mode, when other structures is not shadowing the fetal face.

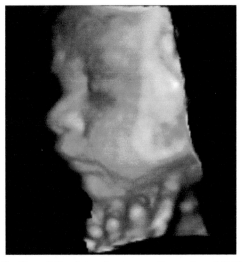

Fig. 30: Profile of the fetus by three-dimensional (3D) surface rendering, with clear visualization of small anatomical features from the fingers.

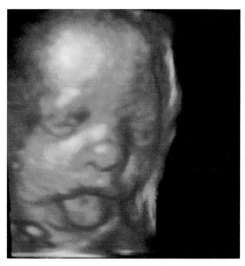

Fig. 33: Three-dimensional (3D) scan of the fetus in semiprofile position showing expulsion of the tongue.

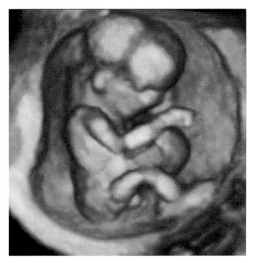

Fig. 31: Three-dimensional (3D) surface rendering of the facial contour in early pregnancy. Facial structures have reached an adequate degree of development in order to start studying them for diagnostic purposes.

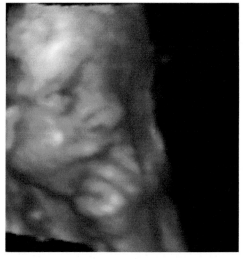

Fig. 34: Three-dimensional (3D) scan of the fetus in semiprofile position, the eyelids are opened and the surfaces of all visible facial features are discernible. The fetus seems to be observing the surrounding environment.

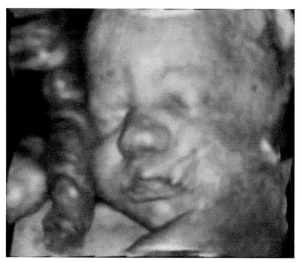

Fig. 35: Three-dimensional (3D) ultrasound of the fetus in the third trimester of gestation. Note clear demonstration of surrounding structure such us umbilical cord.

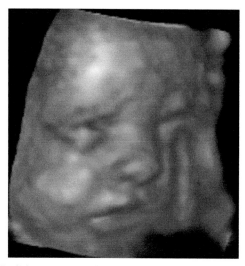

Fig. 38: Eyelids opening and clearly observable anatomy of the eyes such as the eyeballs.

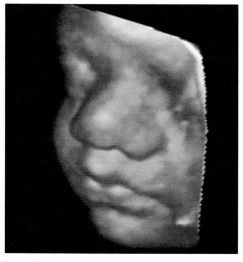

Fig. 36: Three-dimensional (3D) scan of the fetus in semiprofile position demonstrates clearly facial anatomy such as nose, mouth, and eyelids.

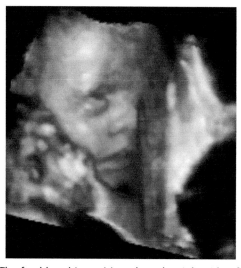

Fig. 39: The fetal hand is positioned on the right side of the fetal cheek and the entire face is discernible, with clear visualization of the eyeballs.

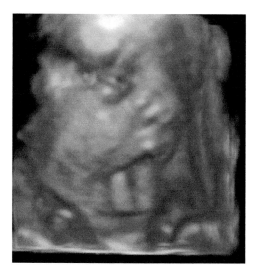

Fig. 37: Three-dimensional (3D) surface rendering shows the expulsion of the tongue and change of the facial expression due to eyelids opening.

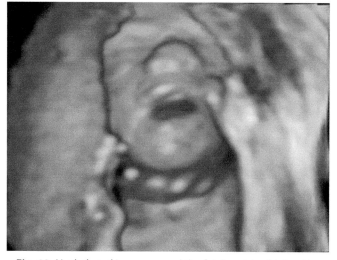

Fig. 40: Nuchal cord image around the fetal neck is obtained by three-dimensional (3D) surface rendering.

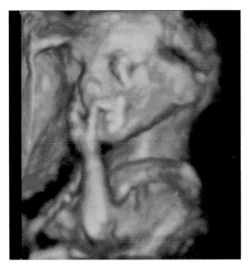

Fig. 41: Change in fetal expressions together with hand-to-mouth movement.

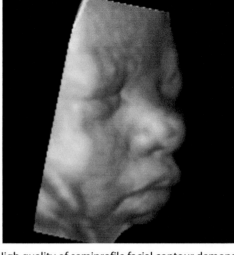

Fig. 44: High quality of semiprofile facial contour demonstrates the lips, nostrils, and forehead.

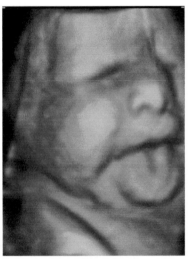

Fig. 42: Change in fetal expression due to expulsion of the tongue.

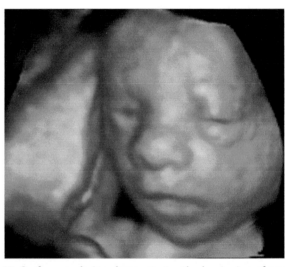

Fig. 45: Surface rendering demonstrates the beginning of opening of the eyelids. Note the fetus seems to be observing something in the left side.

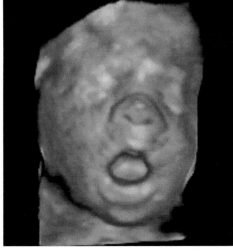

Fig. 43: Opening of the mouth is clearly visible.

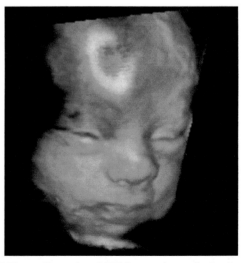

Fig. 46: Three-dimensional (3D) image shows the beginning of opening of the eyelids.

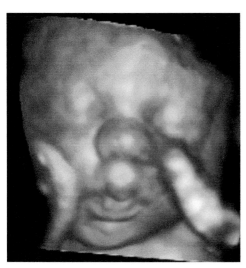

Fig. 47: Alteration of the facial expression is clearly visible on this image which illustrates the surrounding influence, altering the facial expression on one side.

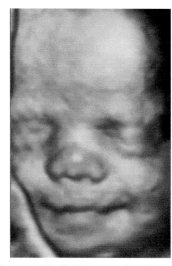

Fig. 50: The change of the facial expression due to turning up the corners of the mouth. The fetus appears to be smiling.

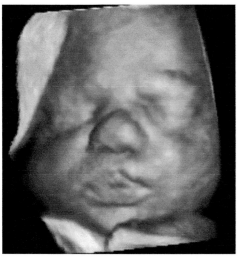

Fig. 48: Three-dimensional (3D) surface rendering of the fetal face shows alteration of the facial expression. Movement of the lateral side of facial musculature causes transient and slight asymmetry. However, it should be differentiated from pathological features such as unilateral paresis.

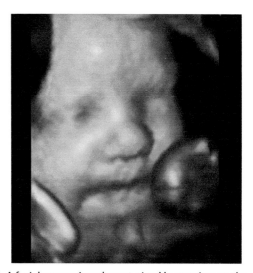

Fig. 51: A facial expression characterized by turning up the corners of the mouth. The fetus seems to be smiling.

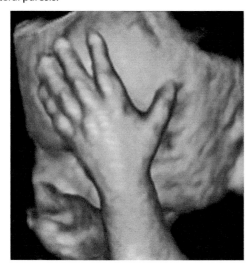

Fig. 49: The subtle alteration of the facial expression is clearly visible on this image with illustrates influence of the fetal hand.

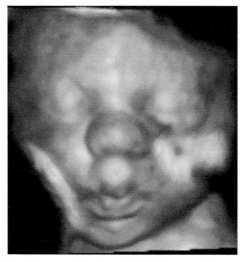

Fig. 52: A facial expression characterized by mouthing expression. This is most common in fetus and it may develop into a persistent, stereotyped behavior pattern.

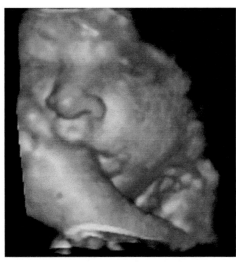

Fig. 53: The fetus is placing the finger or thumb on the roof of the mouth behind the teeth and sucking with lips closed. Thumb sucking is a very frequent fetal behavioral pattern.

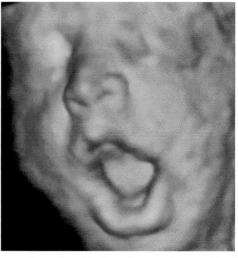

Fig. 56: Three-dimensional (3D) surface rendering of fetal yawning. This movement is often following by retroflexion of the head and sometimes elevation of the arms.

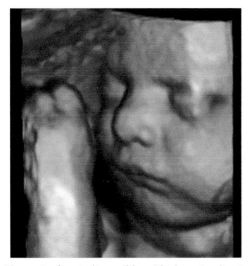

Fig. 54: The entire face is discernible, with clear visualization of the left hand positioned in front of the face.

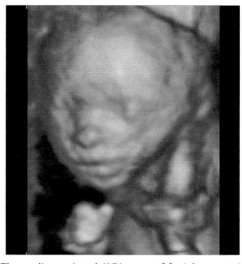

Fig. 57: Three-dimensional (3D) scan of facial expression in the second trimester of gestation is adequate enough for diagnostic purpose.

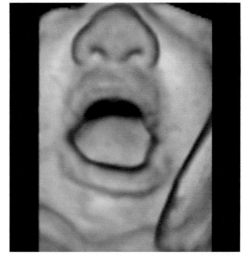

Fig. 55: Yawn expression is defined as an involuntary wide opening of the mouth, with maximal widening of the jaws followed by quick closure.

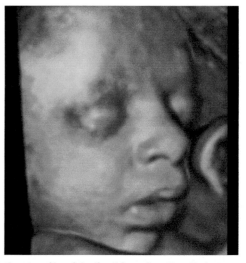

Fig. 58: Semiprofile of the fetal face showing distinct contour of facial musculature.

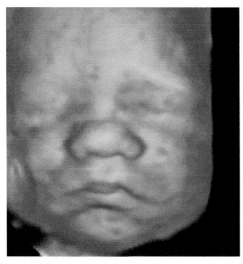

Fig. 59: Both of the eyes and the mouth are closed and the fetus appears calm.

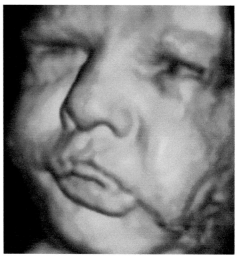

Fig. 62: Surface rendering shows the beginning of eyelids opening. Note clear demonstration of the facial contour of the fetal lips.

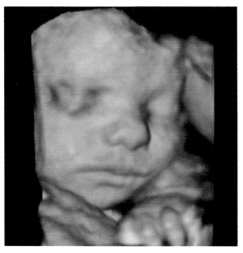

Fig. 60: Calm and tranquil expression of the fetus obtained by three-dimensional (3D) technique.

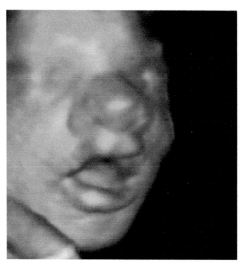

Fig. 63: The beginning of opening of the fetal mouth.

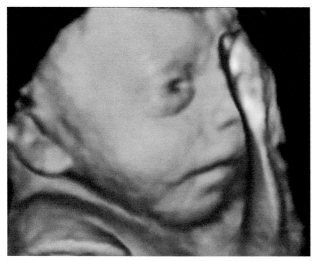

Fig. 61: Three-dimensional (3D) scan of the fetus in semiprofile image. The eyelids are opened and the surfaces of all visible facial features are distinctly clear.

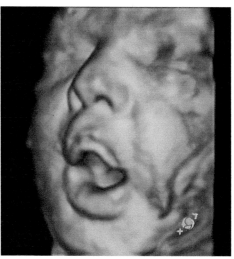

Fig. 64: The ending of maximal opening of the mouth.

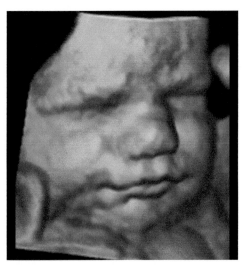

Fig. 65: The change of the facial expression due to movements of the lateral parts of the eyebrows and the facial musculature between them is clearly visible.

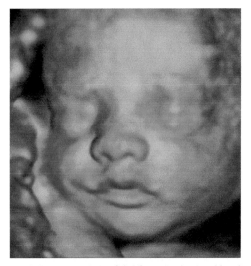

Fig. 66: Calm expression of the fetus is obtained by three-dimensional (3D) surface rendering.

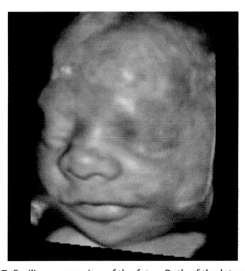

Fig. 67: Smiling expression of the fetus. Both of the lateral side of the mouth is turning up.

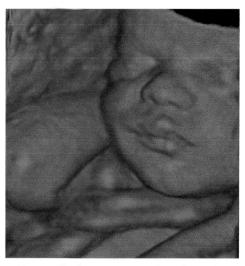

Fig. 68: The fetus appears to be calm in this three-dimensional (3D) image.

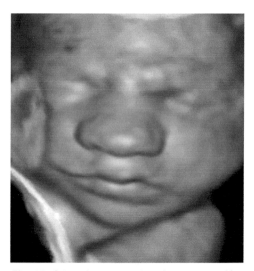

Fig. 69: Grimacing expression demonstrated by three-dimensional (3D) surface rendering.

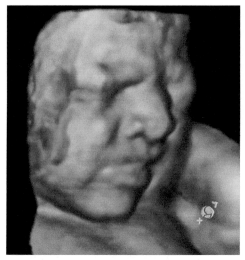

Fig. 70: The frontalis muscle also can be responsible for the appearance of grimacing. However, the main agent responsible for the appearance of scowling is the corrugator muscle. The fetus seems to be sad.

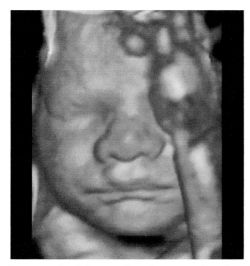

Fig. 71: Both of the mouth and eyes are closed and fetus appears tranquil.

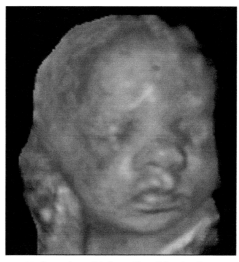

Fig. 74: High quality of full profile of the fetal expression shows sleeping expression.

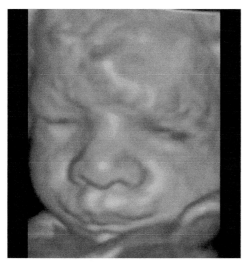

Fig. 72: The fetus seems trying to manipulate something with mouth in this three-dimensional (3D) image.

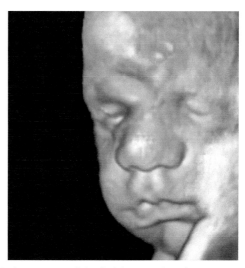

Fig. 75: Asymmetry of the facial expression due to movement of lateral side of the fetal facial musculature.

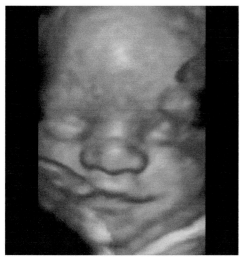

Fig. 73: Smiling expression is obtained by three-dimensional (3D) surface technique.

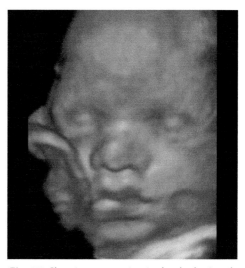

Fig. 76: Sleeping expression is clearly depicted.

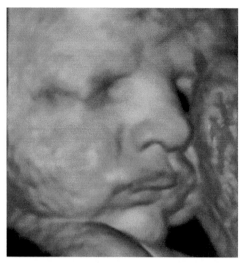

Fig. 77: Grimacing expression is obtained by surface rendering technique.

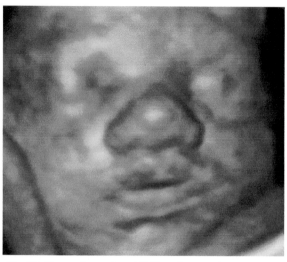

Fig. 80: Three-dimensional (3D) surface rendering shows the clearly contour of fetal face.

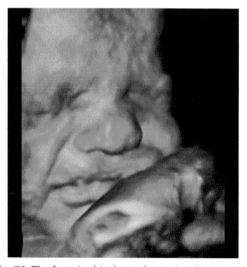

Fig. 78: The fetus in this three-dimensional (3D) image seems to be displeasure.

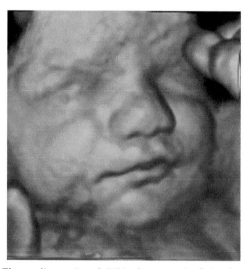

Fig. 81: Three-dimensional (3D) ultrasound of the fetus shows alteration of the facial expression. This kind of asymmetry, however, should be differentiated from pathological features such as unilateral facial paresis.

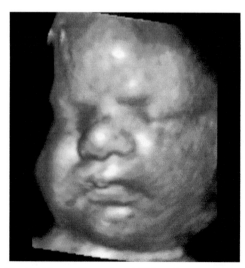

Fig. 79: Three-dimensional (3D) surface rendering demonstrates grimacing expression.

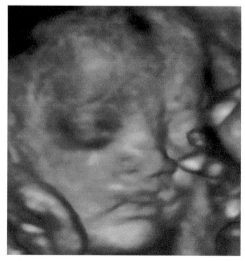

Fig. 82: Three-dimensional (3D) surface rendering of the fetus with trisomy 18 shows the round face.

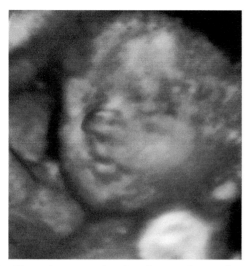

Fig. 83: Three-dimensional (3D) surface rendering of the fetus with trisomy 18.

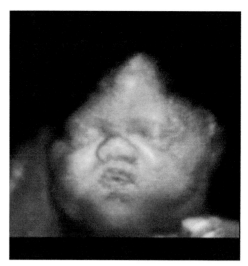

Fig. 86: Three-dimensional (3D) image of the fetus with thanatophoric dysplasia.

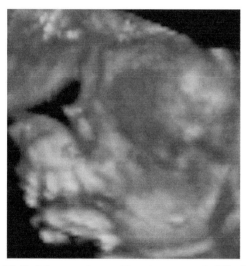

Fig. 84: Facial expression and hand movement of the fetus with trisomy 18.

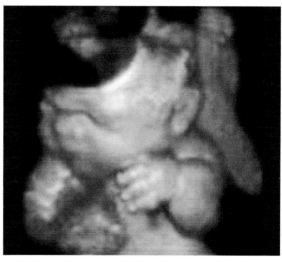

Fig. 87: Three-dimensional (3D) surface rendering of the fetus with osteochondrosis dysplasia.

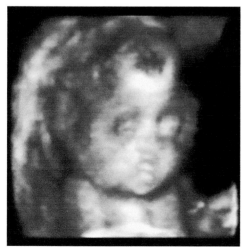

Fig. 85: Three-dimensional (3D) surface rendering of the fetus with thanatophoric dysplasia.

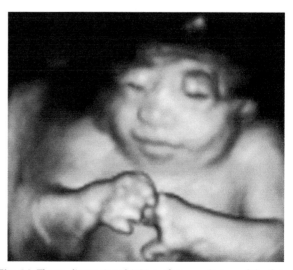

Fig. 88: Three-dimensional (3D) surface rendering of the fetus with anencephaly.

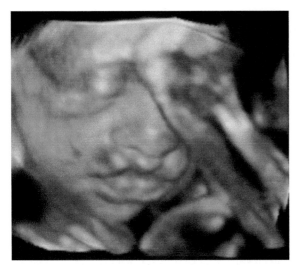

Fig. 89: Three-dimensional (3D) ultrasound image of a fetal face in the fetus with bilateral cleft lip.

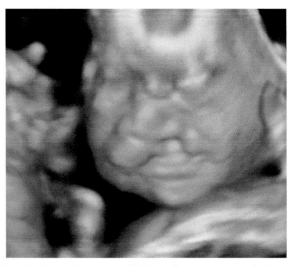

Fig. 92: Three-dimensional (3D) surface rendering of a fetus with unilateral cleft lip.

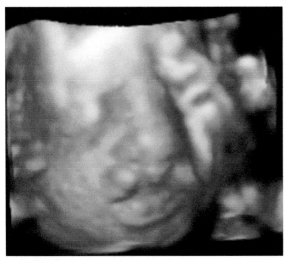

Fig. 90: Three-dimensional (3D) ultrasound of a fetus with bilateral cleft lip.

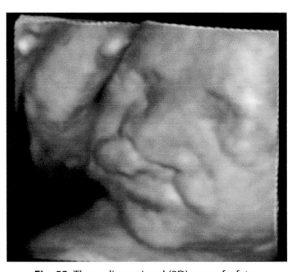

Fig. 93: Three-dimensional (3D) scan of a fetus with a unilateral cleft lips.

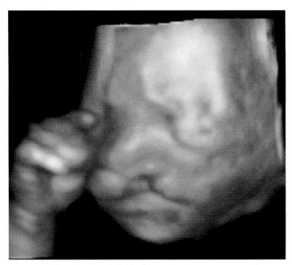

Fig. 91: Cleft lip is clearly visible by three-dimensional (3D) surface rendering. The exact location and surrounding affected structure are visible.

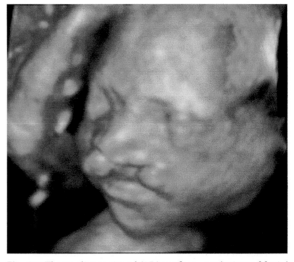

Fig. 94: Three-dimensional (3D) surface rendering of facial expression of the fetus with unilateral cleft lip.

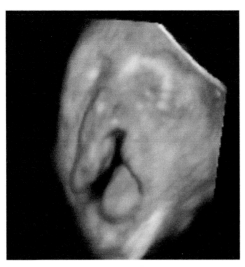

Fig. 95: Three-dimensional (3D) surface rendering demonstrates fetus with labiopalatochizis.

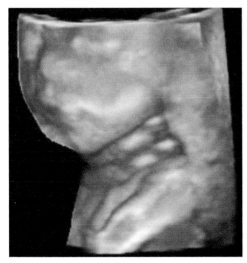

Fig. 96: Three-dimensional (3D) surface rendering of the nuchal cord.

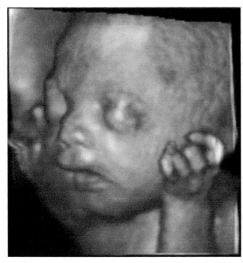

Fig. 97: Three-dimensional (3D) surface rendering shows the facial expression of the fetus with arthrogryposis.

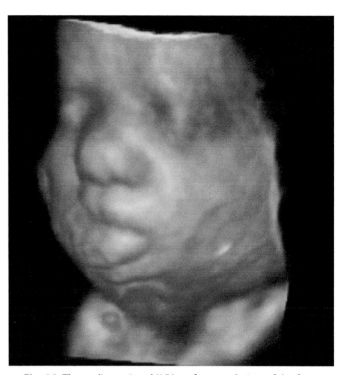

Fig. 98: Three-dimensional (3D) surface rendering of the fetus with macroglossia.

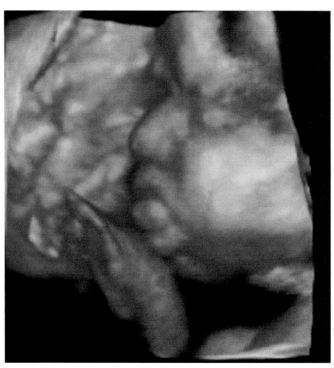

Fig. 99: Three-dimensional (3D) surface imaging showing fetus with macroglossia.

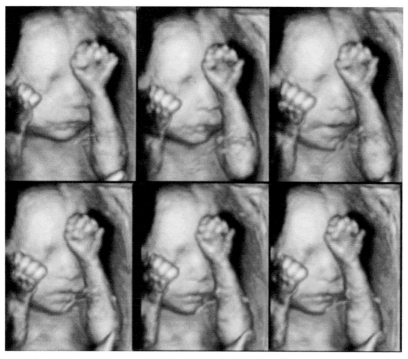

Fig. 100: Four-dimensional (4D) sequence demonstrates alteration in facial expression and movement of the hands beside the head.

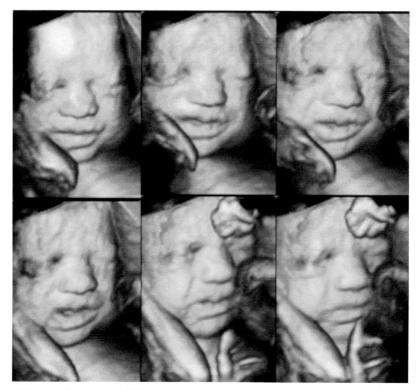

Fig. 101: Four-dimensional (4D) sequence demonstrates grimacing expression of the fetus.

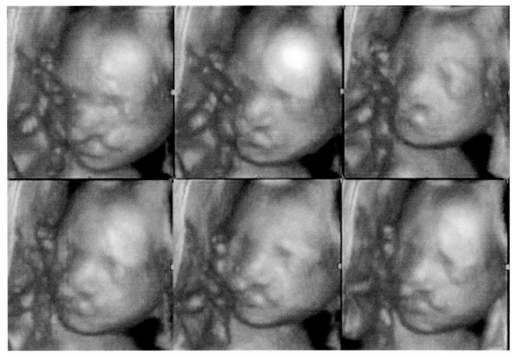

Fig. 102: Four-dimensional (4D) sequence shows changing in the facial expression in the fetus with unilateral cleft lip.

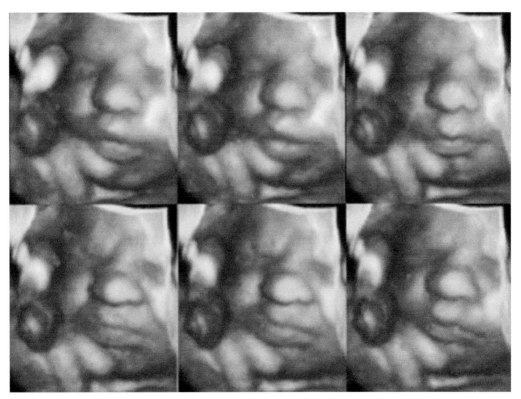

Fig. 103: Grimacing expression of the fetus shows the wrinkling of the brows or face.

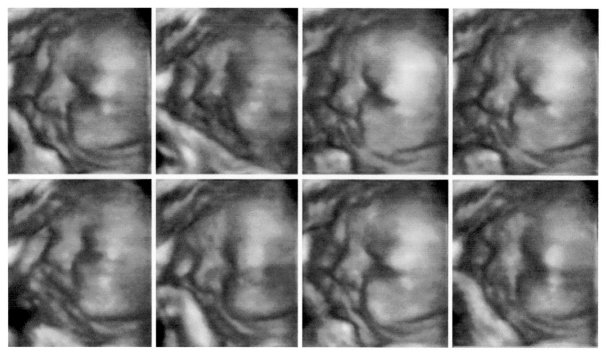

Fig. 104: The fetus seems to express displeasure in this four-dimensional (4D) sequence.

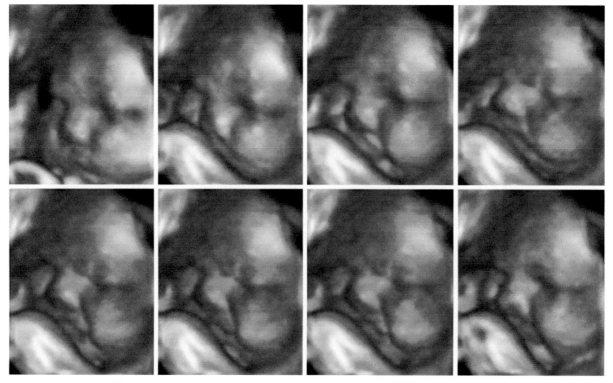

Fig. 105: Four-dimensional (4D) sequence shows wrinkling of the brows or face.

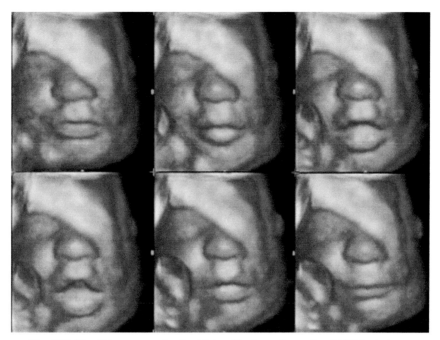

Fig. 106: Mouthing expression is obtained by four-dimensional (4D) technique.

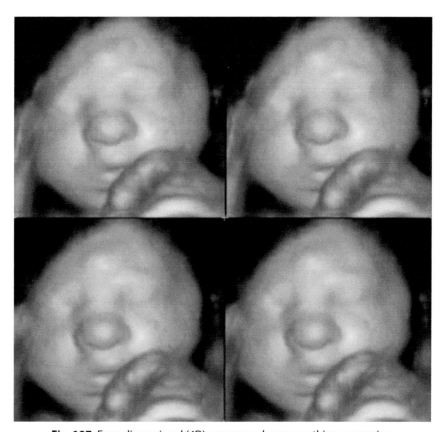

Fig. 107: Four-dimensional (4D) sequence shows mouthing expression.

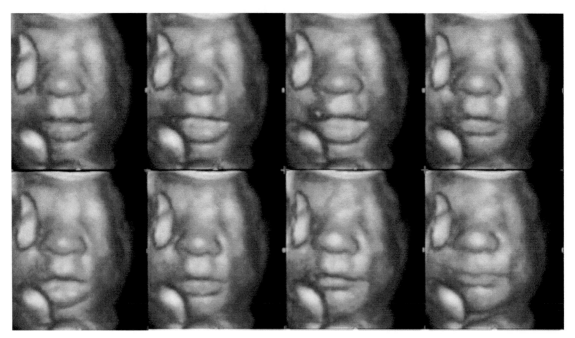

Fig. 108: A facial expression characterized by mouthing expression.

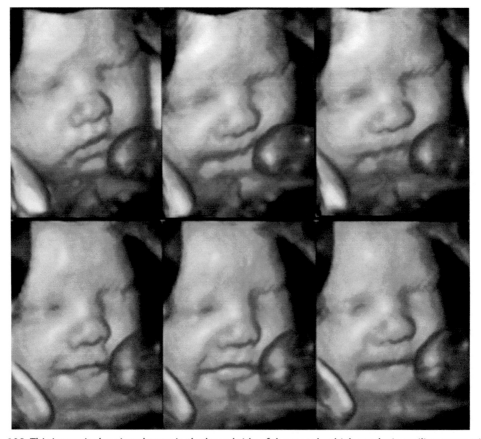

Fig. 109: This image is showing change in the lateral side of the mouth which results in smiling expression.

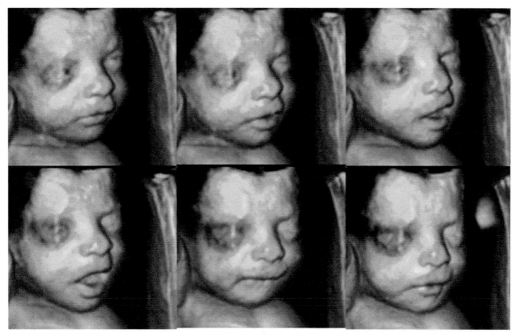

Fig. 110: Four-dimensional (4D) images show a brief closing of the eyelids by involuntary normal periodic closing.

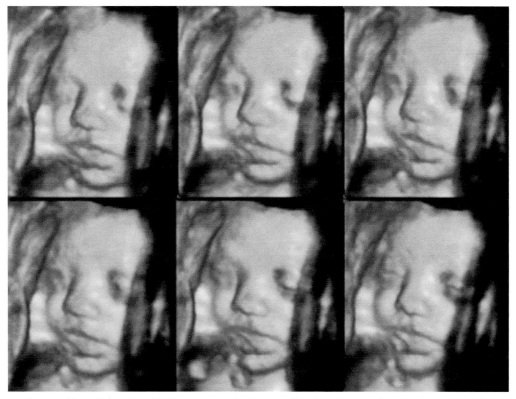

Fig. 111: Four-dimensional (4D) sequence showing a reflex that closes and opens the eyes rapidly.

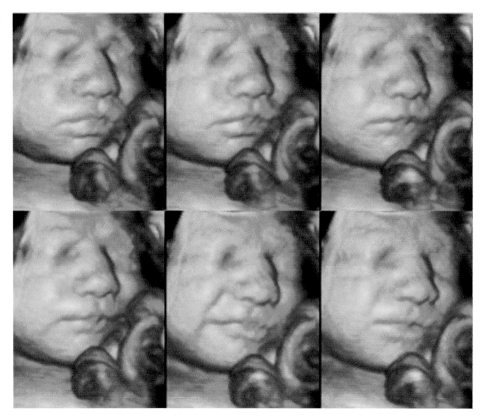

Fig. 112: Four-dimensional (4D) sequence characterized by mouthing expression.

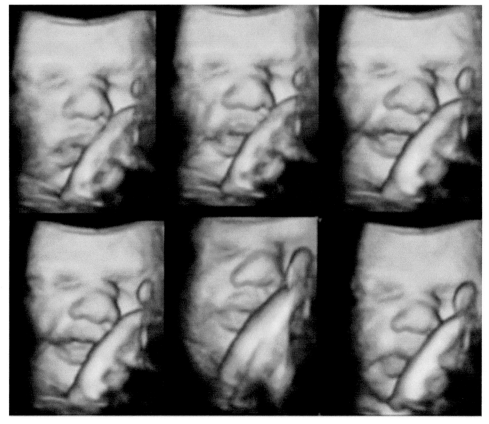

Fig.113: Four-dimensional (4D) imaging characterized by turning up the corners of the mouth. The fetus seems to be smiling.

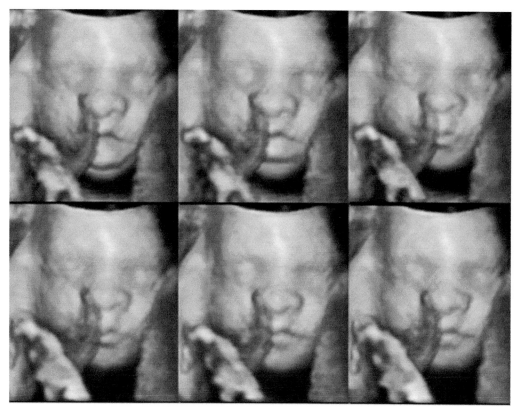

Fig. 114: Four-dimensional (4D) sequence characterized by mouth manipulation to investigate an object. Mouthing is most common in fetus and it may develop into a persistent, stereotyped behavior pattern.

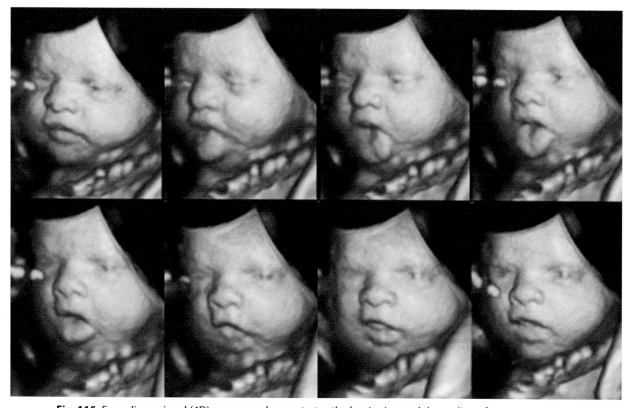

Fig. 115: Four-dimensional (4D) sequence demonstrates the beginning and the ending of tongue expulsion.

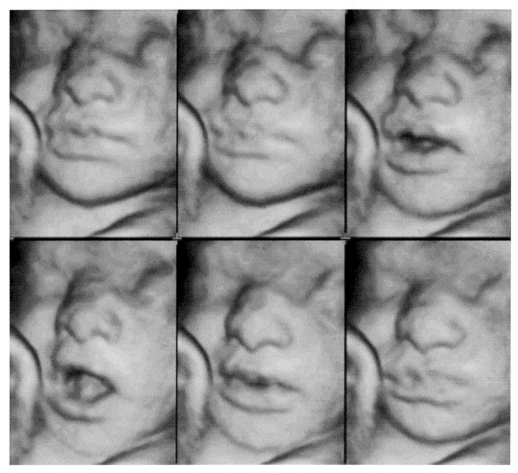

Fig. 116: Four-dimensional (4D) sequence shows mouth opening. The fetus demonstrates drinking and swallowing of the amniotic fluid.

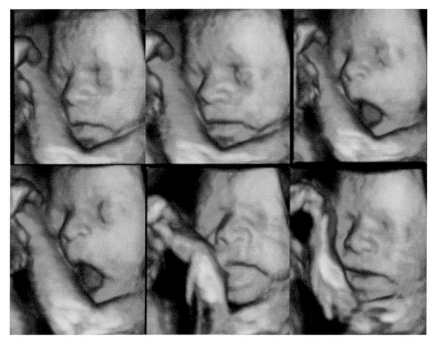

Fig. 117: Four-dimensional (4D) sequence demonstrates mouth opening and hand movement of both of the hands beside the head in the yawning expression.

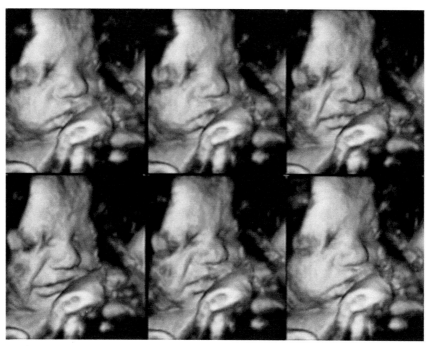

Fig. 118: Four-dimensional (4D) sonography sequence demonstrates changing in the facial expression. The fetus seems to be angry.

OPTIMUM CONDITIONS FOR 3D SCANNING OF THE FETAL FACE

For 3D visualization of the fetal face, the surface mode is generally used. This normally needs a shorter training period with acceptable results in a relatively limited period of time. It must be said, however, that the achievement of appropriate images requires a set of previous conditions without which our results would probably be discouraging. It is clear that one of the great, advantages of 3D ultrasound is that the information remains captured as a volume and it is possible to reconstruct the recorded image and modify all the adjustments as if the patient was still present. This enables us to manipulate the image, re-rotate it three-dimensionally and achieve another 3D reconstruction from the data already taken. There are also electronic scalpels, which assist by cutting off and eliminating all parts that can hide or distort the area we wish to study. With these facilities, we can improve the 3D reconstruction made from an image that is less than favorable.

Appropriate Gestational Age to Visualize the Fetal Face

The appropriate gestational age is neither too early (as the facial structures are not sufficiently developed) nor too late (the relative lack of space available during the last gestational weeks might hinder an appropriate visualization of the fetal face, due to its immediate closeness to the uterine wall, the placenta, or the fetal extremities). From weeks 13 to 14, facial structures have reached an adequate degree of development in order to start studying them for diagnostic purposes.

This may still be too early to show the mother any images if we support, at this stage, the contribution of the scan to reinforce the affective bonds between the fetus and the future parents. Our experience shows that it is counterproductive to show the 3D image of the fetal face to the parents during the first trimester. For most parents, the image appears to be strange and it can create a distorted image of their child, which will not reinforce the affective bonds. It could indeed create anxiety. From weeks 18 to 19, we can obtain 3D reconstruction of the fetal face which is starting to show clear facial features[58] and these can be shown to the parents. From this moment and until week 35 or 36, we can obtain 3D reconstructions of the facial surface in a high percentage of mothers. Experience and much patience are needed to wait for the fetus to adopt an appropriate position for this type of scanning.[59] We think that the most favorable age for 3D scanning of the fetal face is from weeks 23 until 30. During this period of gestation, we have succeeded in visualizing the face three-dimensionally in a high percentage of the cases (higher than 70%) without extending the length of the prenatal 2D ultrasound scan.

Favorable Fetal Position

To obtain the best images, the probe has to be moved so that the face of the fetus is facing the probe surface. In addition, it is very important for the fetal face not to be in contact with other structures such as the uterine wall, the placenta, or fetal extremities. Sometimes, it will be of much assistance to stimulate the fetus using the free hand over the abdominal wall. The fetus may then change position and move away from the structures that prevent correct visualization. Once the correct position is obtained, the capture box is placed over the reference line in the closest possible way to the fetal face. We will have to wait for the baby to keep still, if we seek a static 3D reconstruction, or to make facial movements (yawning, suctioning, lids opening) if we seek a 4D scanning.

Postprocessing of the Image

In addition to these previous requirements, one should not forget that, after capturing the image, there are many adjustment possibilities. Among all the tools we have at the moment, the most useful one is the electronic scalpel, which allows us to eliminate all areas that are of no interest, and also those which disturb the demonstration of the structure that we wish to visualize. This tool can be used in both multiplanar and 3D images. The control of all these adjustments, possibilities and tools does take time, but, the final achievement of images shown will surely compensate for all our efforts.

Once we have acquired this experience, we can verify that, while all the procedures stated here are very complicated and complex, with time they become relatively easy and, in fact, require only a few seconds to adjust the equipment and just a few minutes to retouch the 3D reconstruction. Usually, we start the conventional scanning and, when we acquire a favorable position of the fetal face, we interrupt the 2D exploration and capture the image for 3D reconstruction, following which 2D ultrasound study is then continued. With this procedure, we can achieve 3D visualization of the fetal face without adding >3 or 4 minutes to the complete length of the usual ultrasound scanning.

■ CONCLUSION

Three-dimensional ultrasound offers the possibility of studying the fetal face in a more global way than conventional 2D ultrasound. In normal cases, the images obtained help to transmit a feeling of calmness to the parents and reinforce the affective bonds with their child. In pathological cases, 3D ultrasound can help parents and other doctors involved to take a more realistic view of the problem. It is expected that the use of this novel technology will provide parents with the knowledge to have a better judgment while taking decisions. Four-dimensional ultrasound has enormous potential in perinatal research. This technique is still in its infancy but there is much scope for investigation of fetal anatomy as well as fetal behavior. This technique should assist us in the better understanding of both the somatic and functional development of the early embryo and the fetus.

■ REFERENCES

1. Baba K, Okai T, Kozuma S, Taketani Y, Mochizuki T, Akahane M. Real-time processable three-dimensional US in obstetrics. Radiology. 1997;203:571-4.
2. Baba K, Okai T, Kozuma S. Real-time processable three-dimensional fetal ultrasound. Lancet. 1996;348:1307.
3. Baba K, Satoh K, Sakamoto S, Okai T, Ishi IS. Development of an ultrasonic system for three-dimensional reconstruction of the fetus. J Perinat Med. 1989;17:19-24.
4. Bonilla-Musoles F, Machado L. Ultrasonidos y Reproduccion. Cuadernos de Medicina Reproductiva, No 2. Madrid: Panamericana Ed.; 1999. p. 6.
5. Bonilla-Musoles F, Machado LE, Osborne NC. Ecograha tridimensional en Obstetricia en el nuevo milemo. Madrid: Marco Crafico; 2000.
6. Bonilla-Musoles F, Raga F, Blanes J, Osborne N, Siles CH. Three-dimensional ultrasound in reproductive medicine: preliminary report. Hum Reprod Update. 1995,1:4 item 21 CDRom.
7. Bonilla-Musoles F, Raga F, Osborne N, Blanes J. Ecografia tridimensional en Obstetncia y Ginecologia. Obstet Ginecol Espan. 1994;3:233-50.
8. Campbell S. 4D, or not 4D: that is the question. Ultrasound Obstet Gynecol. 2002,19:1-4.
9. Crane JP, LeFevre ML, Winborn RC, Evans JK, Ewigman BG, Bain RP, et al. A randomized trial of prenatal ultrasonographic screening: impact on the detection, management, and outcome of anomalous fetuses. The RADIUS Study Group. Am J Obstet Gynecol. 1994;171:392-9.
10. Demyer W, Zeman W, Palmer CG. The Face Predicts the Brain: Diagnostic Significance of Median Facial Anomalies for Holoprosencephaly (Arhinencephaly). Pediatrics. 1964;34: 256-63.
11. Devonald KJ, Ellwood DA, Griffiths KA, Kossoff G, Gill RW, Kadi AP, et al. Volume imaging: three-dimensional appreciation of the fetal head and face. J Ultrasound Med. 1995;12:919-25.
12. Hamper UM, Trapanotto V, Sheth S, DeJong MR, Caskey CI. Three-dimensional US: preliminary clinical experience. Radiology. 1994,191:397-401.
13. Hata T, Yonehara T, Aoki S, Manabe A, Hata K, Miyazaki K. Three-dimensional sonographic visualization, of the fetal face. Am J Roentgenol. 1998;170:481-3.
14. Hegge FN, Prescott CH, Watson PT. Fetal facial abnormalities identified during sonography. J Ultrasound Med. 1986;5:679-88.
15. Hepper PC, Shannon FA, Dornan JC. Sex differences in fetal mouth movements. Lancet. 1997;350:1820.
16. Hohlfeld J. Le diagnostic prenatal des feintes labio-palatines. Med Foct Echographie Gynecol. 1995;22:4-15.
17. Hull AD, Pretorius DH. Fetal face: what we can see using two-dimensional and three-dimensional ultrasound. Semin Roentgenol. 1998;33:369-74.
18. Ji EK, Pretorius DH, Newton R, Uyan K, Hull AD, Hollenbach K, et al. Effects of ultrasound on maternal-fetal bonding: a comparison of two- and three-dimensional imaging. Ultrasound Obstet Gynecol. 2005;25:473-7.
19. Kelly IMC, Cardener JE, Brett AD, Richards RR, Lees WR. Three-dimensional US of the fetus. Work in progress. Radiology. 1994;192:253-9.
20. Kelly IMC, Cardener JE, Lees WR. Three-dimensional fetal ultrasound. Lancet. 1991;339:1062-4.
21. Kozuma S, Baba K, Okai T, Taketani Y. Dynamic observation of the fetal face by three-dimensional ultrasound. Ultrasound Obstet Gynecol. 1999,13:283-4.
22. Kozuma S, Okai T, Ryo E, Nishina H, Nemoto A, Kagawa H, et al. Differential developmental process of respective behavioral states in human fetuses. Am J Perinatol. 1998;15:203-8.

23. Kratochwil A. Versuch der 3-dimensionalen Darstellung in der Ceburtshilfe. Ultraschall Med. 1992;13:183-6.

24. Kuno A, Akiyama M, Yamashiro C, Tanaka H, Yamagihara T, Hata T. Three-dimensional sonographic assessment of fetal behavior in the early second trimester of pregnancy. J Ultrasound Med. 2001;20:1271-5.

25. Kuo HC, Chang FM, Wu CH, Yao BL, Liu CH. The primary application of three-dimensional ultrasonography in obstetrics. Am J Obstet Gynecol. 1992;166:880-6.

26. Kurjak A, Azumendi G, Vecek N, Kupesic S, Solak M, Varga D, et al. Fetal hand movements and facial expression in normal pregnancy studied by four-dimensional sonography. J Perinat Med. 2003;31:496-508.

27. Kurjak A, Stanojevic M, Andonotopo W, Salihagic-Kadic A, Carrera JM, Azumendi G. Behavioral pattern continuity from prenatal to postnatal life—a study by four-dimensional (4D) ultrasonography. J Perinat Med. 2004;32:346-53.

28. Kurjak A, Vecek N, Hafner T, Bozek T, Funduk Kurjak B, Ujevic B. Prenatal diagnosis: what does four-dimensional ultrasound add? J Perinat Med. 2002;30:57-62.

29. Kurjak A, Vecek N, Kupesic S, Azumendi C, Solak M. Four-dimensional sonography: how much does it improve perinatal practice. In: Carrera JM, Kurjak A, Chervenak FA (Eds). Controversies in Perinatal Medicine. London: Parthenon Publishing; 2003.

30. Lee A, Deutinger J, Bernaschek C. Three-dimensional ultrasound: abnormalities of the fetal face in surface and volume rendering mode. Br J Obstet Gynaecol. 1995;102:302-6.

31. Lee A. Four-dimensional ultrasound in prenatal diagnosis; leading edge in imaging technology. Ultrasound Rev Obstet Gynecol. 2001;1:194-8.

32. Lees WR, Gardener JE, Gilliams A. Three-dimensional US of the fetus. Radiology. 1991;181:131-2.

33. Levaillant JM, Benoit B, Bady J, Rotten D. Echographie tridimensionelle apport technique et clinique en echographie obstetricale. Reprod Humaine Hormone. 1995;3:341-7.

34. Ludomirski A, Khandelwal M, Uerpairojkit B, Reece EA, Chan L. Three-dimensional ultrasound evaluation of fetal facial and spinal anatomy. Am J Obstets Gynecol. 1996; 174(Suppl):318.

35. Ludomirski A, Ucrpairojkit B, Whiteman VE, Reece EA, Chu GP, Chan L. New technology in three-dimensional obstetrical ultrasonography: technique, advantages, and limitations. Am J Obstet Gynecol. 1996;174(Suppl):328.

36. Maier B, Steiner II, Wienerroither H, Staudach A. The psychological impact of three-dimensional fetal imaging on the fetomaternal relationship. In: Baba K, Jurkovic D (Eds). Three-dimensional Ultrasound in Obstetrics and Gynecology. Lancaster: Parthenon Publishing; 1997. pp. 67-74.

37. Manabe A, Hata T, Aoki S, Matsumoto M, Yanagihara T, Yamada Y, et al. Three-dimensional sonographic visualization of fetal facial anomaly. Acta Obstet Gynecol Scand. 1999,78:917-8.

38. Merz E, Bahlmann F, Weber C, Macchiella D. Three-dimensional ultrasonography in prenatal diagnosis. J Perinat Med. 1995:23:213-22.

39. Merz E, Bahlmann F, Weber C. Volume scanning in the evaluation of fetal malformations: a new dimension in prenatal diagnosis. Ultrasound Obstet Gynecol. 1995;5:222-7.

40. Merz E, Weber C, Bahlmann F, Miric-Tesanic D. Application of transvaginal and abdominal three-dimensional ultrasound for the detection or exclusion of malformations of the fetal face. Ultrasound Obstet Gynecol. 1997;9:237-43.

41. Merz E, Weber G, Bahlmann AF, Macchiella D. Transvaginale 3D-Sonographie in der Gynaekologie. Gynaekologe. 1995; 28:270-5.

42. Merz E. 3-D Ultrasound in Obstetrics and Gynecology. Philadelphia: Lippincott Williams and Wilkins; 1998.

43. Merz E. Einsatz der 3D-Ultraschalltechnik in der pranatalen Diagnostik. Ultraschall Med. 1995;16:154-61.

44. Merz E. Three-dimensional ultrasound in the evaluation of fetal anatomy and fetal malformations. In: Chervenak FA, Kurjak A (Eds). Current Perspectives on the Fetus as a Patient. London: Parthenon Publishing; 1996. pp. 75-87.

45. Mueller CM, Weiner CE, Yankowitz J. Three-dimensional ultrasound in the evaluation of fetal head and spine anomalies. Obstet Gynecol. 1996,88:372-8.

46. Nelson TR, Downey DB, Pretorius DH, Fenster A. Ecografia 3D en Obstetrida en Ecografia 3D. Madrid: Marban; 2000.

47. Nelson TR, Pretorius DH. Three-dimensional ultrasound of fetal surface features. Ultrasound Obstet Gynecol. 1992; 2:166-74.

48. Pretorius DH, House M, Nelson TR, Hollenbach KA. Evaluation of normal and abnormal lips in fetuses: comparison between three and two dimensional sonography. Am J Roentgenol. 1995,165:1233-7.

49. Pretorius DH, Johnson DD, Budonck NE, Jones MC, Lou KV, Nelson TR. Three-dimensional ultrasound of the fetal lip and palate. Radiology. 1997;205(P) (Suppl):245.

50. Pretorius DH, Nelson TR, Jaffe JS. Three-dimensional US of the fetus. Radiology. 1990;177:194.

51. Pretorius DH, Nelson TR. Fetal face visualization using three-dimensional ultrasonography. J Ultrasound Med. 1995;14:349-56.

52. Pretorius DH, Nelson TR. Prenatal visualization of cranial sutures and fontanelles with three-dimensional ultrasonography. J Ultrasound Med. 1994;13:871-6.

53. Pretorius DH, Nelson TR. Three-dimensional ultrasound imaging in patient diagnosis and management: the future. Ultrasound Obstet Gynecol. 1991;1:381-3.

54. Pretorius DH, Richards RD, Budorick NE, Johnson DD, Sklansky MS, Cantrell CJ, et al. Three-dimensional ultrasound in the evaluation of fetal anomalies. Radiology. 1997;205(P) (Suppl):245.

55. Pretorius DH. Maternal smoking habit modification via fetal visualization. University of California Tobacco Related Disease Research Program. Annual Report to the California State Legislature, 1996:76.

56. Roodenburg PJ, Wladimiroff JW, van Es A, Prechtl HF. Classification and quantitative aspect of fetal movements during the second half of normal pregnancy. Early Hum Dev. 1991;25:19-35.

57. Schart A, Chazwiny MF, Steinbom A, Baier P, Sohn C. Evaluation of two-dimensional versus three-dimensional ultrasound in obstetric diagnostics: a prospective study. Fetal Diagn Ther. 2001;16:333-41.

58. Steiner H, Merz E, Staudach A. Three-dimensional fetal facing. Hum Reprod Update. 1995;1:item 6.

59. Ulm MR, Kratochwil A, Ulm B, Solar P, Aro C, Bernaschek G. Three-dimensional ultrasound evaluation of fetal tooth germs. Ultrasound Obstet Gynecol. 1998,12:240-3.

Fetal Echocardiography

Badreldeen Ahmed, Milan Stanojević

■ INTRODUCTION

When introduced in diagnostics, two-dimensional (2D) ultrasound revolutionized many fields of clinical medicine.[1,2] Among them, the cardiology gained a huge advantage of 2D ultrasonography for postnatal diagnostics and treatment of congenital cardiac defects. Jan Donald, the father of the modern obstetrical ultrasonography, could not predict how helpful and significant ultrasonography will become for the prenatal diagnosis of fetal cardiac problems.[1,2] About 25 years ago the significance of prenatal diagnosis of congenital heart defects (CHDs) was considered very important for the prognosis of the fetus, and outcome of pregnancy, possibility of the postnatal correction or lifesaving intervention and prediction of the life quality of the newborn and the family. The incidence of CHD is estimated to be 0.8 in 1,000 live-born infants, and therefore, this new possibility to diagnose them prenatally has also important public-health implications.[3-5] Another question, raised but so far not solved during the development of fetal echocardiography, was that screening of CHD is necessary for all, not only for high-risk pregnancies.[6] Very important criterion for the screening method is its simplicity, good sensitivity, and specificity, acceptable reliability and low costs.[7,8] It was revealed that sensitivity of the fetal echocardiography could be improved by visualization of four-chamber view and depiction of great arteries outflow tracts, three- vessel and three-vessel view and three-vessels-and-trachea (3VT) view in the same fetus, which became a standard of care in low-risk pregnancies.[9,10] Is the education of screeners alone sufficient to achieve that goal of the utmost importance for the improvement of fetal echocardiography as a screening method? The answer to that question is still unequivocal, because improvements of ultrasound technology and telemedicine are opening the new and promising possibilities even for those who are not experts.[11-15]

When introduced, three- and four-dimensional (3D and 4D) echocardiography was quite new and exciting possibility in the fetal cardiology.[13-15] Medications for the rhythm disturbances of the fetal heart have been used successfully for many years. Prenatal interventions, very rarely performed on fetal heart, are becoming more available with development of new nonsurgical methods of the cardiac defect repair.[16] The question is where is development of fetal cardiology headed? At the beginning of 1990s, the first trimester transabdominal or transvaginal route of the assessment of fetal heart was developed in order to define fetal well-being and possible aneuploidy.[6,17-22] An increasing rate of terminations of pregnancies will take place with the earlier diagnosis of CHD. In those who will survive, prenatal interventions will be possible in some cases while in the others, the prognosis will be improved by the early lifesaving postnatal intervention in the cardiac tertiary centers.[16,23]

The aim of the chapter is to give a brief overview on development of promising field of fetal echocardiography.

■ DEVELOPMENT OF FETAL ECHOCARDIOGRAPHY

It was revealed in the 1980s, that fetal echocardiography could correctly predict structural malformations of the heart, and it was concluded that the technique was sufficiently reliable to give an accurate prognosis in early pregnancy and provide the basis for alterations in obstetrical management.[3-6,9] The questions which have been raised from the early years of development of fetal echocardiography for detection of CHD, were:

- To screen or not to screen?
- Whom to screen?
- Who should screen?
- When to screen?

To Screen or Not to Screen for Fetal Congenital Heart Defect

The answer to that question is affirmative, because sufficiently high incidence of CHD is justifying their screening.[3-6,24-26] The screening method is relatively simple and cost-effective, while the intervention after the screening could be effective. Fetal echocardiography has been a useful tool either for the prenatal detection of CHD or for the detection of other heart lesions as arrhythmias or cardiomyopathies.[3-6,9,24-26] Most cases of CHD occur in otherwise normal pregnancies, although the risk of CHD is markedly increased in aneuploidies.[6,12,21,27] It was revealed in the 1980s that fetal echocardiography could predict correctly structural malformations of the heart with the conclusion that the technique is sufficiently reliable to give an accurate prognosis in early pregnancy and provide the basis for alterations in obstetric management.[3] In a series of 1,600 pregnancies, 34 cases of CHD were correctly identified by fetal echocardiography with the confirmation of the diagnosis by anatomical study.[3] It was a great success that 14 pregnancies were terminated electively.[3] Twenty fetuses died subsequently owing either to the complexity of the congenital heart disease or to associated extracardiac abnormalities.[3] They reported eight errors in interpretation of the fetal echocardiogram.[3] There were no reports concerning prenatal intervention on the fetal heart at that time.

In another study, the authors reported their experience with fetal CHD since 1980, when they diagnosed CHD in 1,006 fetuses.[4] Chromosomal anomalies were more frequent in the fetuses with CHD than in the live births.[4] The survival rate after diagnosis was poor because of frequent parental choice to interrupt pregnancy and the complexity of the disease.[4] A large experience with fetal CHD allows good accuracy after postnatal and pathological evaluation of the prenatal findings.[4] Knowledge of the natural history of heart malformations and their treatment allows accurate counseling offered to the parents.[4] The parental decision in this investigation shifted toward termination of pregnancy, which means that smaller number of infants and children with complex cardiac malformations will present in postnatal life.[4]

The 1,589 infants with CHD were identified in a well-defined population.[24] The live-birth prevalence of CHD was 8.1 per 1,000 of which only 6.1% were diagnosed prenatally.[24] The percentage of prenatally diagnosed CHD increased from 2.6% at the beginning of the investigation to 12.7% at the end, and it was lowest for the atrial septal defect (4.7%) and highest for the hypoplastic left heard syndrome (HLHS) (28%).[24] Prenatally diagnosed CHD were associated with the high incidence of infant mortality (30.9%) and fetal wastage (17.5%).[24] Fetal echocardiography has been used increasingly in the prenatal diagnosis of congenital cardiac malformation, and it showed that survival of infants was not improved after prenatal diagnosis with fetal echocardiography.[24]

Chromosomal anomalies were more frequent in fetuses with CHD.[3] This tendency was confirmed by Bronshtein et al. who performed 12,793 transvaginal ultrasound examinations at 12–16 weeks of gestation of which 27% were at high-risk for fetal CHD.[6] Overall detection rate of CHD was 47 of 12,793 (3.6 per 1,000) fetuses, of whom 29 of 9,340 (3.1 per 1,000) belonged to a low-risk population and 18 of 3,453 (5.2 per 1,000) belonged to a high-risk population.[6] Thirty six percent of affected fetuses who underwent karyotyping had abnormal chromosomes.[6]

In a study of 1,040 fetuses at 11–14 weeks of gestation, Doppler velocimetry of the ductus venosus in the combination with nuchal translucency improved predictive capacity of CHD detection in chromosomally normal fetuses.[21] In 29 chromosomally normal fetuses, increased nuchal translucency and reversed or absent flow during atrial contraction of the ductus venosus was found, and in nine fetal echocardiography revealed major CHD.[21] A total of 25 CHD were detected in the whole population, 15 of whom were associated with aneuploidy.[21] They concluded that in chromosomally normal fetuses with increased nuchal translucency, assessment of ductus venosus blood flow velocimetry could improve the predictive capacity for an underlying major cardiac defect.[21]

Extracardiac anomalies are more frequent in the group of fetuses with CHD.[27] In a high-risk group of 334 fetuses, 48 (14.4%) were diagnosed with CHD at 12–17 weeks of gestation, 27 (56.3%) of whom had abnormal karyotype, and 31 (64.6%) had associated extracardiac malformations.[27] In the recently published retrospective study of 9,918 women who were referred for fetal echocardiography, 1,191 (12%) fetuses were diagnosed with CHD, of which 46 (4%) were delivered prematurely.[22] Extracardiac and karyotypic anomalies occurred in 23 (50%). Of those 46 infants 26 (57%) underwent neonatal surgery with the overall mortality rate of 72%.[22]

Whom to Screen: Low-risk or High-risk Population?

The answer to that question is that CHD screening should be offered and performed in all pregnant women.[28] More than 90% of CHD occurs in low-risk population.[28] Prenatal detection rate of CHD in tertiary perinatal centers was 18 and 0% in nontertiary centers.[29] Prenatal detection rate of major CHD was 23.4% in the United Kingdom.[30]

Large retrospective study with 10,806 patients in whom 774 (71.6 per 1,000) cases of structural CHD were detected, revealed that the pattern of indications for fetal echocardiography has changed between 1985 and 2003.[31] There was a significant increase in the proportion of studies for diabetes, maternal structural CHD, suspicious four-chamber heart, and family history of cardiac disease, while decrease of studies was noticed for a previous child with structural CHD, cardiac teratogen exposure, other fetal anomalies, aneuploidy, fetal arrhythmia, and nonimmune hydrops.[31]

It would be interested to investigate what are prenatal detection rates of CHD in developing countries, where antenatal care is far from being satisfactory.[32,33] Postnatal incidence of CHD in Croatia is estimated to be 7.8 in 1,000 live-born infants, of which over 40% were detected in the first month of life and 92% till the end of the second year of life **(Fig. 1)**, while the data concerning prenatal detection rate of CHD are not available.[34] Two hundred and two pregnant women with 208 fetuses of high-risk for fetal CHD, in the year 2002 underwent fetal echocardiography at "Sv. Duh" General Hospital, Zagreb, Croatia. There were 198 live-born infants and 10 perinatal deaths: three still-born, four early neonatal deaths, and three induced abortions.[35] The most frequent indications for fetal echocardiography were: intrauterine growth restriction (IUGR) in 24, polyhydramnios in 22, pyelectasia and/or polycystic kidney disease in 22, mothers' age in 21, ultrasound markers for malformations in 20, CHD

in previous pregnancy in 15, gross fetal malformations in 12, CHD or suspicious cardiac rhythm disturbances on regular ultrasound examination in 9, risk of aneuploidy in 8.[35] In the group of three aborted fetuses with chromosomopathy and cystic hygroma, two CHDs were diagnosed prenatally and confirmed at autopsy postnatally.[35] In three stillborn fetuses neither CHD nor other congenital malformations were diagnosed, while in 10 neonates who died in the early neonatal period, tricuspid regurgitation was diagnosed prenatally in one, not confirmed postnatally.[35]

The most striking issue concerning prenatal screening of CHD is education of gynecologists performing general anomaly scan in pregnancy. As it is well known, four-chamber view detects up to 77% of prenatally developed CHD, while depiction of ventricular outflow tracts increases prenatal detection rate of CHD between 83 and 92%.[6,28,36,37]

The detection of even major malformations seen in the four-chamber view is less than perfect. Some lesions could be overlooked during the examination, because four-chamber view could be normal, which does not exclude existence of CHD.[38,39] Lesions that may be associated with normal or abnormal four-chamber view are given in **Table 1**.[40]

Who Should Screen: General Gynecologists or Pediatric Cardiologists?

In the study, accuracy of prenatal diagnosis of CHD by maternal-fetal medicine specialist and radiologists (MFM/R) in the first group and pediatric cardiologists (PCs) in the second group was investigated.[41] They showed that PC did significantly more fetal echocardiography scans per one normal fetus and per fetus with CHD **(Table 2)**, which resulted in better accuracy of PC **(Table 3)**.[41] They concluded that frequency of fetal echocardiography performed in

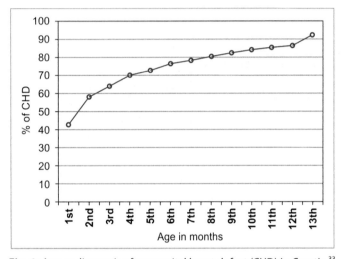

Fig. 1: Age at diagnosis of congenital heart defect (CHD) in Croatia.[33]

TABLE 1: Lesions that may be associated with an abnormal and a normal four-chamber view during fetal echocardiography.[40]		
Lesions that may be associated with:		
An abnormal four-chamber view	*A normal four-chamber view*	*Lesions likely to be overlooked prenatally*
At the venous atrial junction: • Total anomalous pulmonary venous drainage *At the atrioventricular junction:* • Mitral atresia • Tricuspid atresia • Atrioventricular septal defect • Ebstein's anomaly *At the ventriculoarterial junction:* • Aortic atresia • Pulmonary atresia with intact interventricular septum • Critical aortic stenosis • Coarctation of the aorta • Other • Ventricular septal defect • Cardiomyopathy	• Transposition of the great arteries • Double outlet right ventricle • Tetralogy of Fallot • Pulmonary atresia with a ventricular septal defect • Common arterial trunk • Absent pulmonary valve syndrome	• Persistent arterial duct • Secundum atrial septal defect • Milder forms of obstructive lesions of great arteries • Pulmonary stenosis and coarctation of the aorta • Some forms of ventricular septal defects

TABLE 2: Prenatal diagnosis of congenital heart defect (CHD) by maternal fetal specialists and pediatric cardiologists.[41]

Characteristic	Maternal fetal medicine specialist	Pediatric cardiologist	Significance
Number of fetuses	619	2147	–
Echocardiograms/ fetus	1.1 ± 0.6^2	1.6 ± 1.0	<0.0001
Number of fetuses with CHD	**34 (5.5%)**	**88 (4.1%)**	<0.0001
Gestational age at diagnosis	30.4 ± 5.7	29.4 ± 5.6	NS
Extracardiac structural anomalies	35%	34%	NS

^{2}Mean ± standard deviation (SD)

TABLE 3: Postnatal confirmation of diagnosis of congenital heart defect (CHD) after fetal echocardiography.[41]

Facility	Correct/ incorrect	False negative/ positive	Diagnostic accuracy
Maternal-fetal medicine specialist (MFM/R)	25/6	3/2	87%
Pediatric cardiologist (PC)	81/4	3/2	92%*

*Statistically significant

TABLE 4: Detection rate of congenital heart defect (CHD) by routine fetal echocardiography screening using two-dimensional ultrasound by different echocardiography views (four-chamber view, outflow tract view, and three-vessel view).

Echocardiographic view	Detection rate (%)	95% confidence interval
Four-chamber view	52	50–55
Four-chamber + outflow tract view	65	61–69
Four-chamber + outflow tract + three-vessel view	90	86–93

Source: Modified according to reference 42.

BOX 1: High-risk factors for the development of congenital heart defects.[21,40]

Maternal factors:
- Family history (risk 2%)
- Maternal diabetes (2–3%)
- Exposure to teratogens in early pregnancy

Fetal factors:
- Extracardiac fetal anomaly
- Fetal arrhythmias
- Nonimmune fetal hydrops
- Increased nuchal translucency
- Abnormal ductus venosus waveforms

the center may also contribute to the accuracy of the sonographer.[41] The detection rate of CHD depends on the examination protocol and what kind of the views are used during the screening. The data in the **Table 4** are showing that if only four-chamber view is used, the detection rate of CHD would be 52% [confidence interval (CI) 50–55%], if outflow tracts are added to four-chamber, then the detection rate of CHD would be increasing to 65% (CI 61–69%), and if to previous two views three-vessel view is added then detection rate of CHD would be increasing to 90% (CI 86–93%).[42,43]

The level of agreement between obstetric and PC sonographers' diagnosis of fetuses with suspected CHD was studied on 1,037 patients undergoing fetal echocardiography in a 5-year period at the tertiary referral center for fetal echocardiography.[44] The median gestational age at presentation was 21 weeks (range 17–38 weeks) with 49% scans performed at <21 weeks and further, 17% performed at 21–24 weeks.[44] Of 268 fetuses with CHD suspected by obstetric sonographers, 209 had confirmed cardiac defects.[44] Complete correlation between obstetric sonographers' and PCs prenatal cardiac findings was achieved in 62% of cases.[44] The major differences were involving the atrioventricular morphology in 18% and outflow tract anatomy in 20%.[44] Complete agreement between prenatal and postnatal diagnosis in fetuses with complex CHD was achieved in 59% of cases for obstetric sonography and 95% for fetal echocardiography by PCs with special skills in fetal echocardiography.[26,30,44-46]

When appropriately educated gynecologists in a low-risk population were involved in screening of CHD, the detection rate of 77% of all cardiac abnormalities, which would be associated with an abnormal appearance in four-chamber view, was achieved.[47] The maternal and fetal high-risk factors with increased risk of CHD in fetuses are listed in the **Box 1**.[21,40] The existence of risk factors will prompt the gynecologist for referral of every suspicious case to the tertiary echocardiographic center.[21,40,47]

There is a discussion concerning the responsibility for the prenatal screening of CHD: is it PC or gynecologist responsible for the screening?[25,26,45] There is a large discrepancy in study results of second trimester ultrasound screening for fetal malformations, owing to the different level of experience of examiners.[25,26,45] The reported detection rates of fetal CHD were 0–60%.[25] Various screening concepts for more effective detection of CHD are available, and the most recent technique of early echocardiography between 11 and 15 weeks of gestation was considered very useful due to the easier termination of pregnancy if needed.[24,25] It is our opinion that gynecologist is responsible for the screening of CHD and if CHD is suspected, then PC skilled in fetal echocardiography should examine the patient and confirm or make the diagnosis.[30,39,47,48] Gynecologist, PC, geneticist, psychologist, and social worker should be involved in counseling.

When to Screen: The First or the Second Trimester?

The second trimester (usually after 18 weeks) is well-established and valuable investigation for the detection of CHD.[5,9,38,49,50] The first trimester transabdominal and transvaginal fetal echocardiography should be performed in a high-risk population.[6,17-21,27] Weiner et al. performed 329 examinations between 11 and 14 weeks, 438 examinations between 14 and 16 weeks, and 777 examinations between 20 and 24 weeks of gestation.[20] Indications for the early echocardiographic scan were maternal diabetes and/or CHD in previous pregnancy.[20] They diagnosed correctly 6 of 7 major fetal CHD between 11 and 14 weeks, while at that time missed one was correctly diagnosed at 22 weeks of gestation.[20] Only one of five minor CHD was detected between 11 and 14 weeks, and four incorrect diagnoses of minor CHD were made at the same gestational age, excluded on repeated fetal echocardiography examination at 20 and 24 weeks of gestation.[20] According to Simpson JM et al., transabdominal fetal echocardiography can be performed at 12–15 weeks of gestation, permitting accurate early detection of major CHDs in a high-risk population.[17] They detected 13 fetuses with CHD out of 226, and in 11 the CHD was confirmed either postnatally or at autopsy.[17] Of those 213 fetuses with normal prenatal findings, CHD was detected later in pregnancy or postnatally in four (in three ventricular septal defect, and in one cardiomyopathy).[17] Most echocardiographers agreed that fetal echocardiography is feasible prior to 14 weeks' gestation, and when CHD is present, then chromosomal abnormality should be suspected.[6,17-20,27,30,51] In some studies, the shift from the second to the first trimester fetal echocardiography was noted.[7] They conclude that early fetal echocardiography is feasible and allows the detection of most CHD, but should be always followed by echocardiography at midgestation, because CHD vary in appearance at different stages of pregnancy and may evolve in utero with advancing gestational age.[7] According to some investigators, the success rate of early fetal echocardiography depends on gestational age as follows: the complete evaluation of the fetal heart was impossible at 10 weeks, the total success rate was 45% at 11 weeks, 90% between 12 and 14 weeks, and 100% at 15 weeks of gestation.[52] Between 10 and 13 weeks transvaginal approach was superior to transabdominal, at 14 weeks both methods were similar, and at 15 weeks transabdominal sonography enabled visualization of all cardiac structures.[52] Complete evaluation of fetal heart included: total heart diameter, heart area and circumference, right and left ventricular diameter, diameter, area and circumference of the thorax, and diameter of the aorta and pulmonary trunk, visualization of four- and five-chamber view **(Figs. 2 and 3)**, three-vessel view, origin and crossover of the

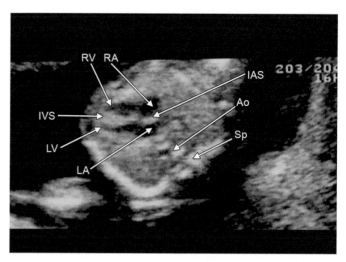

Fig. 2: Lateral four-chamber view (apical long-axis view—17 weeks). (Ao: aorta; IAS: interatrial septum; IVS: intraventricular septum; LA: left atrium; LV: left ventricle; RA: right atrium; RV: right ventricle; Sp: spine)

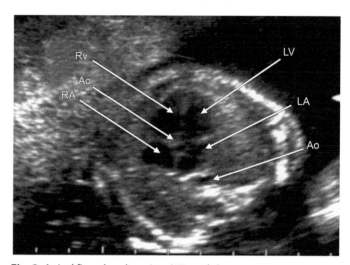

Fig. 3: Apical five-chamber view (17 weeks)
Ao: aorta; LA: left atrium; LV: left ventricle; RA: right atrium; RV: right ventricle)

great arteries, aortic arch **(Fig. 4)**, ductus arteriosus, superior and inferior venae cavae, and pulmonary veins.[52] **Figure 5** shows parasternal short-axis view with depiction of the main pulmonary artery and its' branches and aorta.

3D/4D ultrasound is used in fetal echocardiography with many new assessment techniques and programs for the offline analysis of prerecorded material.[53-55] Application of 3D/4D fetal echocardiography spatiotemporal image correlation (STIC) in so called Omni view and biplane view can depict fetal heart enabling analysis as shown in the **Figure 6**.

Figure 7 showing the new 4D mechanical probe in the left hand with increased resolution and with the possibility to eliminate motion artifacts.

Figures 8A and B showing biplane view used after spatiotemporal image correlation (STIC) which is 4D US technique for depiction of ascending **(Fig. 8A)** and descending aorta **(Fig. 8B)**.

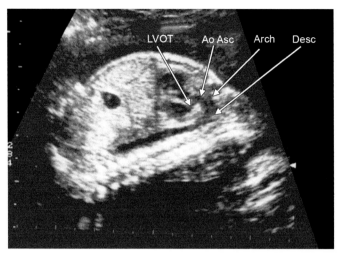

Fig. 4: Aortic arch—sagittal view (18 weeks).
(Ao: aorta; Asc: ascendant; Desc: descendant; LVOT: left ventricular outflow tract)

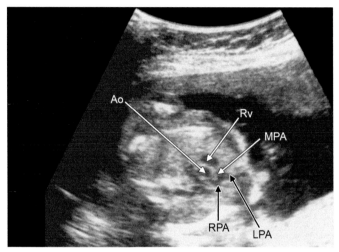

Fig. 5: Parasternal short-axis view of the right ventricle outflow tract (18 weeks).
(Ao: aorta; LPA: left pulmonary artery; MPA: main pulmonary artery; RPA: right pulmonary artery; RV: right ventricle)

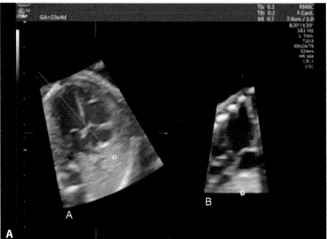
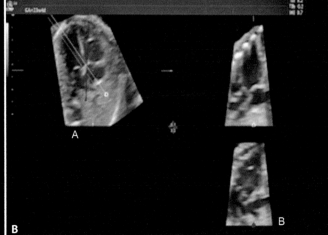

Figs. 6A and B: The mechanical probe of 4D US alows the use of Omniview software with the possibility of postprocessing analysis with placing the line at the site of the aortic outflow (two paralell green lines on the image A) in the 4-chamber view. It is also allowing the visualization of the ascending aorta by placing two paralell green lines in the aortic outflow and two paralell purple lines in the direction towards the ascending aorta, as shown in image B.

What after the Prenatal Diagnosis of Fetal Cardiac Lesion?

Congenital heart defect accounts for 9% of infant mortality in the UK and about 200 infants die each year of undiagnosed CHD.[56] One of the reasons for the growth of fetal echocardiography programs in many developed countries is to decrease the incidence of undiagnosed CHD. It is clear that in the right hands fetal echo has a high sensitivity and specificity. However, it is dependent on an efficient referral system. This necessitates close cooperation between obstetric sonographers and PCs.[56] Fetal echocardiography has its limitations in terms of detection of more minor, yet significant CHD, and is relatively time consuming.[56]

The most common cardiac lesions detected prenatally in the fetus, shown in the **Figure 9**, are: atrioventricular septal defect, hypoplastic left heart syndrome (HLHS), ventricular septal defect, coarctation of the aorta, tricuspid atresia, and other lesions.[40]

The outcome of cardiac malformations diagnosed prenatally, according to Sharland, is in over half of diagnosed fetuses termination of pregnancy, while in the next 30% intrauterine, neonatal or infant death occurred.[40] Overall termination of pregnancy rate is about 80% while survival rate is as low as 20%.[40]

The termination of pregnancy rate is decreasing in the observed period of time, while the opposite tendency is observed with the survival rate of babies from pregnancies that have continued after the diagnosis of CHD **(Figs. 10 and 11)**.[40]

Prenatal diagnosis of structural CHD is associated with a poor prognosis.[48] High mortality rate of 79% has been reported in the study of 222 fetuses, infants, and children in whom prenatal diagnosis of CHD was made.[48] Prenatal death occurred in 57 fetuses, 87 died as neonates, and 31 died in infancy and childhood.[48] Among 47 survivors

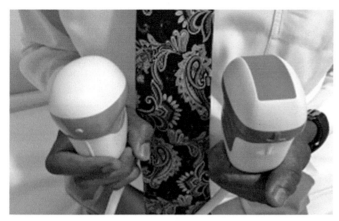

Fig. 7: The new 4D mechanical probe in the left hand with increased resolution and eliminating artifacts.

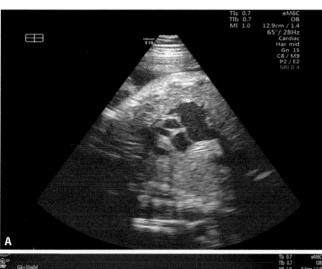

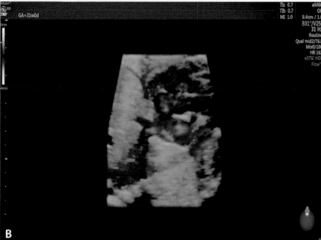

Figs. 8A and B: Biplane view used after spatiotemporal image correlation (STIC) which is four-dimensional ultrasound technique for depiction of ascending aorta (A) and descending aorta (B).

only five have survived beyond 4 years.[48] High mortality was associated with the presence of extracardiac anomalies in 32% and prenatal cardiac failure in 13%.[48,57] Fetal echocardiography has been a useful tool for prenatal detection of CHD and other heart lesions, and in some cases for the treatment of fetal arrhythmias.[38] As the most forms of

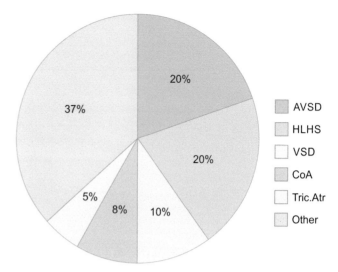

Fig. 9: Incidence of congenital heart defect (CHD) detected by fetal echocardiography.[40]
(AVSD: atrioventricular septal defect; CoA: coarctation of the aorta; HLHS: hypoplastic left heart syndrome; Tric. Atr: tricuspid atresia; VSD: ventricular septal defect)

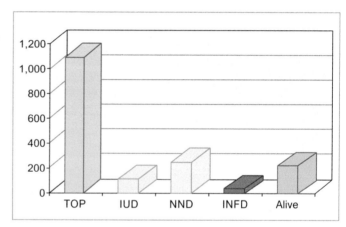

Fig. 10: The outcome of cardiac malformations diagnosed prenatally.[40]
(IUD: intrauterine death; INFD: infant death; NND: neonatal death; TOP: termination of pregnancy)

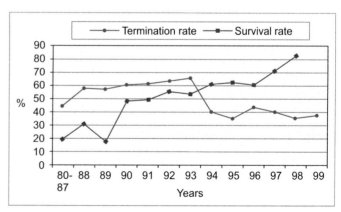

Fig. 11: The outcome of prenatally detected congenital heart defect (CHD).
Source: Modified according to reference 40.

heart disease occur in otherwise normal pregnancies with no high-risk features, detection of these cases is dependent on the skill of the ultrasonographer performing general obstetric scanning.[38] Detection of even major malformations seen in the four-chamber view is still less than perfect.[38,49] It is expected that CHD will be detected earlier in pregnancy and examination will include evaluation of the great artery structure.[49] There is now evidence that prenatal diagnosis of CHD improves perinatal morbidity or mortality.[50] New information about the molecular genetic basis of CHD will help in management and counseling.[50] If extracardiac malformations are excluded, then in utero therapy should be considered for some malformations.[50] It was available for fetal arrhythmias, fetal heart failure, and in some cases for very few structural CHD.[16,40]

The majority of neonates who have CHD will not require delivery room resuscitation in excess of routine care.[23] However, a small number of prenatally diagnosed CHD including transposition of the great arteries with intact ventricular and restrictive atrial septum, HLHS with intact atrial septum, obstructed total anomalous pulmonary venous return, and complete congenital heart block.[23]

The outcome after prenatal diagnosis of the HLHS in 30 fetuses was as follows: 4 of 12 mothers whose fetuses were diagnosed before 24 weeks of gestation choose the termination of pregnancy.[58] Intention to treat was in 24 of the remaining fetuses, of whom 5 were not offered Norwood stage 1 procedure, because of trisomy 18, unfavorable cardiac anatomy or neurological impairment.[58] Of 18 patients who were selected for the operation, nine survived, which means that survival rate was 37.5% from an intention to treat position.[58] It was concluded that survival rate of the patients with the HLHS is poor and discouraging.[58]

The survival after fetal aortic and pulmonary balloon valvuloplasty has been reported and seemed very encouraging approach to the treatment of the fetal CHD.[16,59] The world discouraging experience of percutaneous ultrasound-guided balloon valvuloplasty in human fetuses with severe aortic valve obstruction was reported in 12 fetuses between 27 and 33 weeks of gestation.[60] The range between initial presentation and intervention was 3 days to 9 weeks. Technically successful balloon valvuloplasties were achieved in seven fetuses, none of whom had atretic valve.[60] Only one of these seven fetuses survived, while remaining six died postnatally due to cardiac dysfunction or at surgery in the early postnatal period.[60] The conclusion was that the experience with fetal ultrasound-guided balloon valvuloplasty has been poor due to selection of severe cases and technical problems during the procedure.[60]

NEW IMAGING TECHNIQUES FOR THE EVALUATION OF FETAL HEART

In order to improve fetal cardiac diagnosis, new techniques have been developed for better evaluation of fetal heart.[15] These techniques can provide:

- Sequential assessment of the entire heart using a full 4D dataset
- Four-dimensional delineation of trabeculation patterns on the ventricular walls, en face dynamic shapes of ventricular septal defects and spatially complex malformations
- Derivation of cardiac indices to myocardial contractility and strain rate by Doppler tissue imaging, and/or
- The use of transesophageal ultrasound to guide in utero cardiac intervention.

These techniques are: dynamic 3D or 4D echocardiography, myocardial Doppler imaging, B-flow ultrasonography, endoscopic ultrasound, and magnetic resonance imaging.[15] Of them, 4D echocardiography includes real-time volumetric data acquisition using matrix-array transducer technology, motion artifact elimination using STIC, and various display options. STIC offers an easy-to-use technique to visualize fetal heart in a 4D sequence.[13,53-55] The acquisition is performed in two steps. First, data is acquired by a single, automatic volume sweep. In the second step, the system analyzes the data according to their spatial and temporal domain and processes a 4D sequence.[13] This sequence presents the heart beating in real-time in a multiplanar display.[13] The examiner can navigate within the heart, reslice, and produce all the standard planes necessary for comprehensive diagnosis.[13] This new modality enables to obtain the volume of data which can be manipulated along the X- and Y-axes using reference points from the four-chamber view, five-chamber view, three-vessel view with depiction of ventricular outflow tracts.[61] The multiplanar evaluation of fetal heart allows the easier identification of fetal cardiac structures during "off-line" analysis by a simple technique of heart volume rotation around different axes.[61] A new technology, tomographic ultrasound imaging (TUI), allows the examiner to obtain a volume data set that simultaneously displays multiple images at specific distances from the four-chamber view.[62] TUI technology is capable for identifying normal and abnormal fetal cardiac anatomy with the use of either static or STIC volume data sets **(Figs. 12 and 13)**.[62]

CONCLUSION

Are improvements in the field of the fetal echocardiography possible? The answer should be confirmative, because in the last two decades there were so many new facts concerning the pathophysiology and the management of the cardiac diseases. The shift from the prenatal diagnosis of the structural cardiac anomalies and rhythm disturbances toward the fetal cardiac flow dynamics has been made owing

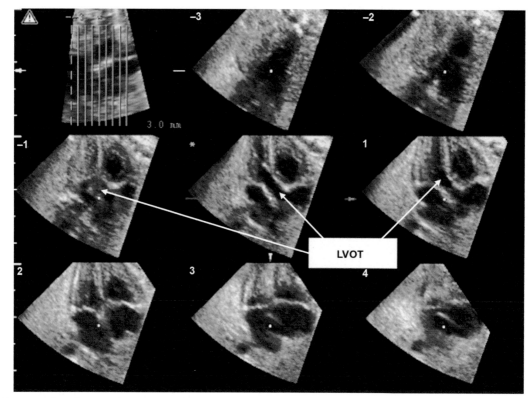

Fig. 12: Tomographic ultrasound imaging—static image correlation volume data set of the left ventricular outflow tract (LVOT).

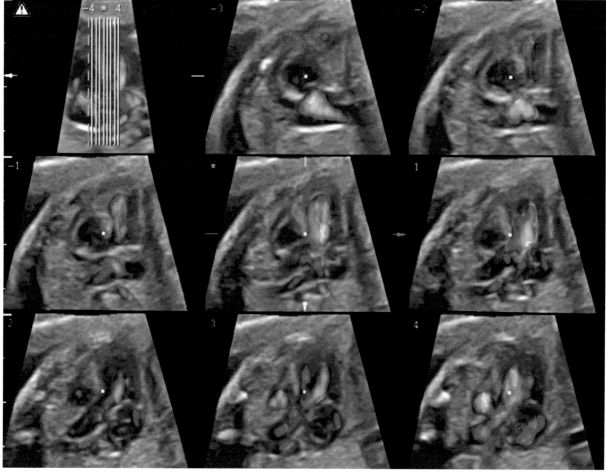

Fig. 13: Tomographic ultrasound imaging with color Doppler—static image correlation volume data set of the left and the right ventricular outflow tracts.

to the development of sophisticated ultrasound techniques in hands of skilled professionals.[28,63] Improvements from the point of view of the public health could be achieved in better screening protocols, broadly performed by more skilled professionals in earlier gestational ages. Increasing role of 3D or live 3D ultrasonography and telemedicine are promising fields of the development of fetal echocardiography, with the possibility to improve detection rate and accuracy of prenatal CHD diagnosis.[9,11,12,64] Goal of the development of fetal echocardiography should be to increase prenatal detection rate of most hemodynamically significant CHD in early pregnancy in order to decrease late diagnosis of CHD postnatally. After the diagnosis of the CHD, the appropriate multidisciplinary counseling should be offered with the development of effective treatment. Genetic counseling and the gene treatment in some cases of CHD are probably the future challenges of the fetal cardiology.[65] The past, when the first diagnosis of CHD was made prenatally, predicted the future of the growing field of fetal cardiology, which is so promising, dynamic, and challenging.

■ REFERENCES

1. Newman PG, Rozycki GS. The history of ultrasound. Surg Clin North Am. 1998;78:179-95.
2. McNay MB, Fleming EE. Forty years of obstetric ultrasound 1957-1997: from A-scope to three dimensions. Ultrasound Med Biol. 1999;25:3-56.
3. Allan LD, Crawford DC, Anderson RH, Tynan MJ. Echocardiographic and anatomical correlations in fetal congenital heart disease. Br Heart J. 1984;52:542-8.
4. Allan LD, Sharland GK, Milburn A, Lockhart SM, Groves AM, Anderson RH, et al. Prospective diagnosis of 1,006 consecutive cases of congenital heart disease in the fetus. J Am Coll Cardiol. 1994;23:1452-8.
5. Barboza JM, Dajani NK, Glenn LG, Angtuaco TL. Prenatal diagnosis of congenital cardiac anomalies: a practical approach using two basic views. Radiographics 2002;22:1125-37.
6. Bronshtein M, Zimmer EZ, Gerlis LM, Lorber A, Drugan A. Early ultrasound diagnosis of fetal congenital heart defects in high-risk and low risk pregnancies. Obstet Gynecol 1993;82:225-9.
7. Smrcek JM, Berg C, Geipel A, Fimmers R, Axt-Fliedner R, Diedrich K, Gembruch U. Detection rate of early fetal echocardiography and in utero development of congenital heart defects. J Ultrasound Med. 2006;25:187-96.
8. Odibo AO, Coassolo KM, Stamilio DM, Ural SH, Macones GA. Should all pregnant diabetic women undergo a fetal echocardiography? A cost-effectiveness analysis comparing four screening strategies. Prenat Diagn. 2006;26:39-44.
9. Carvalho JS, Mavrides E, Shinebourne EA, Campbell S, Thilaganathan B. Improving the effectiveness of routine prenatal screening for major congenital heart defects. Heart. 2002;88:387-91.
10. Yagel S, Moon-Grady AJ. Fetal cardiac evaluation services for low-risk pregnancies: how can we improve? Ultrasound Obstet Gynecol. 2020;55(6):726-727.
11. Jurgens J, Chaoui R. Three-dimensional multiplanar time-motion ultrasound or anatomical M-mode of the fetal heart: a new technique in fetal echocardiography. Ultrasound Obstet Gynecol. 2003;21:119-23.
12. Sharma S, Parness IA, Kamenir SA, Ko H, Haddow S, Steinberg LG, et al. Screening fetal echocardiography by telemedicine: efficacy and community acceptance. J Am Soc Echocardiogr. 2003;16:202-8.
13. DeVore GR, Falkensammer P, Sklansky MS, Platt LD. Spatiotemporal image correlation (STIC): new technology for evaluation of the fetal heart. Ultrasound Obstet Gynecol. 2003;22:380-7.
14. Yagel S, Silverman NH, Gembruch U (Eds). Fetal echocardiography. London, New York: Martin Dunitz Taylor and Francis Group; 2003.
15. Deng J, Rodeck CH. Current applications of fetal cardiac imaging technology. Curr Opin Obstet Gynecol. 2006;18:177-84.
16. Galindo A, Gutierrez-Larraya F, Velasco JM, de la Fuente P. Pulmonary balloon valvuloplasty in a fetus with critical pulmonary stenosis/atresia with intact ventricular septum and heart failure. Fetal Diagn Ther. 2006;21:100-4.
17. Simpson JM, Jones A, Callaghan N, Sharland GK. Accuracy and limitations of transabdominal fetal echocardiography at 12-15 weeks of gestation in a population at high-risk for congenital heart disease. Br J Obstet Gynecol. 2000;107:1492-7.
18. Huggon IC, Ghi T, Cook AC, Zosmer N, Allan LD, Nicolaides KH. Fetal cardiac abnormalities identified prior to 14 weeks' gestation. Ultrasound Obstet Gynecol. 2002;20:22-9.
19. Martinez JM, Gomez O, del Rio M, Puerto B, Borrell A, Cararach V, et al. Early fetal echocardiography: a new challenge in prenatal diagnosis. Ultrasound Rev Obstet Gynecol. 2002;2:251-60.
20. Weiner Z, Lorber A, Shalev E. Diagnosis of congenital cardiac defects between 11 and 14 weeks' gestation in high-risk patients. J Ultrasound Med. 2002;21:23-9.
21. Favre R, Cherif Y, Kohler M, Kohler A, Hunsinger MC, Boufet N, et al. The role of fetal nuchal translucency and ductus venosus Doppler at 11-14 weeks of gestation in the detection of major congenital heart defects. Ultrasound Obstet Gynecol. 2003;21:239-43.
22. Andrews RE, Simpson JM, Sharland GK, Sullivan ID, Yates RW. Outcome after preterm delivery of infants antenatally diagnosed with congenital heart disease. J Pediatr. 2006; 148:213-6.
23. Johnson BA, Ades A. Delivery room and early postnatal management of neonates who have prenatally diagnosed congenital heart disease. Clin Perinatol. 2005;32:921-46.
24. Monatna E, Khoury MJ, Cragan JD, Sharma S, Dhar P, Fyfe D. Trends and outcomes after prenatal diagnosis of congenital cardiac malformations by fetal echocardiography in a well-defined birth population, Atlanta, Georgia, 1990-1994. J Am Coll Cardiol. 1996;28:1805-9.
25. Gambruch U. Prenatal diagnosis of congenital heart disease. Prenat Diagn. 1997;17:1283-98.
26. Allan LD. Fetal congenital heart disease: diagnosis and management. Curr Opin Obstet Gynecol. 1994;6:45-9.
27. Comas Gabriel C, Galindo A, Martinez JM, Carrera JM, Gutierrez-Laraya F, de la Fuente P, et al. Early prenatal diagnosis of major cardiac anomalies in a high-risk population. Prenat Diagn. 2002;22:586-93.
28. Bega G, Kuhlman K, Lev-Toaff A, Kurtz A, Wapner W. Application of three-dimensional ultrasonography in

the evaluation of the fetal heart. J Ultrasound Med. 2001;20: 307-13.

29. American Institute of Ultrasound in Medicine. Performance of basic fetal cardiac ultrasound examination (technical bulletin). J Ultrasound Med. 1998;17:601-7.

30. Friedman AH, Kleinman CS, Copel JA. Diagnosis of cardiac defects: where we've been, where we are and we're going. Prenat Diagn. 2002;22:280-4.

31. Hamar BD, Dziura J, Friedman A, Kleinman CS, Copel JA. Trends in fetal echocardiography and implications for clinical practice: 1985 to 2003. J Ultrasound Med. 2006;25:197-202.

32. Drazancic A. Antenatal care in developing countries. What should be done? J Perinatal Med. 2001;29:188-98.

33. Kurjak A, Bekavac I. Perinatal problems in developing countries: lessons learned and future challenges. J Perinat Med. 2001;29:179-87.

34. Malčić I, Rojnić-Putarek N, Rudan I. Epidemiologija priroðenih srčanih grešaka u Hrvatskoj—multicentrična nacionalna studija; privremeno izvješće. In: Malčić I (Ed). Pedijatrijska kardiologija—odabrana poglavlja. Zagreb: Medicinska naklada; 2001. pp. 30-42.

35. Stanojevic M, Kurjak A. From fetal to neonatal echocardio-graphy: does it predict the future? Ultrasound Rev Obstet Gynecol. 2003;3:150-9.

36. Crane JP, Lefevre ML, Winborn RC. Randomized trial of prenatal ultrasound screening: impact on detection, manage-ment, and outcome of anomalous fetuses. The RADIUS study group. Am J Obstet Gynecol. 1995;172:1641-2.

37. Bull C. Current and potential impact of fetal diagnosis on prevalence and spectrum of serious congenital heart disease at term in the UK. British Paediatric Cardiac Association. Lancet. 1999;354:1242-7ik.

38. Mapp T. Fetal echocardiography and congenital heart disease. Prof Care Mother Child. 2000;10:9-11.

39. Allan LD. A practical approach to fetal heart scanning. Semin Perinatol. 2000;24:324-30.

40. Sharland G. Fetal cardiology. Semin Neonatol. 2001;6:3-15.

41. Berghella V, Pagotto L, Kaufman M, Huhta JC. Accuracy of prenatal diagnosis of congenital heart defects. Fetal Dign Ther. 2001;16:407-12.

42. Zhang YF, Zeng XL, Zhao EF, Lu HW. Diagnostic value of fetal echocardiography for congenital heart disease: a systematic review and meta-analysis. Medicine (Baltimore). 2015;94(42):e1759.

43. van Nisselrooij AEL, Teunissen AKK, Clur SA, Rozendaal L, Pajkrt E, Linskens IH, et al. Why are congenital heart defects being missed? Ultrasound Obstet Gynecol. 2020;55(6):747-57.

44. Mayer-Wittkopf M, Cooper S, Sholler G. Correlation between fetal cardiac diagnosis by obstetric and pediatric cardiologist sonographers and comparison with postnatal findings. Ultrasound Obstet Gynecol. 2001;17:392-7.

45. Tuzler G. Fetal cardiology. Curr Opin Pediatr. 2000;12:492-6.

46. Penny DJ, Weintraub RG. Fetal echocardiography. J Pediatr Child Health. 1995;31:371-4.

47. Sharland G, Allan LD. Screening for congenital heart disease prenatally. Results of a 2 year study in the South East Thames Region. Br J Obstet Gynecol. 1992;99:220-5.

48. Sharland GK, Lockhart SM, Chita SK, Allan LD. Factors influencing the outcome of congenital heart disease detected prenatally. Arch Dis Child. 1991;66:284-7.

49. Allan LD. The outcome of fetal congenital heart disease. Semin Perinatol. 2000;24:380-4.

50. Todros T. Prenatal diagnosis and management of fetal cardiovascular malformations. Curr Opin Obstet Gynecol. 2000;12:105-9.

51. Carvalho JS, Moscoso G, Ville Y. First-trimester transabdominal fetal echocardiography. Lancet. 1998;351:1023-7.

52. Smrcek JM, Berg C, Geipel A, Fimmers R, Diedrich K, Gembruch U. Early fetal echocardiography: heart biometry and visualization of cardiac structures between 10 and 15 weeks' gestation. J Ultrasound Med. 2006;25:173-82.

53. Sen C, Stanojevic M. Fetal heart: Screening, diagnosis and intervention. New Delhi, London, Pnama: Jaypee Brothers Medical Publishers Pvt Ltd.; 2020.

54. Inamura N, Taniguchi T, Yamada T, Tanaka T, Watanabe K, Osaka Fetal Cardiology Group, et al. The Evaluation of fetal cardiac remote screening in the second trimester of pregnancy using the spatio-temporal image correlation method. Pediatr Cardiol. 2020;41(5):979-84.

55. Chaoui R, Abuhamad A, Martins J, Heling KS. Recent development in three and four dimension fetal echo-cardiography. Fetal Diagn Ther. 2020;47(5):345-53.

56. Sands A, Craig B, Mulholland C, Patterson C, Dornan J, Casey F. Echocardiographic screening for congenital heart disease: a randomized study. J Perinat Med. 2002;30:307-12.

57. Lord J, McMullan DJ, Eberhardt RY, Rinck G, Hamilton SJ, Assessment of Genomes and Exomes Consortium, et al. Prenatal exome sequencing analysis in fetal structural anomalies detected by ultrasonography (PAGE): a cohort study. Lancet. 2019;393(10173):747-57.

58. Allan LD, Apfel HD, Printz BF. Outcome after prenatal diagnosis of the hypoplastic left heart syndrome. Heart. 1998;79:371-3.

59. Allan LD, Maxwell DJ, Carminati M, Tynan MJ. Survival after fetal aortic balloon valvuloplasty. Ultrasound Obstet Gynecol. 1995;5:90-1.

60. Kohl T, Sharland G, Allan LD, Gembruch U, Chaoui R, Lopes LM, et al. World experience of percutaneous ultrasound-guided balloon valvuloplasty in human fetuses with severe aortic valve obstruction. Am J Cardiol. 2000; 85:1230-3.

61. Devore GR, Polanco B, Sklansky MS, Platt LD. The 'spin' technique: a new method for examination of the fetal outflow tracts using three-dimensional ultrasound. Ultrasound Obstet Gynecol. 2004;24:72-82.

62. Devore GR, Polanko B. Tomographic ultrasound imaging of the fetal heart: a new technique for identifying normal and abnormal cardiac anatomy. J Ultrasound Med. 2005;24: 1685-96.

63. Michailidis GD, Simpson JM, Karidas C, Economides DL. Detailed three-dimensional fetal echocardiography facilitated by an internet link. Ultrasound Obstet Gynecol. 2001;18:325-8.

64. Cuneo BF, Olson CA, Haxel C, Howley L, Gagnon A, Benson DW, et al. Risk stratification of fetal cardiac anomalies in an underserved population using telecardiology. Obstet Gynecol. 2019;134(5):1096-103.

65. Saiki Y, Rebeyka IM. Fetal cardiac intervention and surgery. Semin Thorac Cardiovasc Surg Pediatr Card Surg Annu. 2001;4:256-70.

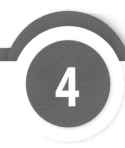

4

Prenatal Diagnostics of Fetal Abnormalities by Ultrasound and Color Doppler

Zehra Nese Kavak, Ertan Ozen, Alin Basgül Yigiter

■ INTRODUCTION

During the last 25 years, the development of increasingly sophisticated equipment [digital techniques, gray scales, color Doppler, and three-dimensional (3D) and four-dimensional (4D) sonography] enabled the diagnosis of a growing number of malformations so that it is now possible to diagnose about 80% of congenital abnormalities with reliable structural images.[1-4]

There is no doubt that ultrasound provides many clinical advantages. The Cochrane database confirms that ultrasound enables the earlier detection of fetal malformations.[2,5]

Professionals expect from routine ultrasound objective information that cannot usually be obtained by clinical procedures.[6] Parents seek reassurance about the absence of fetal congenital anomalies and overall fetal health. Therefore, people view routine ultrasound as a part of obstetrical care, capable of filling important gaps by delivering much key information for improving obstetrical practice.[7] Fetal anomalies screening (FAS) requires higher education and qualifications than obstetrical ultrasound.[8] In most European countries, approximately 98% of pregnant women are examined by ultrasound, frequently 2-3 times (usually once per trimester). Detection rate of congenital anomalies is about 28% in private practice and hospitals, 60-80% in obstetrics and gynecology ultrasound laboratories.[9-11]

While congenital defects constitute 3% of all births, monogenic disorders and chromosomal syndromes constitute 1.4 and 0.6% of all births, respectively.[12]

Progressive improvements in ultrasound equipment within the field of prenatal diagnosis of structural fetal anomalies have permitted to obtain a sensitivity range of 90-95% and specificity range of 95-100%, with utilization of high definition equipment and an expert ultrasonographist in fetal dysmorphology.[13-15]

■ EVALUATION OF ABNORMALITIES OF FETAL CENTRAL NERVOUS SYSTEM

Advanced sonography combined with methodology of approaching the fetal brain has improved the assessment of fetal intracranial structure and diagnosis of the prenatal brain abnormalities.[16,17]

Prenatal assessment of the fetal central nervous system (CNS) is very important as anomalies in this region often determine survival, physical appearance, and function in society.[2,17]

Many malformations of the CNS and fetal neural axis can be detected easily and reliably.[18-22] Such as agenesis of corpus callosum, anencephaly, arachnoid cyst, cranial tumors, craniosynostosis, Dandy–Walker malformations, ventriculomegaly, hydrocephalus, diastematomyelia, encephalocele, holoprosencephaly, hydranencephaly, iniencephaly, intracranial hemorrhage, microcephaly, vein of Galen malformation, spina bifida, meningomyelocele, Arnold–Chiari malformation, and teratomas.

Recent remarkable development of 3D and 4D ultrasound will produce more accurate evaluation of the brain morphology.[3,16]

■ EVALUATION OF FACE AND NECK ABNORMALITIES

It is now possible to make prenatal identification of fetal face and neck malformation with great precision by means of different ultrasonographic proceedings; 2D, 3D, or 4D.[2,3,16,22] Some examples are: cleft lip and palate, ocular abnormalities, nose malformations, ear malformations, micrognathia, facial asymmetry, retrognathia, nuchal translucency and nuchal fold, and various types of cystic lesions and tumors in the neck. The most frequents are: cystic hygroma septated and nonseptated, teratomas, hemangiomas, fetal goiter, and thyroid enlargement.

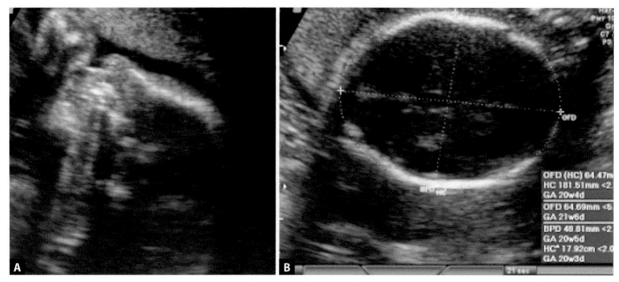

Figs. 1A and B: Microcephaly at 24th gestational weeks. Abnormal fetal profile with small forehead (A) and transverse section of the head (B). Biparietal diameter and head circumference are well below the third percentile. The abdominal circumference was compatible with 24 weeks whereas BPD and HC are measured as 20 weeks. (The abdominal circumference measurement normally about the same size as the head circumference at term is much larger). The head circumference needs to be at least below the fifth percentile before microcephaly is considered, unless there is no ventriculomegaly.

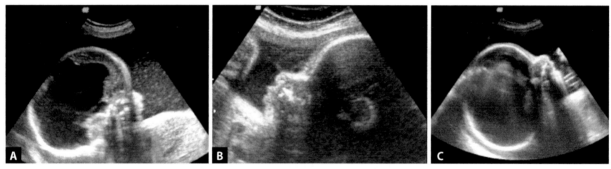

Figs. 2A to C: Communicant hydrocephalus in 28 weeks (A), 30 weeks (B), and 32 weeks fetuses (C).

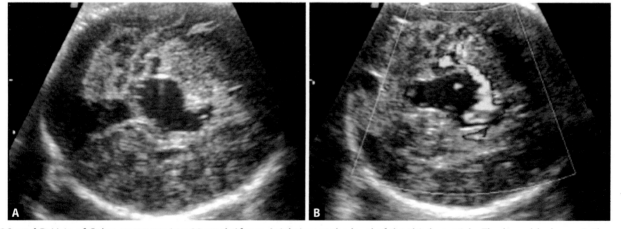

Figs. 3A and B: Vein of Galen aneurysm in a 39 weeks' fetus. Axial view at the level of the third ventricle. The large black area is the vein of Galen aneurysm. The small cystic areas adjacent to the big cystic area represent the feeding arteries [two-dimensional ultrasound (2D-US) in A, power Doppler evaluation in B].

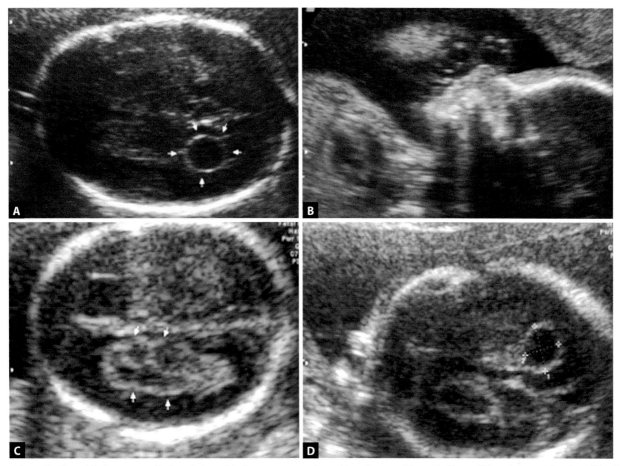

Figs. 4A to D: Choroid plexus cyst. Isolated choroid plexus cyst was found in a fetus at 22 weeks' fetus (A) and normal fetal profile of the fetus (B). Spongy choroid plexuses in a fetus at 16th gestational weeks (C) and choroid plexus cyst in a fetus at 20 weeks of gestation (D).

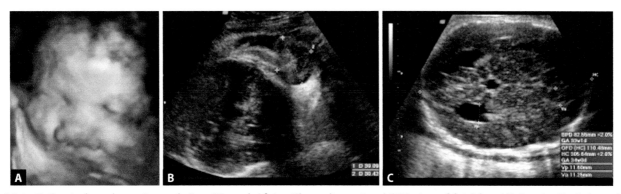

Figs. 5A to C: Cervical myelomeningocele in a 39 weeks' fetus. Three-dimensional (3D) view of fetal face (A), longitudinal view of large myelomeningocele (B), and transverse section of the skull showing mild ventriculomegaly. The head circumference was smaller than his gestational age (C).

■ FETAL THORACIC ABNORMALITIES

The most frequent thoracic anomalies (excluding cardiac malformations) are: the congenital diaphragmatic hernia, congenital cystic adenoid malformation, pleural effusions and sequestration of the lungs, esophageal atresia, tracheal atresia, and tracheoesophageal fistula.[2,23,24]

■ THE GASTROINTESTINAL SYSTEM MALFORMATIONS

The most frequent anomalies that can be detected by ultrasound are: duodenal atresia gastrointestinal atresia or stenosis, gastroschisis, omphalocele, hepatatic tumors, meconium cyst, and meconium ileus.[2,25]

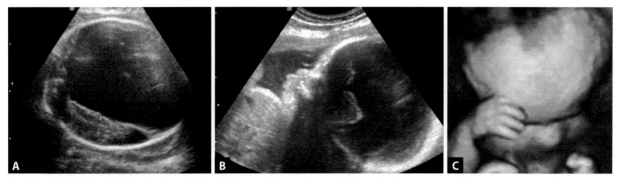

Figs. 6A to C: Alobar holoprosencephaly in a 33-week fetus. The most severe form of holoprosencephaly. Transverse section of the head (A), sagittal section of the fetal profile and the head (B), and three-dimensional (3D) view of the fetal face (C).

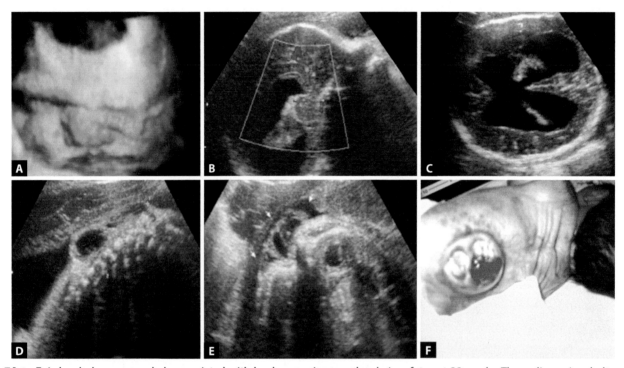

Figs. 7A to F: Labor holoprosencephaly associated with lumbar meningomyelocele in a fetus at 39 weeks. Three-dimensional ultrasound (3D-US) of the fetal face (A), the baby is grimacing. Sagittal view shows the corpus callosum as a hypoechoic semicircular image. Color Doppler shows the pericallosal artery (B), transverse section of the head showing lobar holoprosencephaly with interrupted septum (C), and longitudinal (D) and transverse (E) section of the lumbar myelomeningocele. The newborn (F).

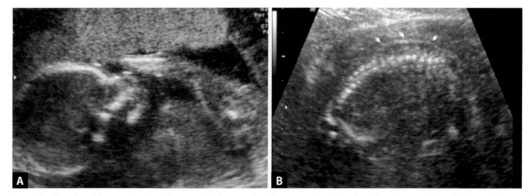

Figs. 8A and B: Arnold–Chiari malformation in a fetus with thoracolumbar meningomyelocele at 19 weeks of gestation. The fetal profile (A), myelomeningocele; the septated cystic mass can be seen in the thoracolumbar area (B).

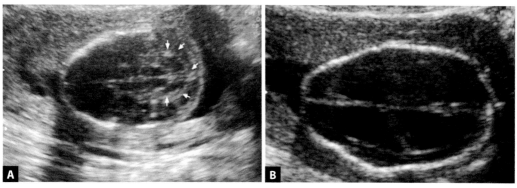

Figs. 9A and B: Arnold–Chiari malformation in a fetus with thoracolumbar meningomyelocele at 19 weeks of gestation. The cerebellum forms a "banana" shape and there is no visible cisterna manga (A). The anterior aspect of the skull is flattened, so the skull assumes a lemon shape (B).

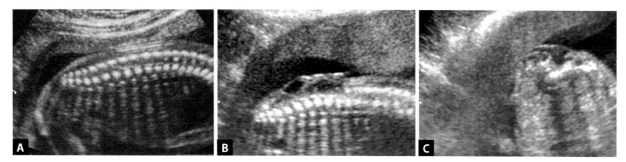

Figs. 10A to C: Lumbosacral spina bifida at 22 weeks. Longitudinal section of a normal spine at 22 weeks (A). Longitudinal (B) and sagittal (C) planes are demonstrating a full-thickness defect of soft tissue overlying the spine in a 22-week fetus with spina bifida.

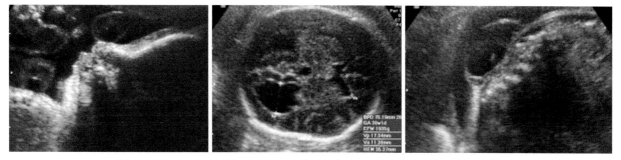

Fig. 11: Moderate ventriculomegaly with lumbosacral meningocele at 30 weeks.

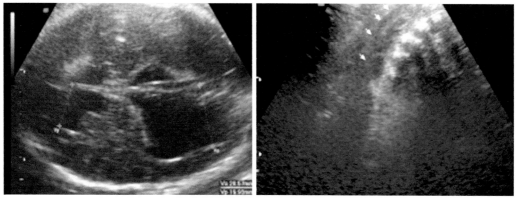

Fig. 12: Moderate to severe ventriculomegaly with lumbar meningocele at 40 weeks.

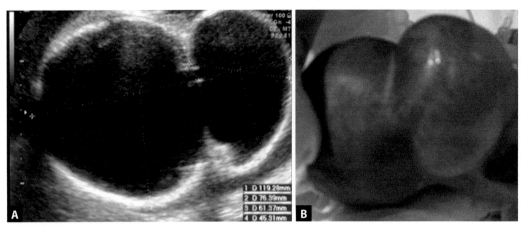

Figs. 13A and B: Large occipital communicating encephalocele in a fetus with a lobar holoprosencephaly at 36 weeks. The transverse view shows the defect of posterior calvaria with protrusion of the brain (A). The baby after birth (B).

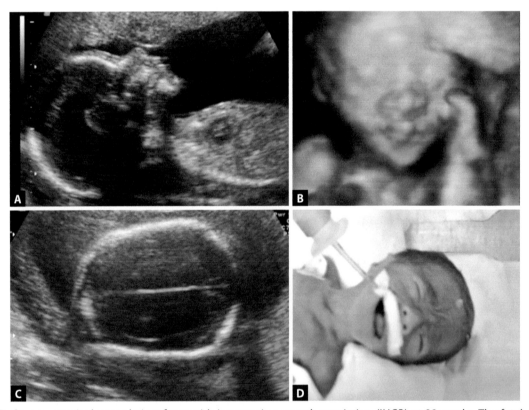

Figs. 14A to D: Severe ventriculomegaly in a fetus with intrauterine growth restriction (IUGR) at 23 weeks. The fetal profile by two-dimensional ultrasound (2D-US) (A), and three-dimensional (3D) view of the fetal face (B). Transverse section of the head (C) showing severe bilateral ventriculomegaly). The baby in the neonatal intensive care unit (D), he died 1 week after birth.

■ GENITOURINARY SYSTEM MALFORMATIONS

Evaluation of the fetal bladder and kidneys is routine practice in obstetric sonography.[26]

Fetal genitalia are also evaluated routinely as the parents frequently ask the fetal gender. Urinary malformations are relatively uncommon.[2,27] The incidence of urinary malformations is found to be 0.65% in a prospective antenatal ultrasound study.[2,28]

The fetal kidney can be visualized ultrasonically as early as 9.5 weeks in optimal circumstances. Kidneys are readily seen at 12th gestational week by abdominal sonography and a week early by transvaginal sonography.[26]

The urinary tract abnormalities are easily recognized as they are invariably accompanied by fluid-filled masses in fetal abdomen. Urinary malformations are suspected if there are following features: decreased amniotic fluid,

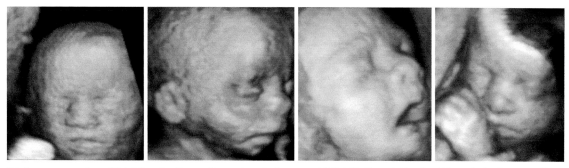

Fig. 15: Some examples of fetal face by three-dimensional ultrasound (3D-US). Especially after 3D and 4D ultrasound imaging has been settled, the images of fetal face are very realistic and impressive.

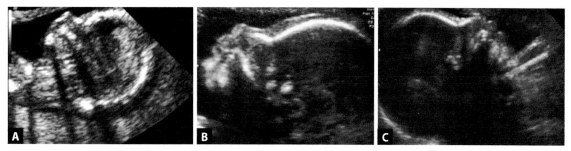

Figs. 16A to C: Normal fetal profile two-dimensional ultrasound (2D-US) at first trimester (A), at second trimester (B), and at third trimester (C).

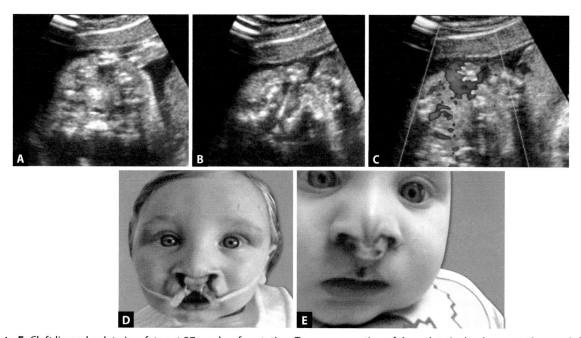

Figs. 17A to E: Cleft lip and palate in a fetus at 27 weeks of gestation. Transverse section of the palate is clearly seen to have a defect in the middle bilaterally (A and B). Color shows in the transverse section of the palate, the amniotic fluid is entering inside the mouth through a full-thickness bilateral defect in the lips and palate (C). The baby is seen at 6 months of age. The palate is repaired and artificial palate replaced (D). The final appearance at 8 months of age with the cleft lip and palate having been repaired (E).

dilatation of the urinary tract (renal pelvicalyceal dilatation, ureteral, or urethral dilatation), presence of a renal cyst, and change in the size, shape, and echogenicity of the kidney, absence or failure to visualize the fetal bladder and any other fetal malformation detected.

The most frequent genitourinary malformations that can be recognized by ultrasound are: renal agenesis, renal dysgenesis infantile polycystic kidney disease; Potter type I, multicystic dysplastic kidney disease (MDKD)—Potter type II, adult polycystic kidney disease (APKD)—Potter type III,

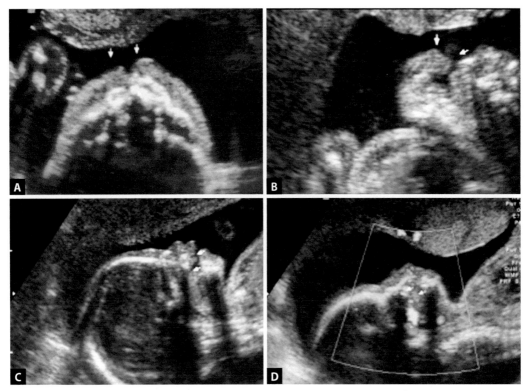

Figs. 18A to D: Unilateral cleft lip and palate at 22 weeks of gestation. Transverse section (A) is showing full thickness, unilateral cleft lip, and palate. Coronal plane (B) showing unilateral cleft lip. The cleft is clear in sagittal section of the fetal profile as well (C). Power Doppler imaging shows with fetal inspiration the amniotic fluid goes up inside the mouth of the fetus through the defect in the palate (D).

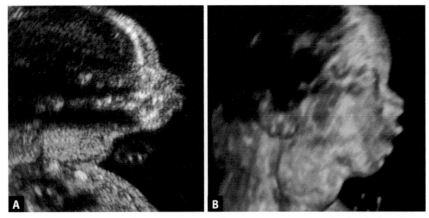

Figs. 19A and B: Fetal goiter at 24 weeks by two-dimensional (2D) (A) and three-dimensional (3D) (B) ultrasound imaging.

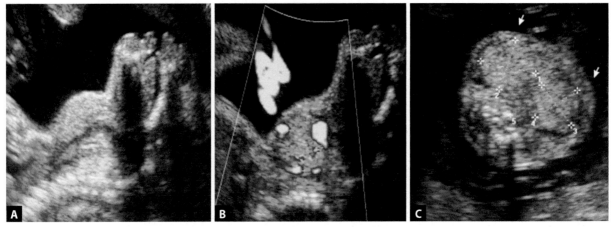

Figs. 20A to C: Fetal goiter at 25 weeks. The fetus is in extension on the sagittal plane, the mass in the neck is clearer (A). Power Doppler sonography shows the presence of blood vessels (B). Transverse section of the fetal neck confirms the bilobed enlarged fetal goiter (C).

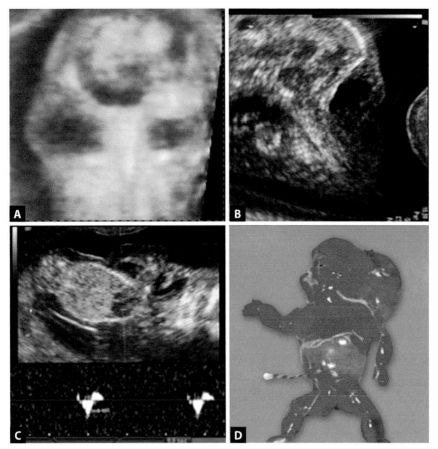

Figs. 21A to D: Bilateral cystic hygromata with diffuse edema in a fetus at 13 weeks of gestation by three-dimensional (3D) scan (A) and two-dimensional (2D) scan (B). The bilateral cystic masses by the neck are the cystic hygroma (A and B) and karyotyping revealed this baby as Turner syndrome. There is skin thickening around the body (C). The fetus had severe bradycardia during the scan (C) and died shortly afterward. The fetus after abortion, note the diffuse edema (D).

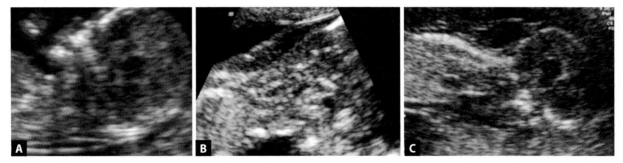

Figs. 22A to C: Increased nuchal translucency in the first trimester. Normal nuchal translucency at 12 weeks (A), moderately increased nuchal translucency (B) and severely increased nuchal translucency at 12 weeks of gestation (C).

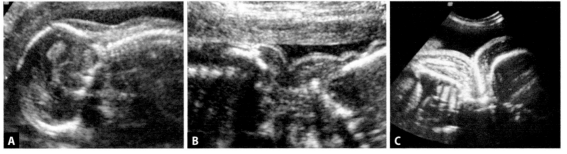

Figs. 23A to C: Increased nuchal fold. Normal nuchal fold at 23rd weeks (A). Increased nuchal fold in a baby with Down's syndrome at 26 weeks (B) and severely increased nuchal edema and hydrops in the last trimester (C).

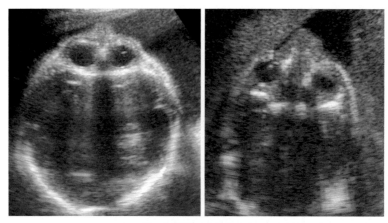

Fig. 24: Hypotelorism.

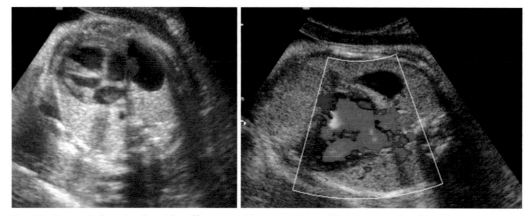

Fig. 25: Congenital cystic adenoid malformation. Transverse view: This is a case of unilateral cystic adenoid malformation of the lungs, macrocyst type.

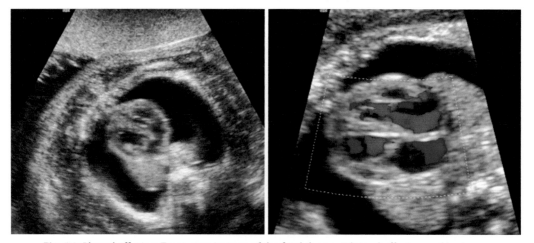

Fig. 26: Pleural effusion. Transverse images of the fetal thorax. Bilateral effusion and hydrops.

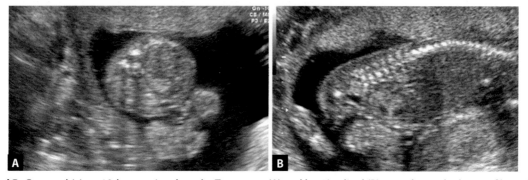

Figs. 27A and B: Gastroschisis at 19th gestational weeks. Transverse (A) and longitudinal (B) scan shows the loops of bowel protruding through a defect in the abdominal wall, not covered by a membrane.

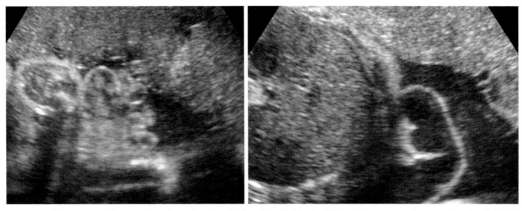

Fig. 28: Gastroschisis at 32nd gestational weeks. Freely floating fluid-filled bowel loops can be seen in the third trimester in a fetus with gastroschisis. Gastroschisis loops can be mistaken for cord loops.[2]

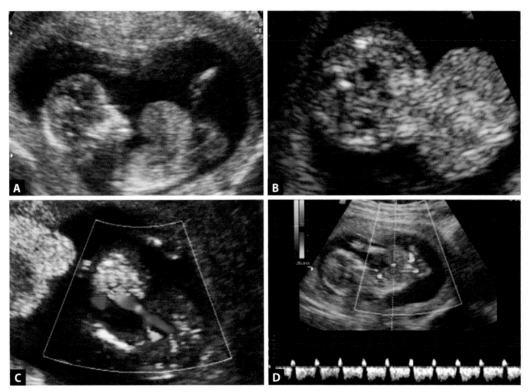

Figs. 29A to D: Omphalocele at 12th gestational weeks. Longitudinal section (A) through the fetal body shows a solid mass protruding from the fetal abdomen. Transverse section (B) shows the omphalocele containing liver with bilateral mild hydronephrosis in the same fetus. Color Doppler examination shows the blood supply (C). Reversed flow in the ductus venosus (D), because of the possible kinking of the ductus as most of the fetal liver is almost outside the abdomen.

cystic renal dysplasia (CRD)—Potter type IV, abnormally distended fetal bladder (megacystis) due to posterior urethral valve, urethral agenesis or stricture, persistence of cloaca and megacystis-microcolon-hypoperistalsis syndrome, bladder extrophy, ureteropelvic junction obstruction, pyelectasis, megaureter, vesicoureteral reflux, horseshoe kidney and empty renal fossa, renal duplication anomalies, tumors of the kidney, adrenal gland tumor, congenital adrenal neuroblastoma, and sacrococcygeal teratoma.[1,2,13,27,28]

Genital anomalies that are recognizable by ultrasound are: fetal ovarian cysts, hydrocolpos and hydrometrocolpos in the case of female fetus, fetal hydrocele, ambiguous genitalia, and hypospadias in the case of male genitals.[27,28]

■ SKELETAL ABNORMALITIES

The fetal skeleton can be visualized by ultrasound very early however, only a small proportion of skeletal malformations can be identified in the early second trimester.[2]

During the scan, it is very important to focus; biometry of the long bone, grade of bone density, fractures or bowing of the bones, fetal spine, appearance and number of digits, and fetal movements.[29]

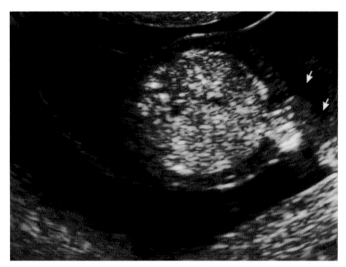

Fig. 30: Omphalocele at 16 weeks. Transverse section shows the extracorporeal bowel surrounded by a membrane.

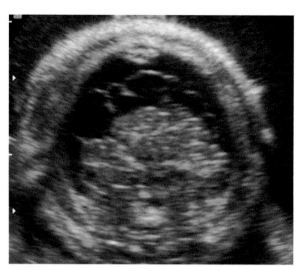

Fig. 33: Abdominal ascites at third trimester.

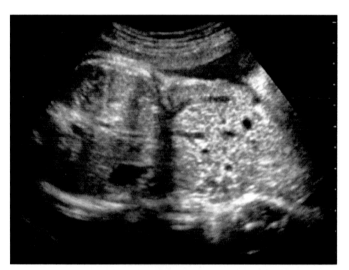

Fig. 31: Large liver—filled omphalocele at 38 weeks.

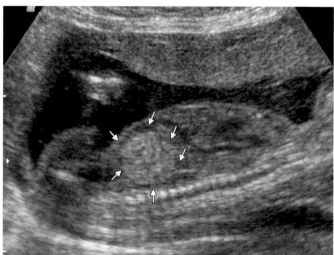

Fig. 34: Hyperechogenic bowel.

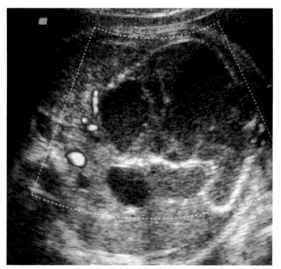

Fig. 32: Intestinal obstruction at third trimester. Dilated loops of the bowel can be seen. The baby had bowel resection after birth.

Numerous abnormalities of skeleton can be detected by ultrasound, some of which are: achondrogenesis, achondroplasia, limb deficiencies, alternations of the hands and feet, thanatophoric dysplasia, osteogenesis imperfecta, arthrogryposis, and campomelic dysplasia.[2,29,30]

■ CARDIAC MALFORMATIONS

Major congenital heart defects (CHDs) account for one-third of all congenital anomalies are the most common severe congenital malformations with an incidence of about 5 in 1,000 live births.[31]

Congenital heart defects are responsible for nearly half of all neonatal and infant deaths due to congenital anomalies.[2] Their incidence is six times greater than chromosomal abnormalities and four times greater than neural tube defects. The majority of the fetuses with CHD occur in the pregnancies with no identifiable risk factors. Therefore,

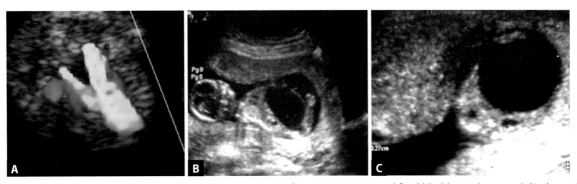

Figs. 35A to C: Posterior urethral valve syndrome. Fetal megacystis at first trimester. Normal fetal bladder and two umbilical arteries around the bladder in the first trimester fetus (A). Sagittal view (B) shows that the bladder is so large that it compresses the chest. Transverse view (C) through fetal abdomen show bilateral mild hydronephrosis together with huge fetal bladder.

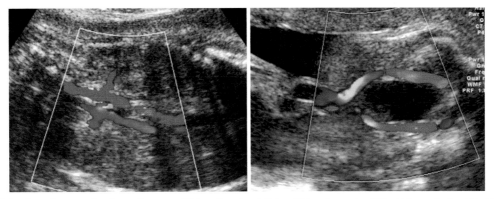

Fig. 36: Color Doppler examination of a normal fetus showing bilateral blood supply of the kidneys in the third trimester; coronal plane (on the left). Two umbilical arteries are running around the fetal bladder.

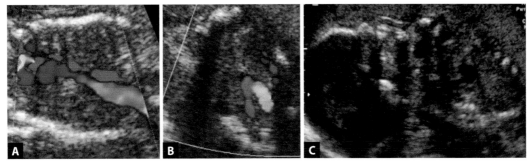

Figs. 37A to C: Bilateral renal agenesis. Color Doppler examination confirms the renal agenesis by the failure to demonstrate bilateral renal arteries (coronal section in A and kidneys are not visualized. Empty fetal bladder and two umbilical arteries running around (transverse section in B). Anhydramnios as a result of bilateral renal agenesis can be visualized in sagittal section (C).

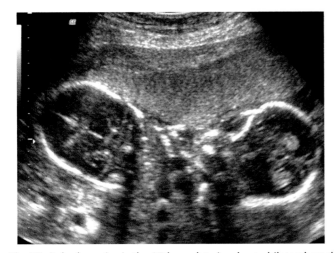

Fig. 38: Anhydramnios in the 17th week twins due to bilateral renal agenesis in both of the fetuses.

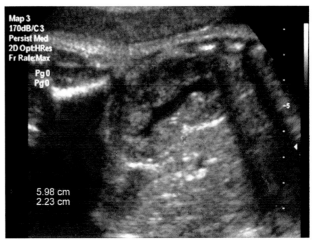

Fig. 39: Unilateral renal agenesis at third trimester. Coronal view demonstrates single kidney. Note the large single kidney.

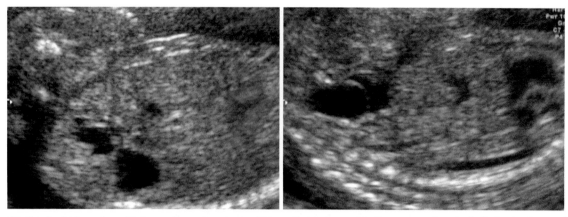

Fig. 40: Duplex kidney. A sagittal scan through a duplex kidney shows two collecting system (on the left). Sagittal scan of the fetal bladder shows the ureterocele due to duplex system.

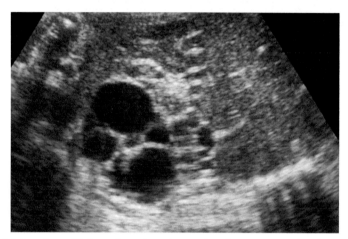

Fig. 41: Renal cyst. Unilateral renal cyst is seen in a fetus at 28 weeks of gestation.

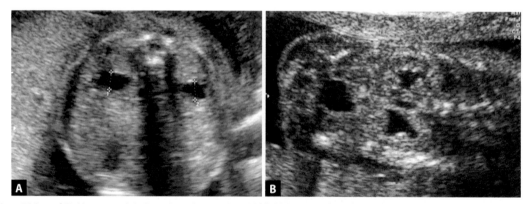

Figs. 42A and B: Ureteropelvic junction obstruction. Mild dilatation of the fetal kidneys at 23rd gestational weeks [transverse (A) and sagittal (B) sections].

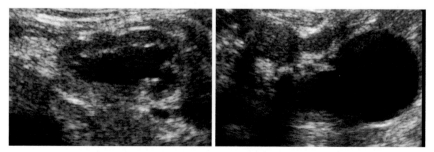

Fig. 43: Distal obstruction. The kidney had moderate dilatation on the sagittal section (on the left) and dilated bladder has a key hole deformity, the posterior urethra.

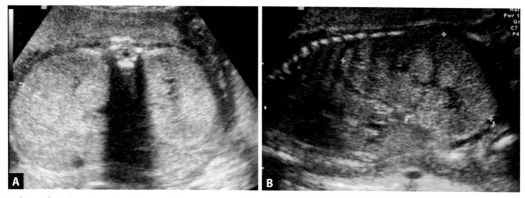

Figs. 44A and B: Infantile polycystic kidney, 27 weeks' sonogram. Transverse section (A) shows bilateral large kidneys with almost the same echogenicity as the remainder of abdomen. Sagittal section (B) shows the enlarged kidney.

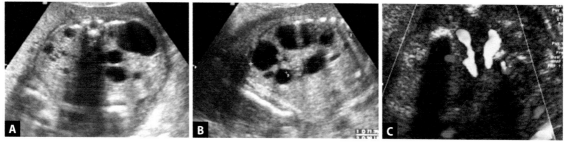

Figs. 45A to C: Multicystic dysplastic kidney disease. The kidney (s) appear (s) enlarged with multiple cysts (A and B) which are variable in size, noncommunicating most randomly positioned but sometimes peripheral. The sizes of the kidneys are proportional to the number of visible cysts. Empty fetal bladder, transverse section (C).

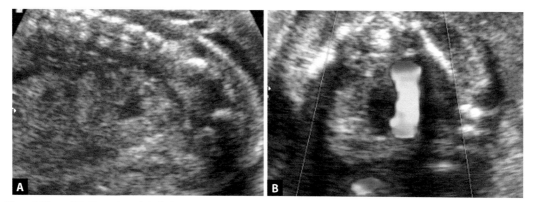

Figs. 46A and B: Ectopic pelvic kidney (A) and single umbilical artery (B) in the same fetus at 22 weeks of age.

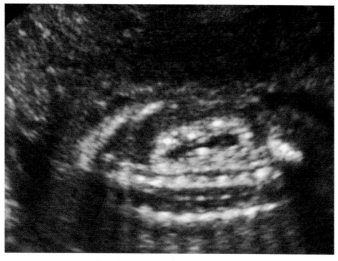

Fig. 47: Hyperechogenic kidney.

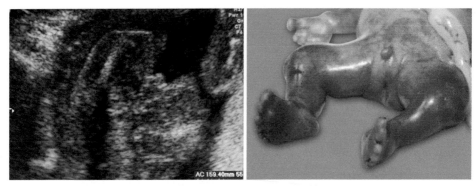

Fig. 48: Ambiguous genitalia in the male fetus.

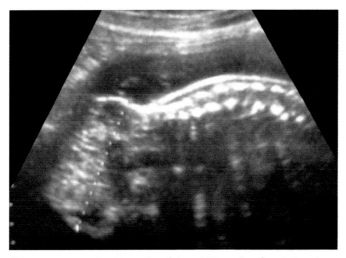

Fig. 49: Type 2 (mainly external), solid sacrococcygeal teratoma in a fetus at 30 weeks of gestation. Laser ablation therapy was successfully done. Teratoma weighing 1,300 g was excised after birth.

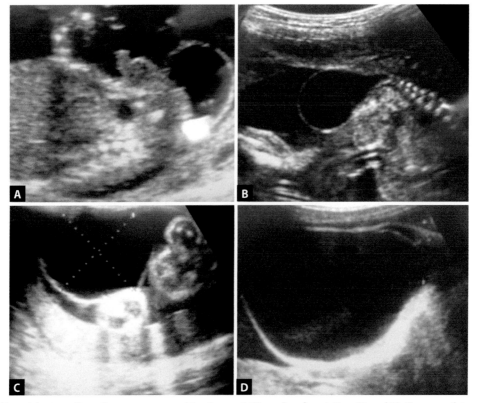

Figs. 50A to D: Type 1 (external), cystic sacrococcygeal teratoma at 18 weeks of gestation (A and B), the same fetus at 33 weeks (C) and 37 weeks (D). The baby born alive and operated in 1 week of delivery.

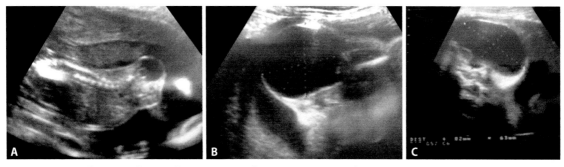

Figs. 51A to C: Type 2 (mainly external), mixed sacrococcygeal teratoma at 22 weeks (A) measuring 4 × 3.5 cm, at 31 weeks (B), 33 weeks (C) measuring 10 × 9 cm. The baby born at 39 weeks. She weighed 4,000 g and operated successfully 3 days after delivery.

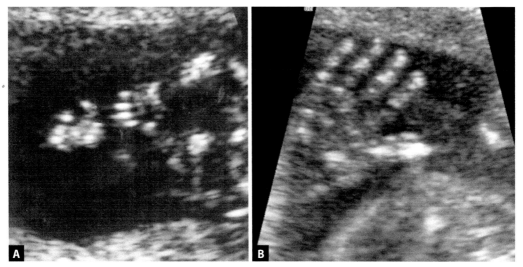

Figs. 52A and B: Normal fetal hand at first trimester (A) and second trimester (B).

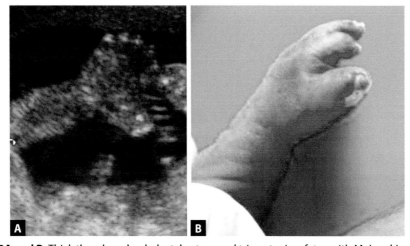

Figs. 53A and B: Thick thumb and polydactyly at second trimester in a fetus with Majewski syndrome (short rib polydactyly syndrome) (A), the fetus after birth at autopsy (B).

there is wide agreement that cardiac ultrasound screening should be introduced as an integral part of the routine scan, especially between 20th and 23rd gestational weeks.[2,32,33] Recently, every fetal echocardiography has been studied extensively by using high-frequency transvaginal probe between 11 and 13 weeks. However, the detection rate of CHD of the first trimester is low and varies according to the experience of the center and population studied. A large study involving 44,859 singleton pregnancies reported that the detection rate of major CHDs was 34%.[34]

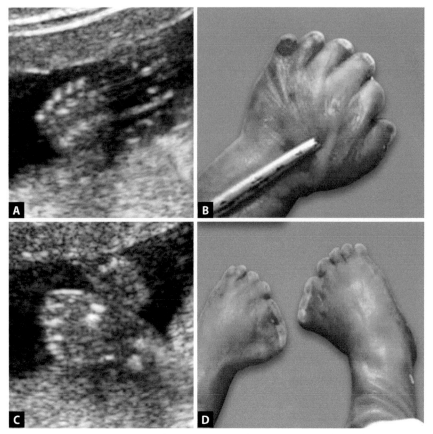

Figs. 54A to D: Polydactyly in the hands (A and B) and feet (C and D) at 16th weeks in this fetus with short rib polydactyly syndrome. Note that there is also syndactyly of the first and second toes in both feet (C and D).

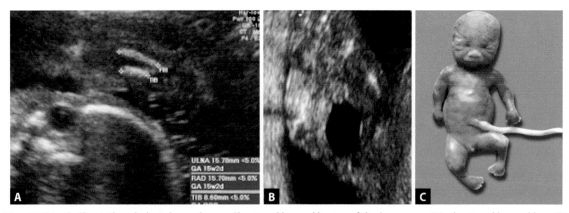

Figs. 55A to C: Short rib polydactyly syndrome. Short and bowed bones of the lower arm (A), short and bowed legs (B), and the fetus after abortion (C).

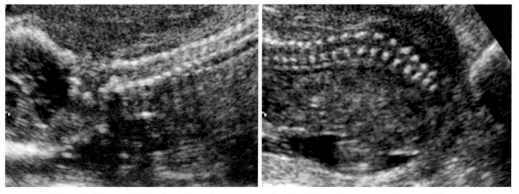

Fig. 56: Platypelloid spine. Note the elongated spine in both images in the same fetus.

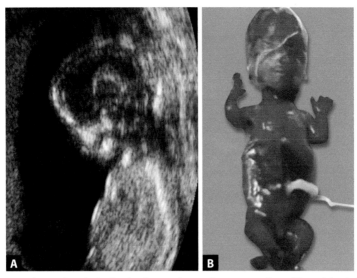

Figs. 57A and B: Thanatophoric dysplasia. Sagittal scan shows the narrow chest (A) and the baby after abortion (B).

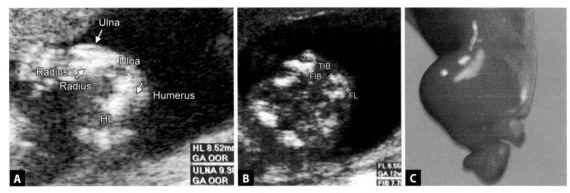

Figs. 58A to C: Thanatophoric dysplasia. Short and bowed upper (A) and lower (B) extremities are seen. Note severe micromelia of the limbs. The lower extremity of the baby after abortion (C).

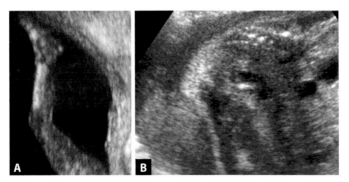

Figs. 59A and B: Normal fetal leg (A), unilateral talipes equinovarus (B) in a second trimester fetus.

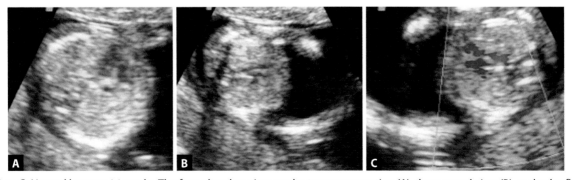

Figs. 60A to C: Normal heart at 14 weeks. The four-chamber view on the transverse section (A), three-vessel view (B), and color flow in the three-vessel view showing the same flow direction of pulmonary artery, aorta, and superior vena cava (C).

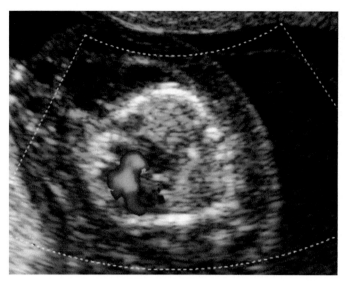

Fig. 61: Large ventricular septal defect at 14 weeks.

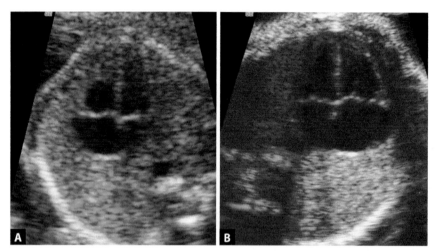

Figs. 62A and B: Four-chamber view of normal heart in the second (A) and third (B) trimester.

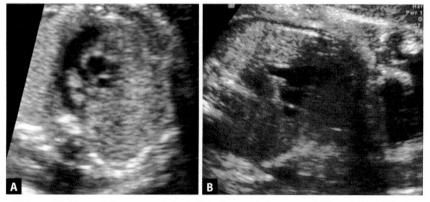

Figs. 63A and B: Normal three-vessel view of the heart in the second (A) and third (B) trimester.

During cardiac scan, visualization of intact four-chamber view allows the detection of 40% of anomalies while additional visualization of the outflow tracts and the great arteries increase the rate up to 60–70% in general low-risk population.[32]

Color and pulsed Doppler are particularly useful to confirm normal inflow to the ventricles and to detect turbulent flow or jets suggesting valve regurgitation. Color Doppler helps in confirming presence of intact septum and in diagnosing atrial septal defects and

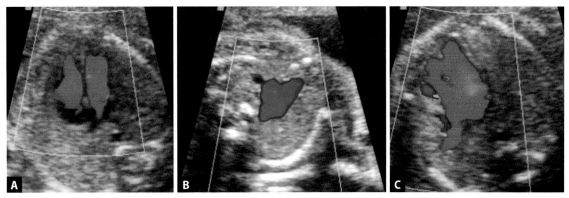

Figs. 64A to C: Color Doppler evaluation of the normal heart showing the intact ventricles (A), normal three-vessel flow (B) and normal pulmonary venous return (C).

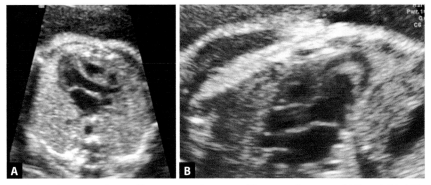

Figs. 65A and B: Left ventricular outflow tract in the normal heart at the second (A) and third (B) trimester.

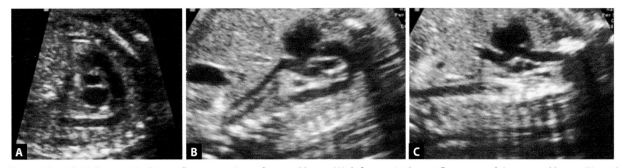

Figs. 66A to C: Right ventricular outflow tract view of normal heart (A), left ventricular outflow tract of the normal heart (B), and superior and inferior vena cava and right atrium (C).

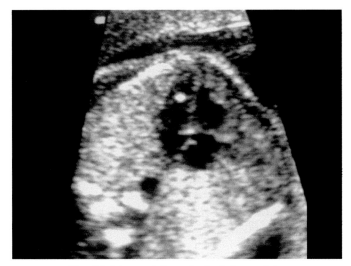

Fig. 67: Echogenic focus in the left ventricle.

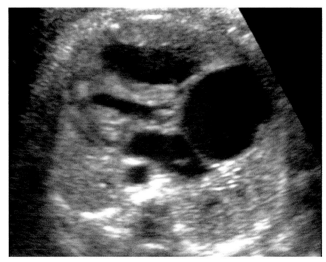

Fig. 68: Cardiomegaly in a fetus with Galen vein aneurysm at third trimester due to hyperdynamic circulation.

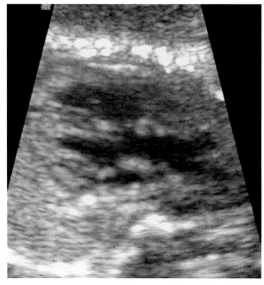

Fig. 69: Overriding aorta in a fetus with Fallot tetralogy.

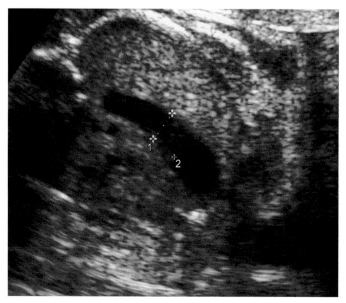

Fig. 72: Aorta in the three-vessel view of a fetus with transposition of the great arteries.

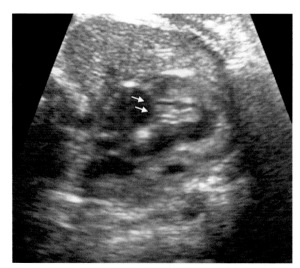

Fig. 70: Hypoplastic left ventricle.

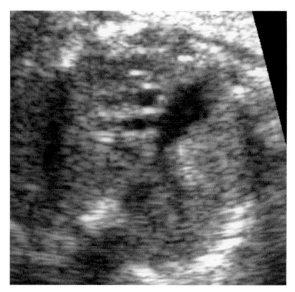

Fig. 71: Narrow aorta in a fetus with interrupted aortic arch.

ventricular septal defects. It also helps to better visualization of the outflow tracts confirming antegrade flow through the semilunar valves and great arteries and makes easier the examination of aortic and ductal arches. Color Doppler is also useful in identifying systemic and pulmonary venous return.[2,32,33,35,36]

The most frequent fetal heart anomalies diagnosed at routine echocardiography are: ventricular septal defects, atrial septal defects, abnormal venoatrial connections, tricuspid atresia or dysplasia, atrioventricular septal defects, single ventricle, aortic atresia, aortic stenosis, hypoplastic left heart, pulmonary atresia, and stenosis, tetralogy of Fallot, transposition of great arteries, truncus arteriosus, double outlet right ventricle, aortic arch anomalies, isomerism, myocardiopathy, and complex cardiac defects.[2,32]

There are also malformations that can be detected in twins [conjoined twins, intrauterine growth restriction (IUGR) in twins, acardiac twin, twin-to-twin transfusion syndrome, etc.], syndromes [Beckwith–Wiedemann syndrome, deletion of 22q 11.2 syndrome, DiGeorge syndrome, Meckel–Gruber syndrome, Pena–Shokeir syndrome (fetal akinesia-hypokinesia sequence), tuberous sclerosis, VACTERL association, Fryns syndrome, etc.], abnormalities caused by infections (Cytomegalic inclusion disease, parvovirus, congenital syphilis, toxoplasmosis, varicella infection), abnormalities caused by drug usage [fetal alcohol syndrome, anti-seizure drugs (phenytoin, carbamazepine, valproic acid, and phenobarbital], and illegal drugs (cocaine and heroin).[1,2,7,11-13,15]

Miscellaneous abnormalities such as chorioangioma, nonimmune hydrops fetalis, rhesus incompatibility,

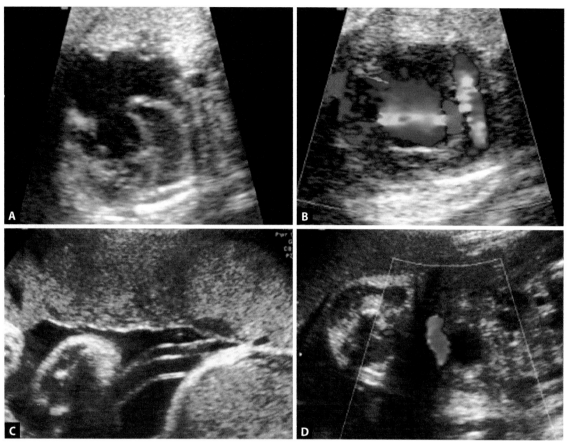

Figs. 73A to D: Ebstein's anomaly in the third trimester. Note the marked tricuspid valve displacement. The hinge point of the septal leaflet of the tricuspid valve is displaced from the crux (A), severe tricuspid regurgitation in Ebstein anomaly (B), single umbilical artery visualization in the same fetus by two-dimensional ultrasound (2D-US) (C) and color flow (D).

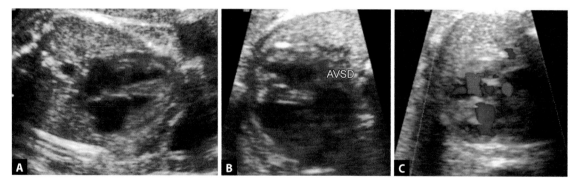

Figs. 74A to C: Atrioventricular septal defect (AVSD). Intact ventricular septum of a normal heart at the third trimester (A), atrioventricular septal defect by two-dimensional ultrasound (2D-US) (B), color flow visualization of AVSD in the third trimester (C).

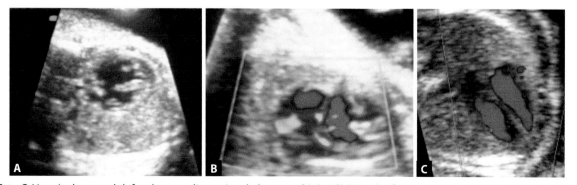

Figs. 75A to C: Ventricular septal defect by two-dimensional ultrasound (2D-US) (A), color flow showing the shifting of the blood through the defect in the ventricular septum (B), color flow examination of an intact ventricular septum (C).

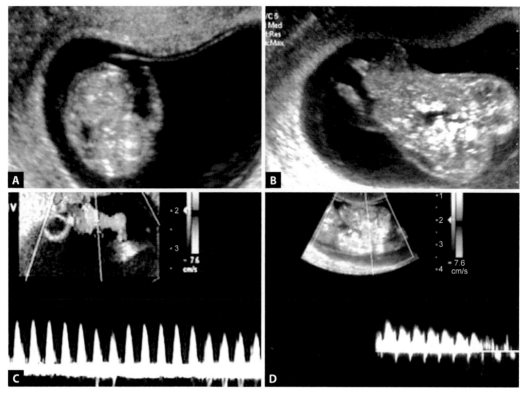

Figs. 76A to D: Conjoint twins at 9 weeks of gestation. Twin babies are seen to be conjoined at thorax and abdomen (A). Thoracal union with two separately looking hearts on transverse cross-sectional view on transvaginal ultrasound scan (B). Doppler flow pattern of umbilical artery (above) and vein (below) (C), Doppler flow waveform at the single ductus venosus showing reversed flow (D).

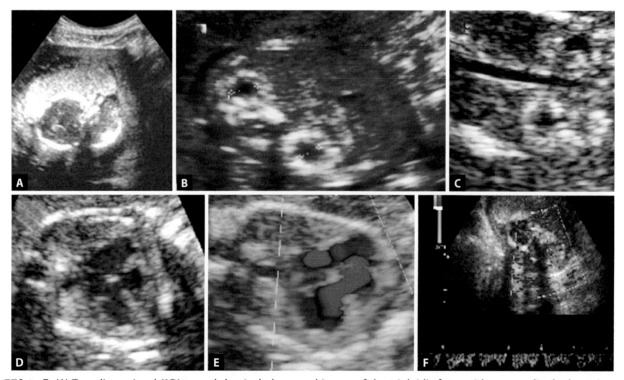

Figs. 77A to F: (A) Two-dimensional (2D) transabdominal ultrasound image of the triploidic fetus with severe oligohydramnios can be visualized; (B and C) Transverse and coronal sections of hyperechogenic kidneys with pelvic dilatation are visualized by transvaginal scan; (D and E) 2D transvaginal scan with color Doppler; a large ventricular septal defect (VSD) can be seen easily; (F) Reversed flow in the ductus venosus indicating severe decompensated intrauterine growth restriction (IUGR).

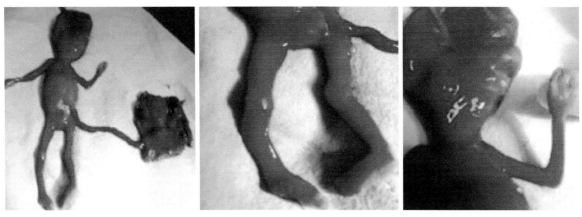

Fig. 78: Postmortem images of this 19-week fetus with triploidy (69,XXX). Note bilateral talipes and syndactyly in the hand fingers.

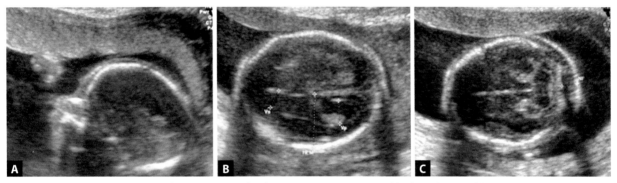

Figs. 79A to C: Down's syndrome. The fetus karyotyped as having trisomy 21. Normal looking fetal profile (A), mild ventriculomegaly (B), increased nuchal fold (C) at 18 weeks of gestation.

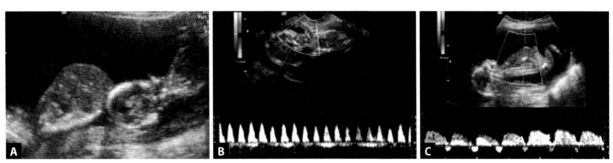

Figs. 80A to C: Twin-to-twin transfusion syndrome. Twins are seen in the sagittal plane (A), Doppler flow examination showed absent end diastolic flow in the donor twin (B) and reversed flow in the ductus venosus of the recipient twin (C).

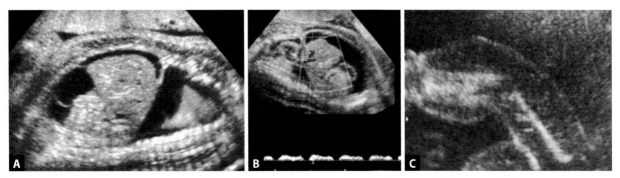

Figs. 81A to C: Fetal hydrops. Sagittal section of the fetus shows the severe pleural effusion and fetal ascites (A), Doppler flow pattern shows absent a wave in the ductus venosus (B), edematous upper extremity of the fetus with generalized hydrops (C).

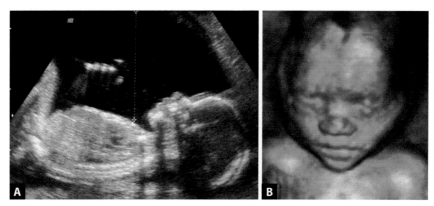

Figs. 82A and B: Polyhydramnios. Deepest vertical pocket of the amniotic fluid was >10 cm (A), the three-dimensional (3D) view of the fetus (B).

cord cysts, and abnormal sonographic findings such as macrosomia, IUGR, oligohydramnios, anhydramnios, and polyhydramnios can also be detected by ultrasonography.[1,2,13,15]

■ REFERENCES

1. Kurjak A, Kirkinen P, Latin V, Rajhvajn B. Diagnosis and assessment of fetal malformation and abnormalities by ultrasound. J Perinat Med. 1980;8:219-35.

2. Carrera JM, Torrents M, Munog A, Maiz N, Millan C, Scazzochio E, Ruiz M, Rodriguez MA. Prenatal diagnosis of congenital defects. In: Kurjak A, Carrera JM (Eds). Donald School Atlas of Clinical Application of Ultrasound in Obstetrics and Gynecology. New Delhi: Jaypee Brothers Medical Publishers (P) Ltd.; 2006. pp. 166-239.

3. Kurjak A. 3D ultrasound and perinatal medicine. J Perinat Med. 2002;30:5-7.

4. Leung KY, Ngai CS, Chan BC, Leung WC, Lee CP, Tang MH. Three-dimensional extended imaging: a new display modality for three-dimensional ultrasound examination. Ultrasound Obstet Gynecol. 2005;263:244-51.

5. Kurjak A, Chervenak FA. Ultrasound in perinatal medicine: Editorial. Ultr Rev Obst Gynecol. 2001;1:193-4.

6. Carrera JM. Fetal ultrasonography: the first 40 years: Editorial, Ultr Rev Obst Gynecol. 2004;4:193-4.

7. Levi S, Hyjazi Y, Schaapst JP, Defoort P, Coulon R, Buekens P. Sensitivity and specificity of routine antenatal screening for congenital anomalies by ultrasound: the Belgian Multicentric Study. Ultrasound Obstet Gynecol. 1991;1:102-10.

8. Levi S. Routine ultrasound screening of congenital anomalies. An overview of the European experience. Ann N Y Acad Sci. 1998;18;847:86-98.

9. Zimmer EZ, Avraham Z, Sujoy P, Goldstein I, Bronshtein M. The influence of prenatal ultrasound on the prevalence of congenital anomalies at birth. Prenat Diagn. 1997;17:623-8.

10. Grandjean H, Larroque D, Levi S. Sensitivity of routine ultrasound screening of pregnancies in the Eurofetus database. The Eurofetus Team. Ann N Y Acad Sci. 1998;18; 847:118-24.

11. Levi S. Ultrasound in prenatal diagnosis: polemics around routine ultrasound screening for second trimester fetal malformations. Prenat Diagn. 2002;22:285-95.

12. Grandjean H, Larroque D, Levi S. Detection of chromosomal abnormalities, an outcome of ultrasound screening. The Eurofetus Team. Ann N Y Acad Sci. 1998;18;847:136-40.

13. Lys F, De Wals P, Borlee-Grimee I, Billiet A, Vincotte-Mols M, Levi S. Evaluation of routine ultrasound examination for the prenatal diagnosis of malformation. Eur J Obstet Gynecol Reprod Biol. 1989;30(2):101-9.

14. Kurjak A, Bekavac I. Perinatal problems in developing countries: lessons learned and future challenges. J Perinat Med. 2001;293:179-87.

15. Bronshtein M, Zimmer EZ, Blumenfeld Z. Early sonographic detection of fetal anomalies. In: Kurjak A (Ed). Textbook of Perinatal Medicine. London: Parthenon Publishing; 1998. pp. 263-80.

16. Kurjak A, Vecek N, Hafner T, Bozek T, Funduk-Kurjak B, Ujevic B. Prenatal diagnosis: what does four-dimensional ultrasound add? J Perinat Med. 2002;30(1):57-62.

17. Johnson ML, Dunne MG, Mack LA, Rashbaum CL. Evaluation of fetal intracranial anatomy by static and real-time ultrasound. J Clin Ultrasound. 1980;8(4):311-8.

18. Chervenak FA, Berkowitz RL, Romeo R, Tortora M, Mayden K, Duncan C, et al. The diagnosis of fetal hydrocephalus. Am J Obstet Gynecol. 1983;1476:703-16.

19. Chervenak FA, Isaacson G, Mahoney MJ, Berkowitz RL, Tortora M, Hobbins JC. Diagnosis and management of fetal cephalocele. Obstet Gynecol. 1984;64(1):86-91.

20. Chervenak FA, Duncan C, Ment LR, Tortora M, McClure M, Hobbins JC. Perinatal management of meningomyelocele. Obstet Gynecol. 1984;63(3):376-80.

21. Chervenak FA, Isaacson G, Mahoney MJ, Tortora M, Mesologites T, Hobbins JC. The obstetric significance of holoprosencephaly. Obstet Gynecol. 1984;63(1):115-21.

22. Chervenak FA, Isaacson G, Blakemore KJ, Breg WR, Hobbins JC, Berkowitz RL, et al. Fetal cystic hygroma. Cause and natural history. N Engl J Med. 1983;309(14):822-5.

23. Papp Z. Ultrasound examination of the fetal thorax. In: Kurjak A, Chervenak FA (Eds). Textbook of Ultrasound in Obstetrics and Gynecology. New Delhi: Jaypee Brothers Medical Publishers (P) Ltd.; 2004. pp. 272-9.

24. Ruano R. Recent advances in sonographic imaging of fetal thoracic structures. Expert Rev Med Devices. 2005;2(2):217-22.

25. D'addario V, Di Cagno L, Tamburo R. Malformations of the gastrointestinal system. In Kurjak A, Chervenak FA (Eds).

Textbook of Ultrasound in Obstetrics and Gynecology. New Delhi: Jaypee Brothers Medical Publishers (P) Ltd.; 2004. pp. 290-7.

26. Kurjak A, Kirkinen P, Latin V, Ivankovic D. Ultrasonic assessment of fetal kidney function in normal complicated pregnancies. Am J Obstet Gynecol. 1981;14(13):266-70.

27. Kurjak A, Latin V, Mandruzzato G, D'Addario V, Rajhvajn B. Ultrasound diagnosis and perinatal management of fetal genitourinary abnormalities. J Perinat Med. 1984;12(6): 291-312.

28. Livera KN, Brookfield DS, Egginton JA, Hawnaur JM. Antenatal ultrasonography to detect fetal renal abnormalities: a prospective screening programme. BMJ. 1989;298(6685): 1421-3.

29. Bronshtein M, Keret D, Deutsch M, Liberson A, Bar Chava. Transvaginal sonographic detection of skeletal anomalies in the first and early second trimesters. Prenat Diagn. 1993; 13(7):597-601.

30. Chervenak FA, Isaacson G, Lorber J. Anomalies of the fetal head neck and spine: ultrasound, diagnosis, and management. Philadelphia: WB Saunders; 1988. pp. 17-36.

31. Mensah GA, Brown DW. An overview of cardiovascular disease burden in the United States. Health Affairs. 2007;26:38-48.

32. Allan LD. Fetal cardiology. Curr Opin Obstet Gynecol. 1996;2: 142-7.

33. Todros T. Prenatal diagnosis and management of fetal cardiovascular malformations. Curr Opin Obstet Gynecol. 2000;12:105-9.

34. Syngelaki A, Chelemen T, Dagklis T, Allan L, Nicolaides KH. Challenges in the diagnosis of fetal non-chromosomal abnormalities at 11-13 weeks. Prenat Diagn. 2011;31:90-102.

35. Haak MC, Twisk JW, Van Vugt JM. How successful is fetal echocardiographic examination in the first trimester of pregnancy? Ultrasound Obstet Gynecol. 2002;20:9-13.

36. Campbell S. Isolated major congenital heart disease (Opinion). Ultrasound Obstet Gynecol. 2001;17:370-9.

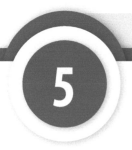

The Advantages of Three-dimensional Sonography in the Diagnosis and Assessment of Fetal Abnormalities

Zehra Nese Kavak, Ertan Ozen, Alin Basgül Yigiter, Alexandra Shera Lieb

■ INTRODUCTION

Three-dimensional ultrasound (3D-US) is a natural development of the imaging technology.[1,2] Our purpose is to increase awareness of its present clinical usefulness in detecting and evaluating abnormalities.

Three-dimensional ultrasound provides a very clear look on the fetal anatomy, makes anomalies easier to recognize, facilitates maternal-fetal bonding, and helps families better understand fetal abnormalities.[3,4] While, the images obtained help parents feel great relief and reinforce the affective bonds with their child in normal cases, in fetuses with abnormalities 3D-US can help parents and other doctors involved, to take a more realistic view of the problem.[5,6] Additionally, in pathological cases, the use of 3D-US will also provide parents with the knowledge to have a better judgment while taking decision about continuing or terminating the ongoing pregnancy.[7,8] Moreover, consulting specialists understand fetal pathology better and can better plan postnatal interventions.[1,8] They can be more objective in counseling of the family.[6,7]

■ OTHER ADVANTAGES OF THREE-DIMENSIONAL ULTRASOUND

It is clear that one of the great advantages of 3D-US is that the information remains captured as a volume and it is possible to reconstruct the recorded image and modify all the adjustments as if the patient was still present.[1,9,10] This enables us to manipulate the image, re-rotate it three-dimensionally and achieve another 3D reconstruction from the data already taken.[11,12] There are also electronic scalpels, which assist by cutting off and eliminating all parts that can hide or distort the area we wish to study. With these facilities, we can improve the 3D reconstruction made from an image that is less than favorable.[1,11]

Three-dimensional ultrasound can observe a region of interest from any orientation. 3D-US obtains a volume data set composed of a series of two-dimensional (2D) images

and thus is able to conveniently demonstrate the features of the lesions and their spatial relationships. The different display modalities like transparency mode, maximum intensity mode, surface rendering mode enable operator to evaluate the pathology in the structures of the fetal cranium/face, spine/extremities, and body surface. Multiplanar mode can be used to observe internal structures from various orientations simultaneously.[1,13]

■ ADVANTAGES OF THREE-DIMENSIONAL ULTRASOUND IN COMPARING TWO-DIMENSIONAL ULTRASOUND TO SCAN FETAL ABNORMALITY

Although conventional two-dimensional sonography (2D-US) is able to detect many kinds of fetal malformations, some studies[14,15] have shown that the 2D-US detection rate for fetal anomalies in low-risk pregnancies is poor in the primary care setting. Even in tertiary care centers, only 40–50% of cases of fetal malformations are detected prenatally by 2D-US.[14,8] Therefore, the adjunctive use of 3D-US will increase the detection rate and quality of assessment of fetal anomalies.[8] Moreover, the demonstration of a fetal defect in the third-dimension is impossible by the conventional technique. Three-dimensional ultrasound allows visualization of the fetal malformations in all three dimensions at the same time, providing an improved overview and a more clearly defined demonstration of adjusted anatomical planes. In many studies, it has been shown that 3D-US was able to discover some complicated fetal malformations that were missed by 2D-US and to determine the fetal malformations more precisely than 2D-US did.[7,8] The advancement of 3D volume sonography is enormously exciting and gives us control over the subject we are imaging, which goes well further than 2D imaging.[16] We can manipulate that volume, rescan the fetus using the volume, and display any part of it. However, we have much to learn to determine where the applications will be as this technology leaps forward in the future.[17] The 3D technique is superior to the traditional 2D biometries, without the common limitations such as fetal position.[18] Merz et al. examined 204 patients with 3D-US and proved that 3D-US is advantageous in demonstrating fetal defects.[2]

EVALUATION IN THE CENTRAL NERVOUS SYSTEM ABNORMALITIES BY 3D/4D ULTRASONOGRAPHY

Transvaginal high-resolution ultrasound and 3D-US enable detailed assessment of fetal central nervous system (CNS) development and CNS abnormalities in the first trimester. However, fetal brain develops rapidly in the second trimester, therefore early scanning covers only selected CNS anomalies and serial continuing observation in the second trimester will be required.[19-21]

Combination of both transvaginal high-resolution sonography and 3D-US may be a great diagnostic tool for evaluation of 3D structure of the fetal CNS during the second and third trimester.[22]

Kurjak's antenatal neurodevelopmental test (KANET) can be used to evaluate fetal brain function to detect the fetuses at risk for neurological impairment between 28 and 38 gestational weeks.[23]

In the recent years, HD live, HDlive silhouette, and flow technology enhance the visualization of the 3D images. Comparing the 2D and 3D techniques, 3D-US showed superiority with 60.8% of detected anomalies.[24]

FOUR-DIMENSIONAL ULTRASOUND: CLINICAL APPLICATIONS IN FETAL ABNORMALITIES

Real-time 3D-US is called four-dimensional ultrasound (4D-US). This technology enables the user to see fetal motion in almost real-time. The time vector is the fourth dimension.[1] This technique should assist us in the better understanding of both the somatic and functional development of the fetus.[25] Fetal behavior can be studied by observing the various body movements.[26] The introduction of 4D-US was a turning point in the assessment of fetal behavior.[27] Behavioral study of the fetus will be necessary to understand the origins of motor and sensory capabilities of infants and the mechanisms of altered developmental outcomes.[28] Ahmet et al. studied 120 cases of abnormal fetuses and described preliminarily behavior of eight abnormal fetuses.[29] 4D-US can evaluate precisely the function of the hand, i.e., opening and closing of the fist. Moreover, observing fetal tone as the building blocks of the biophysical profile will probably now be possible.[30,31]

Four-dimensional ultrasound will undoubtedly enable an even closer look at various fetal anomalies in which motion plays a significant part.[29]

EVALUATION OF THE ABNORMALITY BY 3D-US IN THE FETAL FACE, NECK, AND CRANIUM

Three-dimensional ultrasound offers the possibility of studying the fetal face in a more global way than conventional 2D-US. This part of the fetal body was, and still is, the most documented structure in 3D-US.[32,33]

A diagnosis of a cleft of the palate and lip are at times hard to make using 2D-US. Using multiplanar imaging the simultaneously evaluated orthogonal planes will enable the hard to image axial planes to be seen and in other planes, the alveolar ridge and upper lip appear at the same time.[34] Lee et al. analyzed 7 fetuses with confirmed facial cleft anomalies and found that surface rendering of the face may allow increased diagnostic confidence for normal and abnormal lips.[32,35] Cephaloceles have been located and described better than by 2D-US.[36] The cranial sutures fontanels were also successfully evaluated using 3D-US.[37] Monteagudo et al.[38] worked on 24 fetuses with brain pathology. Three-dimensional ultrasound technology can effectively be used to examine the fetal brain. The ability to simultaneously view and review a brain volume in all three scanning planes, by navigating back and forth through digitally stored data was found to be clinically important.

EVALUATION OF THE ABNORMALITY BY 3D-US IN THE FETAL SKELETON AND EXTREMITIES

Using X-ray mode and the maximum mode the bony structures such as bones and extremities can be visualized.[39] Skeletal dysplasias also can be evaluated by 3D-US in conjunction with 2D-US successfully.[40] Developmental anomalies of the skeleton are identified with a high degree of reliability.[41-43] The vertebrae, ribs, and clavicle can be demonstrated as well as the general appearance of the fetal body.[40-43] As far as the extremities are concerned, 3D-US is almost the ideal tool to evaluate the hands and feet. 3D-US performed better than 2D-US in evaluating fetal digits. It can accurately delineate flexion deformities such as clubfoot and overlapping fingers.[44,45]

EVALUATION OF THE ABNORMALITY BY 3D-US IN THE THORAX AND GASTROINTESTINAL SYSTEM

Anterior abdominal wall defects (omphalocele, gastroschisis), congenital diaphragmatic hernias intra-abdominal and intrathoracic masses, their composition, vascularity, and inner wall of the cysts can be advantageously evaluated with 3D surface-rendered and multiplanar modes.[1,3,46-48] However, some authors suggested that 3D-US added little value in diagnosing malformations of the fetal thorax and abdomen.[8,9]

EVALUATION OF THE ABNORMALITY BY 3D-US IN GENITOURINARY SYSTEM

Fetal sex can be assessed by 3D-US, therefore diagnosing anomalies of the genitalia is a real possibility.[49] It is possible to assess the volume of the urinary bladder and to evaluate better some anomalies like bladder extrophy.[50] However, there are reports suggesting only a small improvement in diagnosing genitourinary anomalies by 3D-US.[2,3]

COLOR AND POWER DOPPLER IMAGING AND THREE-DIMENSIONAL ULTRASOUND

Three-dimensional power Doppler sonographic imaging provides a 3D view of the blood vessels.[51] This technique reportedly has advantages over other forms of sonography in visualizing normal and abnormal fetal vascular anatomy.[51,52] Additionally vascular structures of structural defects and tumoral pathologies in the fetus can be evaluated entirely with glass body appearance and 3D color or power Doppler angiography mode very clearly.[1-3,51,53]

CARDIOVASCULAR EVALUATION BY THREE-DIMENSIONAL SPATIOTEMPORAL IMAGE CORRELATION TECHNOLOGY

Spatiotemporal image correlation (STIC) is a new approach for the clinical assessment of the cardiac malformations. It offers an easy to use technique to acquire data from the fetal heart and to aid in visualization with both 2D and 3D cine sequences.[54] Once the volume data are processed and displayed, examination of cardiovascular structures can be accomplished by rotating 2D images in an infinite number of planes. In addition, 3D surface-rendered anatomy of the heart and great vessels can be accomplished. It has a potential to shorten the evaluation time, especially when the complex heart defects are suspected.[54,55] 3D-US gives a new perspective to fetal heart scanning, especially in cardiac defects.[54-56]

CONCLUSION

Three-dimensional sonography (3D-US) has been demonstrated to be a promising technique for detecting fetal malformations. It is now clear that in the near future 3D technology will be present on all (probably even on portable) ultrasound machines. 3D-US can be a powerful adjunctive tool to 2D-US in providing a more comprehensible, 3D-US impression of congenital anomalies. Although there are still some problems like surface rendering in oligohydramnios and movement artifacts during volume acquisition that need to be resolved, 3D-US opens up a new dimension in ultrasound investigations.

CASE SERIES

Case 1

A 34-week fetus with holoprosencephaly, encephalocele, facial dysmorphism, spina bifida, and single umbilical artery. The fetus died soon after birth and was confirmed to have velocardiofacial syndrome. 3D-US images have made the pathology extremely clear both for the parents and for the consulting physicians (**Figs. 1 to 9**).

Case 2

A 32-week fetus with holoprosencephaly and hydrocephaly. Fetal karyotype was normal. The baby died few days after birth (**Figs. 10 to 14**).

Case 3

A 22-week fetus with unilateral cleft lip and palate. Fetal karyotype was normal. The baby was operated 3 months after birth (**Figs. 15 to 17**).

Case 4

A 23-week fetus with unilateral small cleft lip. The baby operated soon after birth (**Fig. 18**).

Case 5

A 28-week fetus was referred with a mass in the anterior part of the neck. Detailed 3D multiplanar and rendered images revealed fetal goiter. After confirming low levels of thyroid hormones with cordocentesis the baby had intra-amniotic thyroxine injection. He/she did not need treatment after birth (**Figs. 19 to 23**).

Case 6

Isolated hydrocephalus (**Figs. 24 to 26**).

Case Report

A 28-year-old, multiparous, was referred to our center at 31st week of gestation. Severe ventriculomegaly has been detected. The dilatation of the ventricles increased and the baby born by cesarean section. The karyotype of the baby was 46XX and the baby operated for shunting soon after birth. She is 8 months old and doing well at the moment.

Case 7

Isolated choroid plexus cyst (**Fig. 27**).

Case Report

A 32-year-old multiparous woman was referred to our clinic at 19th week of gestation. Isolated bilateral choroids plexus cysts were detected. The patient had amniocentesis and waiting for the results.

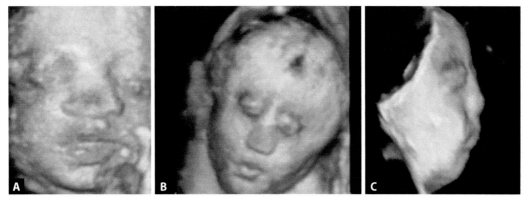

Figs. 1A to C: Three-dimensional (3D) surface-rendered image of fetal face at 34th week of gestation. Normal face by 3D-US is shown (A) triangular-shaped face with dysmorphic features (small mouth, long face, and nose, hypotelorism are clearly visible) in a fetus with velocardiofacial syndrome at 32nd week of gestation (B and C).

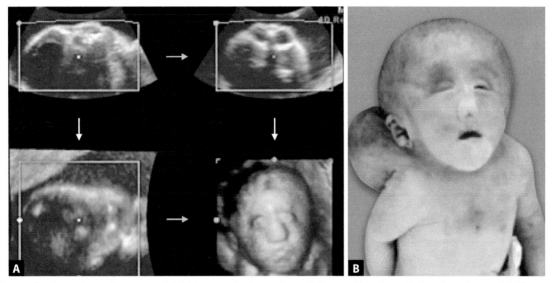

Figs. 2A and B: Multiplanar three-dimensional (3D) images in the 34th week fetus with velocardiofacial syndrome (A). These simultaneous views are not typically provided by 2D-US systems. Diagnostic clues provided by the interactive review of multiplanar images and 3D surface-rendered images may allow better characterization of facial features. Postmortem photograph demonstrating dysmorphic fetal face (B).

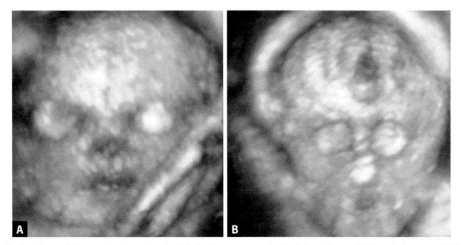

Figs. 3A and B: Evaluation of the metopic suture in this holoprosencephalic fetus. Normal (A) and abnormal (B) metopic suture at 34th week. The cranial sutures and fontanels were also successfully evaluated using three-dimensional (3D) ultrasound.

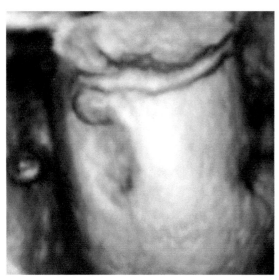

Fig. 4: Three-dimensional (3D) surface-rendered image of spina bifida at 34th week of gestation.

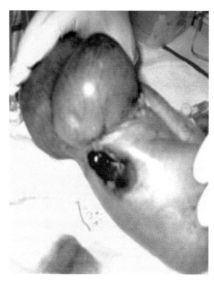

Fig. 5: Photograph of the neonate just after birth, demonstrating spina bifida, and posterior skin covered occipital encephalocele.

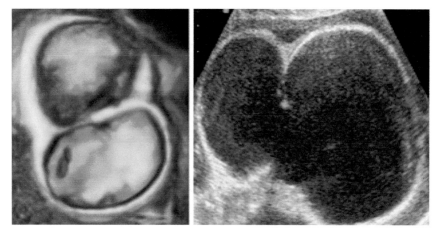

Fig. 6: Three-dimensional ultrasound (3D-US) image demonstrating connecting posterior encephalocele (on the left). 2D image of the bulging cystic mass with calvarial defect in the posterior region of the head. Cephaloceles have been located and described better than by 2D ultrasound.

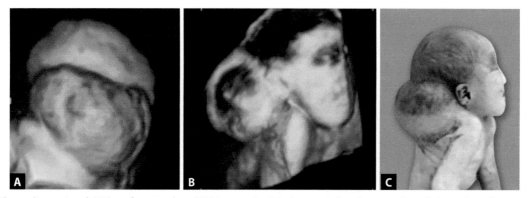

Figs. 7A to C: Three-dimensional (3D) surface-rendered US image. Occipital encephalocele at 33rd week (A and B). This image is presented to demonstrate the ease with which the 3D display enables pinpointing of the location of the bony gap in the skull through which brain protrudes and postmortem image lateral view (C).

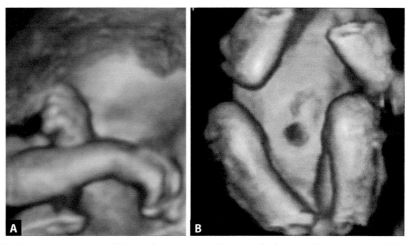

Figs. 8A and B: Three-dimensional (3D) surface-rendered image of a fetus with normal tone (A) and hypotonic sitting position of the fetus with holoprosencephaly (B).

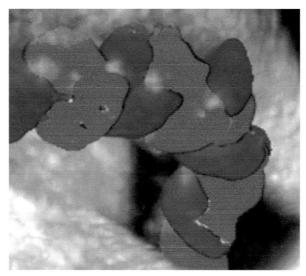

Fig. 9: Three-dimensional ultrasound (3D-US) glass body appearance of single umbilical artery.

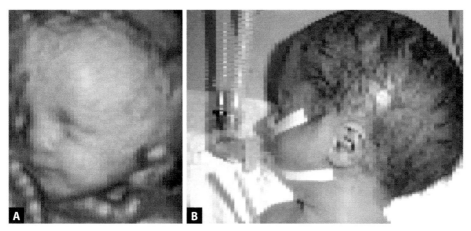

Figs. 10A and B: Three-dimensional (3D) surface-rendered image of a fetus with hydrocephaly and holoprosencephaly (A) and picture of the newborn in the neonatal intensive unit and intubated (B).

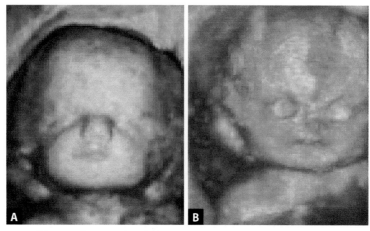

Figs. 11A and B: Three-dimensional (3D) surface-rendered (A) and transparency maximum mode (B) of the fetal face in this fetus with hydrocephaly and holoprosencephaly. Note the perfectly clear facial features and metopic suture of the face and cranium.

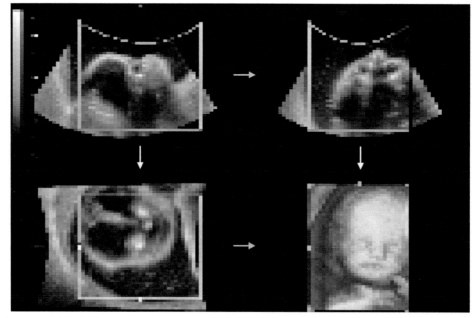

Fig. 12: Three-dimensional multiplanar and rendered images of the 32nd week fetus with hydrocephaly and holoprosencephaly. It is easier to evaluate the pathology with different planes simultaneously.

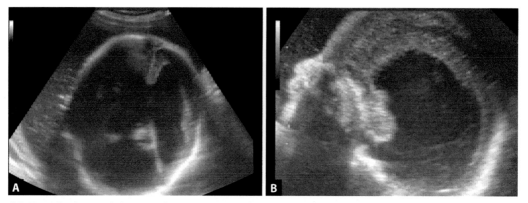

Figs. 13A and B: Two-dimensional ultrasound (2D-US) image of this 32 weeks fetus. Transverse (A) and sagittal (B) sections show the holoprosencephaly and hydrocephaly. To be able to get these images, sonographer has to wait the most appropriate fetal position.

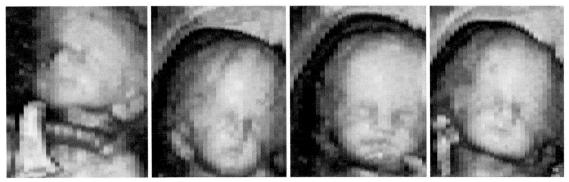

Fig. 14: Four-dimensional (4D) sequence demonstrated behavior of fetus complicated by holoprosencephaly and hydrocephaly at 32nd week of gestation.

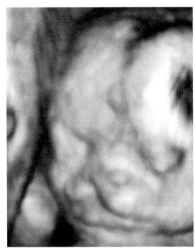

Fig. 15: Three-dimensional (3D) surface-rendered image of the cleft lip. Three-dimensional sonogram in surface mode visualizes the extent and shape of the cleft lip. Surface rendering of facial clefting is very helpful for prenatal counseling and planning obstetrical and neonatal management.

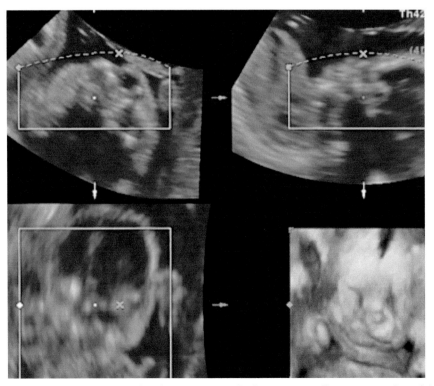

Fig. 16: Three-dimensional (3D) volume data and rendered images: 3D multiplanar images allow one to evaluate labial defects abnormalities of the maxillary tooth bearing alveolar ridge. 3D-US may provide additional benefit by allowing visualization of these structures in a manner that is complementary to two-dimensional ultrasonography.

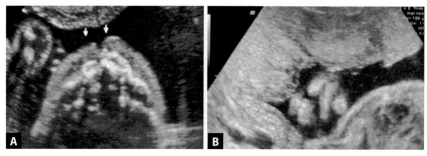

Figs. 17A and B: Two-dimensional (2D) sonogram displays the location of the unilateral cleft palate (A) and cleft lip (B). The operator has to try hard to be able to get these images by 2D-US.

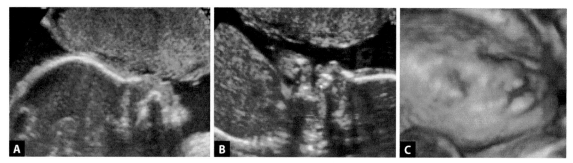

Figs. 18A to C: A 22-week fetus with unilateral small cleft lip. The profile of the fetus looks perfect when the mouth is closed in the sagittal section (A) whereas when the baby opened his mouth the effect is visible in the lip (B). However, three-dimensional ultrasound (3D-US) surface-rendered image clearly shows the defect in the lip (C).

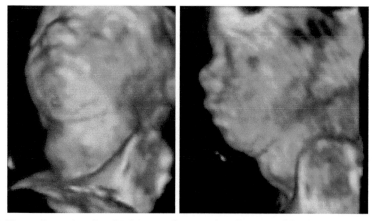

Fig. 19: Three-dimensional multiplanar surface-rendered image of the fetal face and neck at 28th week demonstrating fetal goiter very clearly.

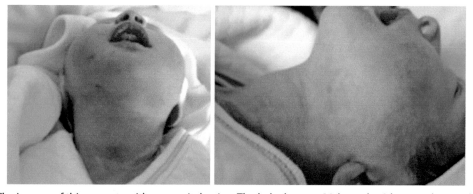

Fig. 20: The images of this neonate with congenital goiter. The baby born at 39th week with normal vaginal delivery.

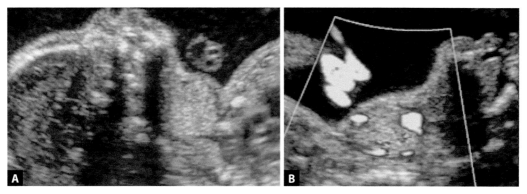

Figs. 21A and B: Two-dimensional ultrasound (2D-US) image (A) and 2D power US (B) evaluation of the sagittal section of the fetus with goiter at 28th week.

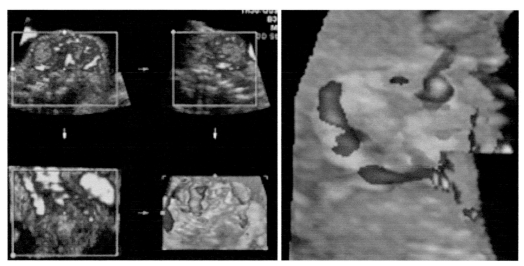

Fig. 22: Three-dimensional (3D) multiplanar power Doppler angiography of the goiter at 28th week demonstrating markedly increased vascular flow. 3D sonography, especially when combined with power Doppler angiography may play a very important role in the evaluation and management of the fetus with goiter.

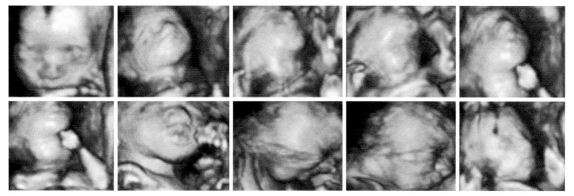

Fig. 23: Four-dimensional ultrasound (4D-US) image sequence demonstrated behavior of the fetus complicated by fetal goiter at 28th week of gestation.

Case 8

Alobar holoprosencephaly associated with Fallot tetralogy **(Figs. 28 to 30)**.

Case Report

A 39-year-old multiparous lady was referred at 33rd week of gestation. She had first-degree consanguinity with her husband. A detailed 3D transabdominal ultrasound evaluation revealed alobar holoprosencephaly and Fallot tetralogy in the fetus. The parents were informed about the high mortality and morbidity of the expected baby but they decided to continue the pregnancy, due to religious reasons. The baby died 1 hour after birth.

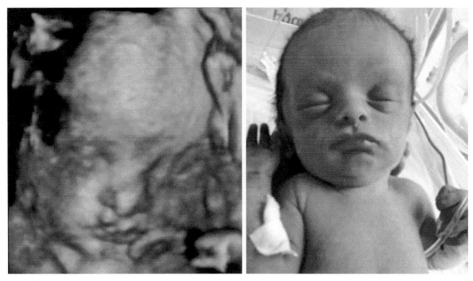

Fig. 24: Three-dimensional (3D) surface-rendered image of a fetus with hydrocephaly at 31st week (on the left) and picture of the neonate.

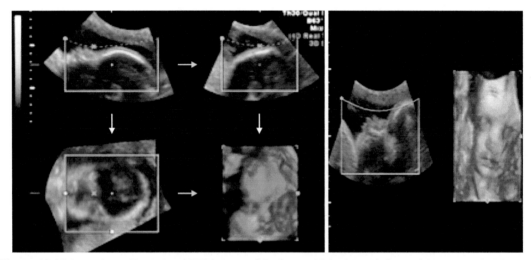

Fig. 25: Multiplanar three-dimensional (3D) images of the fetus with hydrocephalus and constructed 3D image.

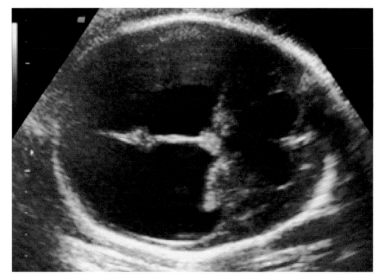

Fig. 26: Two-dimensional ultrasound of the fetus with hydrocephaly at 31st week. Transverse section of the head showing severely dilated ventricles with intact septum.

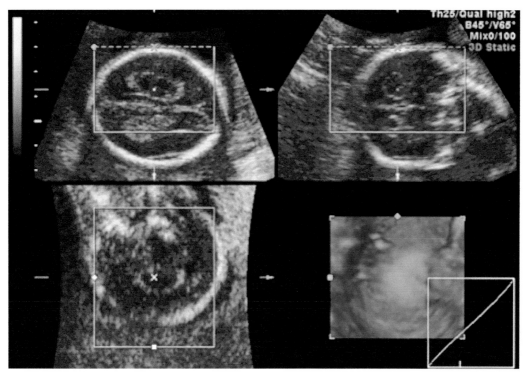

Fig. 27: Multiplanar three-dimensional ultrasound (3D-US) image of the fetus with bilateral choroids plexus cyst at 19 weeks of gestation.

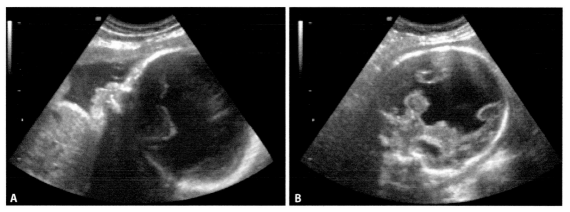

Figs. 28A and B: Two-dimensional ultrasound (2D-US) sagittal (A) and transverse (B) section of the fetal head, showing alobar holoprosencephaly.

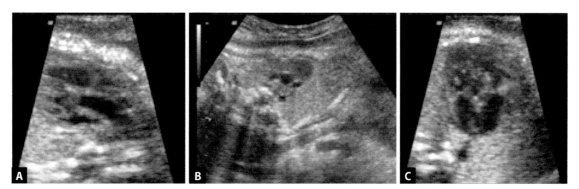

Figs. 29A to C: Two-dimensional ultrasound (2D-US) image of the heart of a fetus with Fallot's tetralogy. Overriding aorta (A), pulmonary stenosis in the three-vessel view (B) and normal looking four-chamber view (C). However, in the 3D-US spatiotemporal image correlation (STIC) mode with color Doppler revealed ventricular septal defect (VSD).

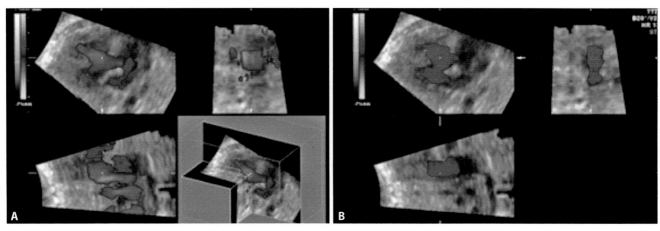

Figs. 30A and B: Three-dimensional (3D) spatiotemporal image correlation (STIC) technology with color Doppler niche mode showing aorta supplying blood to both ventricles (A) and ventricular septal defect (B) in a fetus with Fallot tetralogy at 32nd week.

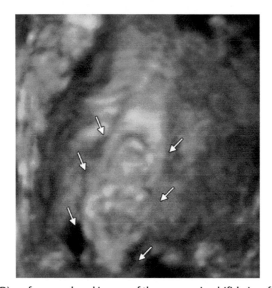

Fig. 31: Three-dimensional (3D) surface-rendered image of the open spina bifida in a fetus at 24th week of gestation.

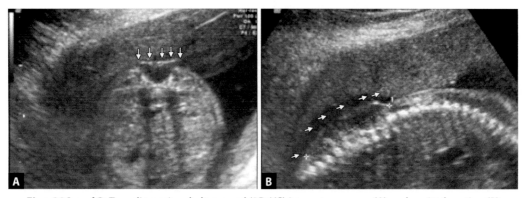

Figs. 32A and B: Two-dimensional ultrasound (2D-US) image transverse (A) and sagittal section (B) showing spinal defect at 23rd week of gestation.

Case 9

Spina bifida **(Figs. 31 and 32)**.

Case Report

A 20-year-old lady was referred to our clinic at 23rd-week of gestation. Three-dimensional surface-rendered and multiplanar images and 2D-US evaluation revealed large open spina bifida. After counseling about the high morbidity of the expected baby the parents opted continuing the pregnancy.

Case 10

Lumbar meningomyelocele **(Figs. 33 and 34)**.

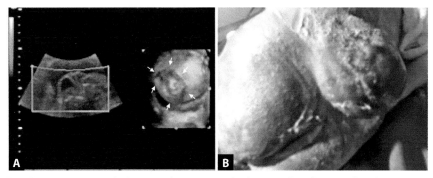

Figs. 33A and B: Three-dimensional ultrasound (3D-US) multiplanar and surface-rendered image (A) of a fetus with meningomyelocele at 30th week of gestation. Image of the neonate (B) with meningomyelocele just after birth.

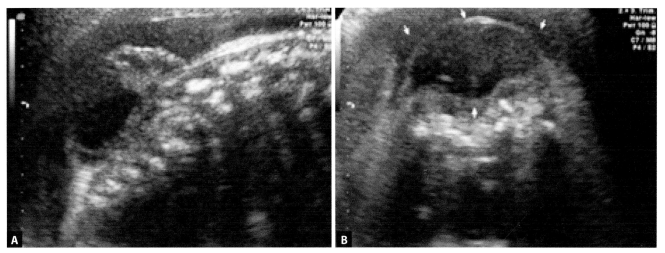

Figs. 34A and B: Two-dimensional ultrasound (2D-US) images of sagittal (A) and transverse (B) sections showing meningomyelocele.

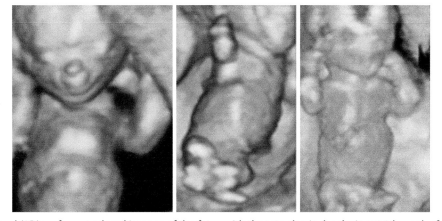

Fig. 35: Three-dimensional (3D) surface-rendered images of the fetus with thanatophoric dysplasia at 16th week of gestation. Note marked difference between chest and abdomen. All the extremities are clearly seen to be extremely small.

Case Report

A 35-year-old multiparous was referred to our hospital at 30th week of gestation. The three-dimensional and 2D-US evaluation of the fetus revealed a lumbar meningomyelocele measuring 5 × 5 × 6 cm. The baby born with cesarean section at 39th week of gestation. The baby operated soon after birth.

Case 11

Thanatophoric dysplasia **(Figs. 35 to 39)**.

Case Report

A 20-year-old primiparous woman referred to our center at 16th week of gestation. 3D and 2D-US examination revealed

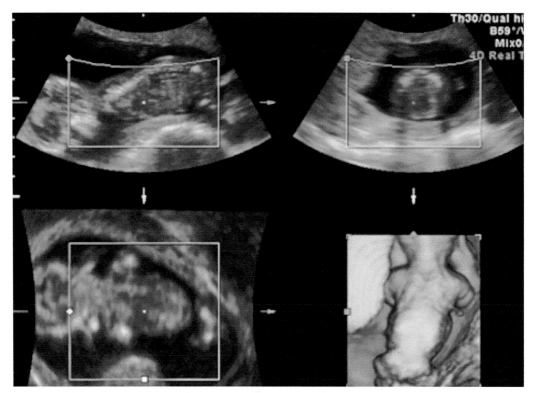

Fig. 36: Three orthogonal plane sections are displayed simultaneously in a fetus with thanatophoric dysplasia at 16th week.

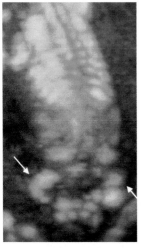

Fig. 37: Three-dimensional (3D) skeleton mode showing short bowed femurs and narrow chest of the fetus with thanatophoric dysplasia.

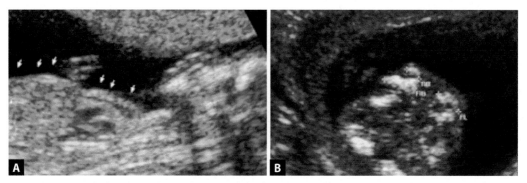

Figs. 38A and B: Two-dimensional ultrasound (2D-US) image of the fetus with thanatophoric dysplasia. Sagittal section (A) shows narrow chest. Marked difference in the size of chest and abdomen can be seen. Extremely short and bowed (B) femur, tibia, and fibula can be visualized.

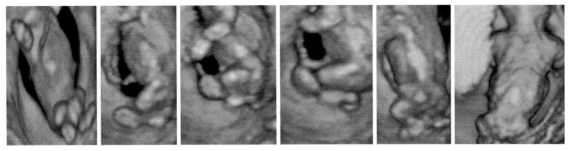

Fig. 39: Four-dimensional ultrasound (4D-US) sequence demonstrated behavior of the fetus complicated by thanatophoric dysplasia at 16th week.

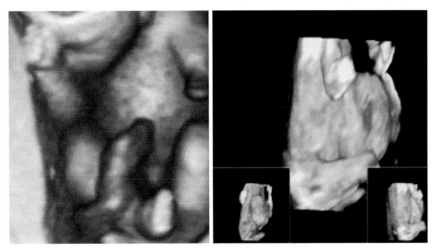

Fig. 40: Three-dimensional (3D) surface-rendered image shows normal abdominal wall and umbilical cord entrance (on the left). 3D surface-rendered images with transvaginal 3D rotation cine mode show the fetus with large omphalocele with simultaneous different angles at 12th week of gestation. During counseling of the parents about the continuation of the pregnancy these images helped the family to imagine what kind of pathology their baby has and effected their decision positively about continuing the pregnancy.

narrow chest and severe micromelia of the limbs. All long bones of the extremity were very short and bowed. The fetus was diagnosed as having thanatophoric dysplasia. After counseling the parents elected the termination of the pregnancy.

Case 12

Omphalocele **(Figs. 40 to 42)**.

Case Report

A 22-year-old G1P0 woman was referred to our hospital at 12th week of gestation. Detailed 2D and 3D multiplanar and surface-rendered and color Doppler evaluation revealed a large omphalocele containing liver. Fetal karyotype was found to be normal. After counseling the parents elected continuing the pregnancy. Follow-up of the case has been done in another center.

Case 13

Gastroschisis **(Figs. 43 to 45)**.

Case Report

A 19-year-old G1P0 woman was referred to our center at 18th week of gestation. Detailed 2D and 3D-US examination

revealed left-sided gastroschisis. After counseling the parents opted for continuing the pregnancy. The baby born by cesarean section at 35th week of gestation. She had six consecutive closure operations 1 month apart by pediatric surgeons as planned before birth after our 3D-US evaluations.

Case 14

Intestinal obstruction **(Figs. 46 to 49)**.

Case Report

A 37-year-old pregnant woman, gravida 3, para 2, was referred to our center at 35th week of gestational age because of suspected renal pathology. We performed 3D power Doppler sonography with simultaneous multiplanar imaging and 2D-US examination. Kidneys were normal but dilated bowel loop measuring 6 × 4 × 7 cm was diagnosed. The vascular supply of the dilated bowel was examined and superior mesenteric artery and superior mesenteric vein were wound counterclockwise forming the "barber-pole" sign. Previous research suggests that the counterclockwise barber-pole sign is a normal finding. This "negative finding" has been suggested before that it might be used to exclude the diagnosis of midgut volvulus, a dangerous

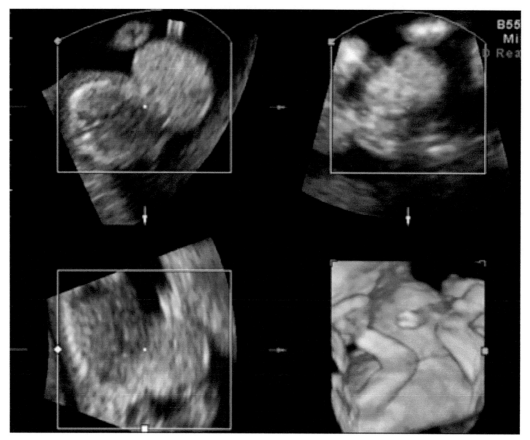

Fig. 41: Multiplanar and rendered three-dimensional (3D) images of a fetus with omphalocele at 12th week of gestation. 3D sonogram clearly demonstrates the exact location and extends of the defect and also relationship between the mass and the body.

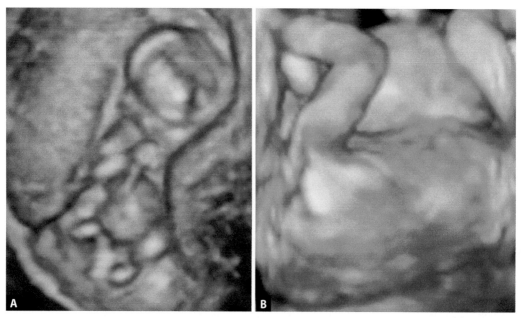

Figs. 42A and B: Three-dimensional (3D) surface-rendered image of the fetus with omphalocele at 12th week of gestation by transabdominal (A) and transvaginal (B) approach. Although both demonstrate the mass very well. Transvaginal route shows the pathology undoubtfully clearer and more impressive investigation for the possible systemic disease and waiting for the operation.

condition that would be expected to cause three vessels to wrap around in a clockwise direction. The baby born at 40th week of gestation. Intestinal obstruction in the ileocecal region was diagnosed and resection and reanastomosis of the obstructed bowel has been done. The baby is 6 months old and doing very well at the moment.

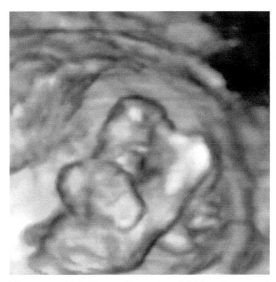

Fig. 43: An 18-week fetus with gastroschisis. Three-dimensional (3D) surface-rendered image of the trunk and lower extremity clearly show the nature and localization of the defect.

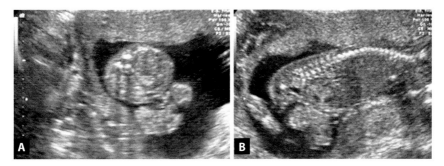

Figs. 44A and B: An 18-week fetus with gastroschisis. Two-dimensional (2D) transverse (A) and sagittal (B) images show the pathology.

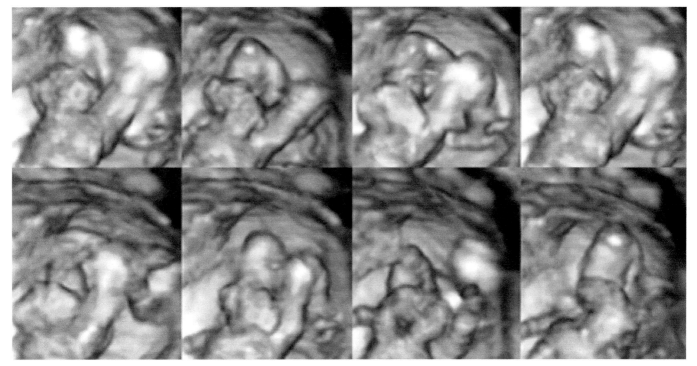

Fig. 45: Four-dimensional (4D) sequence of the trunk and lower extremity of the fetus with gastroschisis at 18th week of gestation.

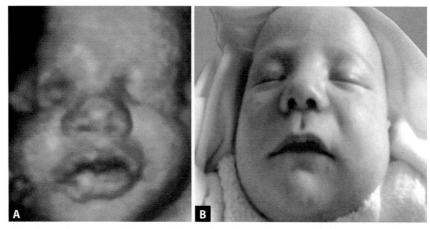

Figs. 46A and B: Three-dimensional ultrasound (3D-US) surface-rendered image of the face (A) of the fetus with intestinal obstruction and neonate 1 month after the operation (B).

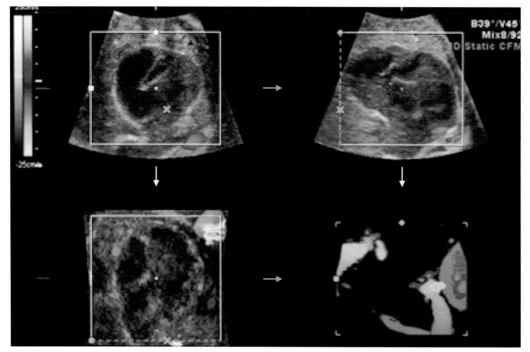

Fig. 47: Three-dimensional (3D) multiplanar color Doppler imaging of a fetus with intestinal obstruction at 35th week. 3D color Doppler sonography can demonstrate vascular changes in the fetal intestine to investigate the obstruction.

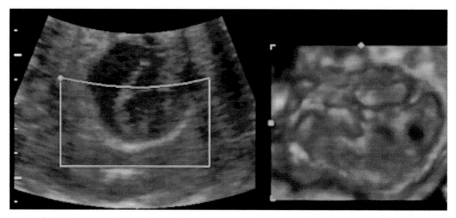

Fig. 48: Three-dimensional (3D) sonography with simultaneous gray-scale image showing inside the dilated conglomerous bowel.

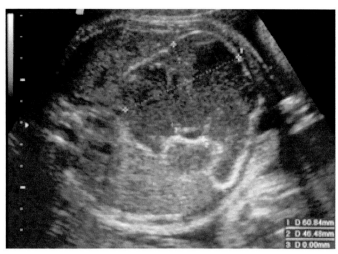

Fig. 49: Two-dimensional ultrasound (2D-US) image showing a mass in the abdominal region in a fetus with intestinal obstruction at 35th week of gestation.

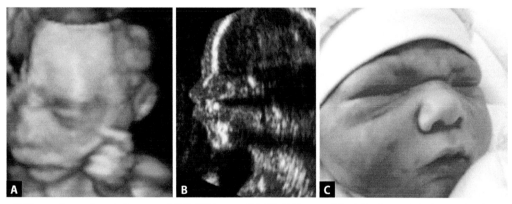

Figs. 50A to C: Three-dimensional ultrasound (3D-US) image (A), 2D-US image (B) of the fetus with thoracolumbar hemangioma at 21st week. Picture of the newborn (C).

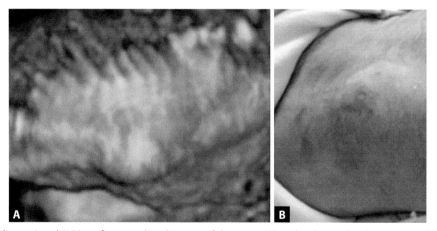

Figs. 51A and B: Three-dimensional (3D) surface-rendered image of the mass (A) at the thoracolumbar region of the fetus. It was very clear to evaluate the location and nature of the vascular mass with multiplanar view and 3D color Doppler. Picture of the hemangioma 1 day after the birth of the baby (B).

Case 15

Thoracolumbar hemangioma **(Figs. 50 to 52)**.

Case Report

A 28-year-old, gravida 3, parity 1, woman was referred to our center with the suspicion of the spina bifida at 21st week of gestation. After evaluation with 3D rendered and color Doppler and 2D sonogram, hemangioma at the thoracolumbar region was diagnosed. The baby born with normal vaginal delivery. Pediatric surgeons confirmed the diagnosis of hemangioma and the baby is under observation.

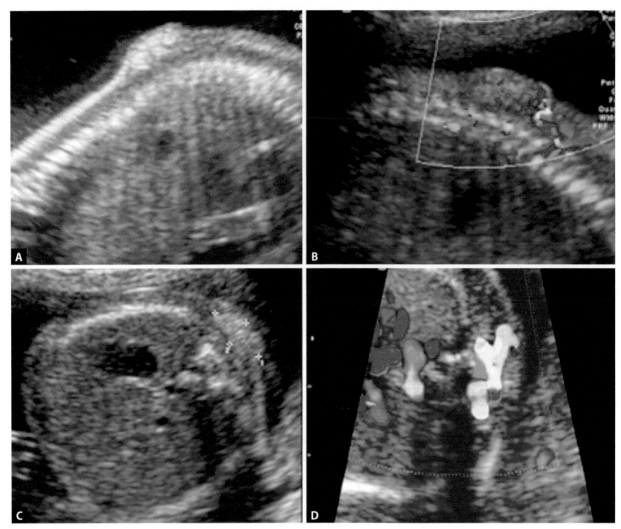

Figs. 52A to D: Two-dimensional ultrasound (2D-US) sagittal section (A) of a fetus with hemangioma at 21st week of gestation. It looks more like a lipoma or a solid mass without color Doppler evaluation. Color Doppler evaluation sagittal section (B). Gray scale (C) and color Doppler (D) in transverse sections almost confirmed that the mass was composed of vessels.

Case 16

Nonimmune hydrops **(Figs. 53 to 57)**.

Case Report

A 29-year-old, gravida 1, parity 0, woman was referred to our center at 32nd week of gestation. Two-dimensional (2D) and 3D-US evaluation confirmed generalized hydrops. The blood tests could not find Rh incompatibility and other blood antigens that could cause hydrops. Serum samples could not find anything but IgG positivity. Cordocentesis ruled out anemia. Thoracocentesis was done to evaluate the possible infection. PCR evaluation of the CMV was negative in the thoracentesis material. Karyotyping of the fetus was normal. The fetus died in utero at 34th week of gestation.

Case 17

Twin-to-twin transfusion syndrome **(Figs. 58 to 59)**.

Case Report

A 32-year-old G1P0 woman with monochorionic diamniotic twin pregnancy was detected to have severe twin-to-twin transfusion syndrome at 22nd week of gestation. The parents understood the situation by 3D surface-rendered images of these fetuses. Cord occlusion of the stucked (donor) twin with laser was done in another center. Recipient twin was born alive at term and 5 months old at the moment.

Case 18

Cystic adenoid malformation of the lung **(Figs. 60 to 62)**.

Case Report

A 30-year-old woman G3P2 was diagnosed as having cystic adenoid malformation of the lung of the fetus at 33rd week of gestation. The cystic mass was measuring 3 × 4 × 3 cm in the right lung. 3D multiplanar evaluation confirmed that the cystic mass

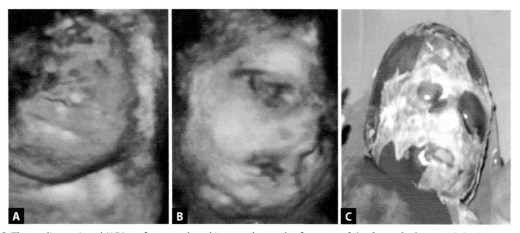

Figs. 53A to C: Three-dimensional (3D) surface-rendered image shows the features of the face of a fetus with hydrops at 32nd week of gestation (A and B). Postmortem macerated face of the hydropic baby (C).

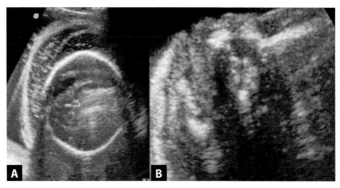

Figs. 54A and B: A 32-week fetus with hydrops. Two-dimensional (2D) sonogram shows the scalp edema (transverse section, in A) but does not delineate the fetal face (sagittal section of the fetal profile, in B).

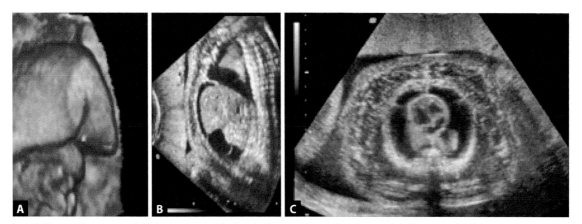

Figs. 55A to C: Three-dimensional (3D) sonogram (A) clearly demonstrates the shape of the liver, gallbladder, bowel, and the affiliated ligaments. 2D sonogram of the fetal viscera and thorax shows marked ascites and pleural effusion (B and C).

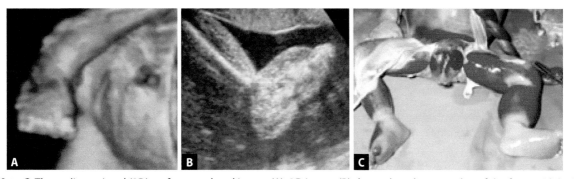

Figs. 56A to C: Three-dimensional (3D) surface-rendered image (A), 2D image (B) shows the edematous leg of the fetus with hydrops at 32nd week of gestation. Postmortem picture of the edematous legs of the baby (C).

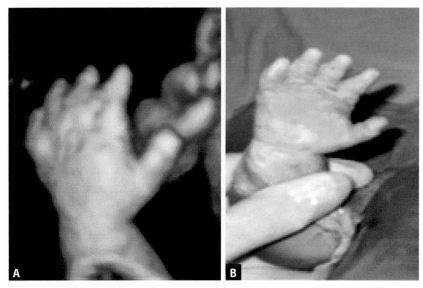

Figs. 57A and B: Three-dimensional (3D) surface-rendered image of the fetal hand of the fetus with hydrops at 32nd week (A) clearly demonstrates the features of the hand. Postmortem picture of the hand of the fetus with hydrops (B).

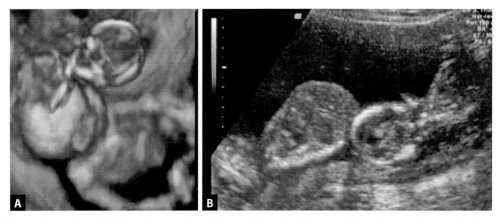

Figs. 58A and B: Three-dimensional (3D) surface-rendered image (A) in the fetuses with twin-to-twin transfusion syndrome at 22nd week. The difference in size between recipient twin and the donor (stucked) twin is striking with these images. 2D image (B) shows the polyhydramnios.

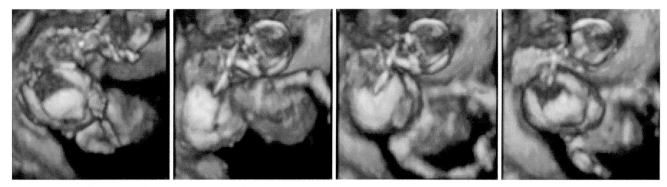

Fig. 59: Four-dimensional (4D) sequence of the fetuses with twin-to-twin transfusion syndrome in a monochorionic diamniotic twin pregnancy. Freely moving recipient twin is seen very clearly whereas the donor twin (stucked) cannot move because of severe oligohydramnios.

was in the lung itself and it was very difficult by 3D multiplanar mode to differentiate it from the congenital diaphragmatic hernia in which stomach bubble can be seen in the thorax. The baby had partial lobectomy of the lung after birth.

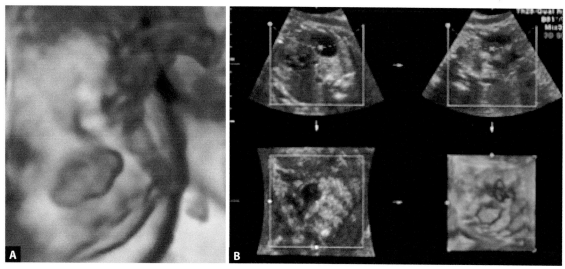

Figs. 60A and B: Three-dimensional (3D) surface-rendered face image (A) and multiplanar image of the thorax (B) of a fetus with cystic adenoid malformation of the lung at 33rd week of gestation. The nature of the cystic mass and its exact localization in the right lung can be seen easily.

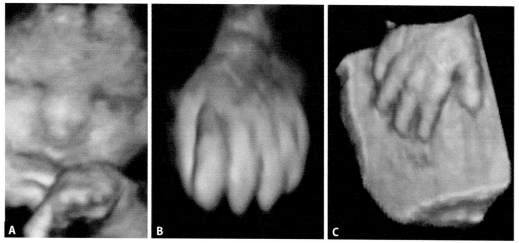

Figs. 61A to C: Normal fetal face (A), hand is closed (B) and open (C). Anatomical and functional pathology and the tone in the fetal hand and digits can be evaluated clearly and easily by three-dimensional ultrasound (3D-US).

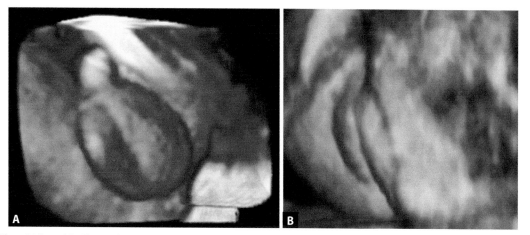

Figs. 62A and B: Three-dimensional (3D) surface-rendered image of a normal male (A) and female (B) genitalia. Abnormalities of the fetal gender are also easy to detect by 3D-US.

■ REFERENCES

1. Timor-Tritsch IE, Platt LD. Three-dimensional ultrasound experience in obstetrics. Curr Opin Obstet Gynecol. 2002; 14(6):569-75.

2. Merz E, Bahlmann F, Weber C, Macchiella D. Three-dimensional ultrasonography in prenatal diagnosis. J Perinat Med. 1995;23:213-22.

3. Merz E. Three-dimensional ultrasound in the evaluation of fetal anatomy and fetal malformations. In: Chervenak FA, Kurjak A (Eds). Current Perspectives on the Fetus as a Patient. London: Parthenon Publishing; 1996. pp. 75-87.

4. Lee W. 3D fetal ultrasonography. Clin Obstet Gynecol. 2003;46(4):850-67.

5. Maier B, Steiner H, Wienerroither H, Staudach A. The psychological impact of three-dimensional fetal imaging on the fetomaternal relationship. In: Baba K, Jurkovic D (Eds). Three-dimensional Ultrasound in Obstetrics and Gynecology. New York: Parthenon Publishing; 1997. pp. 67-74.

6. Kurjak A, Hafner T, Kos M, Kupesic S, Stanojevic M. Three-dimensional sonography in prenatal diagnosis: a luxury or a necessity? J Perinat Med. 2000;28:194-209.

7. Dyson RL, Pretorius DH, Budorick NE, Johnson DD, Sklansky MS, et al. Three-dimensional ultrasound in the evaluation of fetal anomalies. Ultrasound Obstet Gynecol. 2000;16(4):321-8.

8. Xu HX, Zhang QP, Lu MD, Xiao XT. Comparison of two-dimensional and three-dimensional sonography in evaluating fetal malformations. J Clin Ultrasound. 2002;30(9):515-25.

9. Merz E, Bahlmann F, Weber C. Volume scanning in the evaluation of fetal malformations: a new dimension in prenatal diagnosis. Ultrasound Obstet Gynecol. 1995;5:222-7.

10. Gregg AR, Steiner H, Staudach A, Weiner CP. Accuracy of 3D sonographic volume measurements. Am J Obstet Gynecol. 1993;168:348.

11. Baba K, Satoh K, Sakamoto S, Okai T, Ishi IS. Development of an ultrasonic system for three-dimensional reconstruction of the fetus. J Perinat Med. 1989;17:24.

12. Kelly IM, Gardener JE, Brett AD, Richards R, Lees WR. Three-dimensional US of the fetus. Work in progress. Radiology 1994;192:253.

13. Merz E. 3-D Ultrasound in Obstetrics and Gynecology. Philadelphia, PA: Lippincott Williams and Wilkins; 1988.

14. Ewigman BC, Crane JP, Frigoletto FD, LeFevre ML, Bain RP, McNellis D. Effect of prenatal sonography screening on prenatal outcome. N Engl J Med. 1993;12:821-7.

15. Crane JP, LeFevre ML, Winborn RC, Evans JK, Ewigman BG, Bain RP, et al. A randomized trial of prenatal ultrasonographic screening: impact on the detection, management, and outcome of anomalous fetuses. The RADIUS Study Group. Am J Obstet Gynecol. 1994;171(2):392-9.

16. Baba K, Okai T, Kozuma S, Taketani Y, Mochizuki T, Akahane M. Real-time processable three-dimensional US in obstetrics. Radiology. 1997;203:571-4.

17. Nelson TR, Downey DB, Pretorius DH, Feuster A. Three-dimensional Ultrasound. Philadephia, PA: Lippincott Williams and Wilkins; 1999.

18. Baba K, Okai T, Kozuma S, Taketani Y. Fetal abnormalities: evaluation with real-time processable three-dimensional US—preliminary report. Radiology. 1999;211:441-6.

19. Pooh RK. Neurosonoembryology by three-dimensional ultrasound. Semin Fetal Neonatal Med. 2012;17:261-8.

20. Kim MS, Jeanty P, Turner C, Benoit B. Three-dimensional sonographic evaluations of embryonic brain development. J Ultrasound Med. 2008;27(1):119-24.

21. Engels AC, Joyeux L, Brantner C, De Keersmaecker B, De Catte L, Baud D, et al. Sonographic detection of central nervous system defects in the first trimester of pregnancy. Prenat Diagn. 2016;36(3):266-73.

22. Pooh RK. Contribution of Trans-vaginal high-resolution ultrasound in fetal neurology. Donald School J Ultrasound Obstet Gynecol. 2011;5(2):93-9.

23. Miskovic B, Predojevic M, Stanojevic M, Tikvica A, Kurjak A, Ivankovic D, et al. KANET test: Experience of Zagrep group. Donald School J Ultrasound Obstet Gynecol. 2012; 6(2): 166-70.

24. Merz E, Welter C. 2D and 3D Ultrasound in the evaluation of normal and abnormal fetal anatomy in the second and third trimesters in a level III center. Ultraschall Med. 2005;26(1):9-16.

25. Kurjak A, Vecek N, Hafner T, Bozek T, Funduk-Kurjak B, Ujevic B. Prenatal diagnosis: what does four-dimensional ultrasound add? J Perinat Med. 2002;30(1):57-62.

26. Kuno A, Akiyama M, Yamashiro C, Tanaka H, Yamagihara T, Hata T. Three-dimensional sonographic assessment of fetal behavior in the early second trimester of pregnancy. J Ultrasound Med. 2001;20:1271-5.

27. Kurjak A, Vecek N, Kupesic S, Azumendi C, Solak M. Four-dimensional sonography: how much does it improve prenatal practice. In: Carrera JM, Kurjak A, Chervenak FA (Eds). Controversies in Perinatal Medicine. London: Parthenon Publishing; 2003.

28. Kurjak A, Azumendi F, Vecek N, Kupesic S, Solak M, Varga D, et al. Fetal hand movements and facial expression in normal pregnancy studied by four-dimensional sonography. J Perinat Med. 2003;31:496-508.

29. Ahmed B, Kurjak A, Andonotopo W, Khenyab N, Saleh N, Al-Mansoori Z. Fetal behavioral and structural abnormalities in high risk fetuses assessed by 4D sonography. Ult Rev Obs Gyn. 2005;5:275-87.

30. Kurjak A, Stanojevic M, Andonotopo W, Salihagic-Kadic A, Carrera JM, Azumendi G. Behavioral pattern continuity from prenatal to postnatal life-a study by four-dimensional (4D) ultrasonography. J Perinat Med. 2004;32:346-53.

31. Campbell S. 4D or not 4D: that is the question (Editorial). Ultrasound Obstet Gynecol. 2002;19:1-4.

32. Lee A, Deutinger J, Bernaschek C. Three-dimensional ultrasound: abnormalities of the fetal face in surface and volume rendering mode. Br J Obstet Gynaecol. 1995;102:305-6.

33. Pretorius DH, Nelson TR. Fetal face visualization using three-dimensional ultrasonography. J Ultrasound Med. 1995; 14:349-56.

34. Pretorius DH, House M, Nelson TR, Hollenbach KA. Evaluation of normal and abnormal lips in fetuses: comparison between three and two-dimensional sonography. Am J Roentgenol. 1995;165:1233-7.

35. Lee W, Kirk JS, Shaheen KW, Romero R, Hodges AN, Comstock CH. Fetal cleft lip and palate detection by three-dimensional ultrasonography. Ultrasound Obstet Gynecol. 2000;16:314-20.

36. Timor-Tritsch IE, Monteagudo A, Mayberry P. Three-dimensional ultrasound of the fetal brain: the three horn view. Ultrasound Obstet Gynecol. 2000;16:302-6.
37. Pretorius DH, Nelson TR. Prenatal visualization of cranial sutures and fontanelles with three-dimensional ultrasonography. J Ultrasound Obstet Gynecol. 2000;16:302-6.
38. Monteagudo A, Timor-Tritsch IE, Mayberry P. Three-dimensional transvaginal neurosonography of the fetal brain: 'navigating' in the volume scan. Ultrasound Obstet Gynecol. 2000;16(4):307-13.
39. Ludomirski A, Khandelwal M, Uerpairojkit B, Reece EA, Chan L. Three-dimensional ultrasound evaluation of fetal facial and spinal anatomy. Am J Obstets Gynecol. 1996;174(Suppl):318.
40. Hull AD, Pretorius DH, Lev-Toaff A, Budorick NE, Salerno CC, Johnson MM, et al. Artifacts and the visualization of fetal distal extremities using three-dimensional ultrasound. Ultrasound Obstet Gynecol. 2000;16(4):341-4.
41. Steiner H, Spitzer D, Weiss-Wichert PH, Graf AH, Staudack A. Three-dimensional ultrasound in prenatal diagnosis of skeletal dysplasia. Prenat Diagn. 1995;15:373-7.
42. Garjian KV, Pretorius DH, Budorick NE, Cantrell CJ, Johnson DD, Nelson TR. Fetal skeletal dysplasia: three-dimensional US initial experience. Radiology. 2000;214:717-23.
43. Yanagihara T, Hata T. Three-dimensional sonographic visualization of fetal skeleton in the second trimester of pregnancy. Gynecol Obstet Invest. 2000;49:12-6.
44. Ploeckinger-Ulm B, Ulm MR, Lee A, Kratochwil A, Bernaschek G. Antenatal depiction of fetal digits with three-dimensional ultrasonography. Am J Obstet Gynecol. 1996;175:571-4.
45. Budorick NE, Pretorius DH, Johnson DD, Tartar MK, Lou KV, Nelson TR. Three-dimensional ultrasound examination of the fetal hands: normal and abnormal. Ultrasound Obstet Gynecol. 1998;12:227-34.
46. Riccabona M, Johnson D, Pretorius DH, Nelson TR. Three dimensional ultrasound: display modalities in the fetal spine and thorax. Eur J Radiol. 1996;22:141-5.
47. Lee AL, Kratochwill A, Stümpflen I, Deutinger J, Bernaschek G. Fetal lung volume determination by three-dimensional ultrasonography. Am J Obstet Gynecol. 1996;175:588-92.
48. Hsu CY, Chiba Y, Fukui O, Sasaki Y, Miyashita S. Counterclockwise barber-pole sign on prenatal three-dimensional power Doppler sonography in a case of duodenal obstruction without intestinal malrotation. J Clin Ultrasound. 2004;32(2):86-90.
49. Lev-Toaff AS, Ozhan S, Pretorius D, Bega G, Kurtz AB, Kuhlman K. Three-dimensional multiplanar ultrasound for fetal gender assignment: value of the mid-sagittal plane. Ultrasound Obstet Gynecol. 2000;16:345-50.
50. Riccabona M, Nelson TR, Pretorius DH, Davidson TE. In vivo three-dimensional sonographic measurement of organ volume: validation in the urinary bladder. J Ultrasound Med. 1996;15:627-32.
51. Ritchie CJ, Edwards WS, Mack LA, Cyr DR, Kim Y. Three-dimensional ultrasonic angiography using power-mode Doppler. Ultrasound Med Biol. 1996;22:277-86.
52. Matijevic R, Kurjak A. The assessment of placental blood vessels by three-dimensional Power Doppler ultrasound. J Perinat Med. 2002;30:26-32.
53. Downey DB, Fenster A, Williams JC. Clinical utility of three-dimensional US. Radiographics. 2000;20:559-71.
54. DeVore GR, Falkensammer P, Sklansky MS, Platt LD. Spatio-temporal image correlation (STIC): new technology for evaluation of the fetal heart. Ultrasound Obstet Gynecol. 2003;22(4):380-7.
55. Guerra FA, Isla AI, Aguilar RC, Fritz EG. Use of free-hand three-dimensional ultrasound software in the study of the fetal heart. Ultrasound Obstet Gynecol. 2000;16(4):329-34.
56. Snyder JE, Kisslo J, von Ramm OT. Real-time orthogonal mode scanning of the heart. I. System design. J Am Coll Cardiol. 1986;7:1279-85.

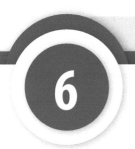
Prenatal Ultrasound Diagnosis in Turner Syndrome and Triploidy

Radu Vladareanu, Alina Veduta, Simona Vladareanu

■ INTRODUCTION

Turner syndrome (Ullrich–Turner) is a genetic disease, caused by the absence or abnormality of one of the sex chromosomes. The usual postnatal presentation is a form of genetically determined nanism, with exclusively feminine phenotype and characteristic gonadic dysgenesis (gonadal streaks) in over 90% of the cases.[1,2] Triploidy is a chromosomal abnormality where three complete sets of the haploid genome instead of the normal two sets are present. Triploidy syndrome is rare at birth but is estimated to occur in about 2% of human conceptuses.[1] Prevalence of triploidy is 1/2,000 at 12 weeks, and very rare at term. Prevalence of Turner syndrome is about 1/1,200 at 12 weeks, and <1/4,000 at 40 weeks.

The incidence of various chromosomal anomalies **(Table 1)**, including triploidy and Turner syndrome, has been estimated in recent studies.[1,3]

Triploidy is known as probably the most frequent human genetic defect; over 25% of genetic abortions are being triploid. The 69 XXY karyotype is the most frequent (about 60%); 37% of triploid embryos are 69 XXX and 3% are 69 XYY. It has no correlation with the maternal age, and livebirth incidence is about 1/50,000.

Triploidy is characterized by general dysmaturity, muscular hypotonia, large posterior fontanel, low set dysmorphic auricles, hypertelorism, microphthalmia and coloboma, cutaneous syndactyly of third and fourth fingers, simian crease, hypospadias and/or maldeveloped external genitalia.[4]

The prenatal appearance of digynic triploidy is different from that of diandric triploidy. Early severe asymmetric growth restriction and fetal malformations (mostly cerebral and cardiac) are seen in digynic triploidy. In diandric triploidy, a malformed embryo is either present or absent, the placenta has a characteristic molar appearance, and the ovaries of the mother are often enlarged, with multiple cysts. If maternal serum levels of pregnancy-associated plasma protein A (PAPP-A) and β-human chorionic gonadotropin

TABLE 1: The incidence of chromosomal anomalies in early spontaneous abortion.	
Chromosomal anomaly	**Incidence (%)**
Turner syndrome, 45X0	18
Triploidy	17
Trisomy 16	16
Other polyploidies	6.1
Trisomy 22	5.7
Trisomy 21	4.7
Trisomy 15	4.2
Trisomy 14	3.7
Trisomy 13	3.5
Trisomy 18	3.1
Other trisomies	14

Source: Adapted from references 3 and 22.

(β-hCG) are checked, they are both very low in digynic triploidy, while β-hCG level is markedly increased in diandric triploidy (diandric triploidy is a form of molar pregnancy).

The incidence of the X chromosome defects is estimated at 1:2,000–2,500 live births; more recent studies show an incidence of about 1:5,000–6,000 of the female live births.[3] Monosomy for the X chromosome is probably the most frequent genetic abnormality in humans, but it is accompanied by a very high embryo-fetal lethality; the incidence of the 45X0 zygotes is almost 2% from the total of the conceptive products, but <1% of them survive to the term; 7–15% of all the spontaneous abortions have 45X0 karyotype. The embryos with mosaicism or with structural defects of an X chromosome survive more frequently than those with 45X0 karyotype. It is likely that most individuals which survive the neonatal period are Turner mosaics.

The phenotype in Turner syndrome is caused by a defect of the sexual X chromosome; this chromosome may be absent from the entire or from a part of the cell lines of the respective organism or may have an abnormal structure. The classical karyotype described is aneuploid, 45X0, but it can also be a mosaicism 45X/46XX, 45X/47XXX, 45X/46XX/47XXX (Turner gonadal dysgenesis—like with positive sexual chromatin), 45X/46XY, 45X/47XYY, 45X/46XY/47XYY mosaicism (Turner gonadal dysgenesis—like with negative sexual chromatin and with the deletion, in many cases, of the SRY gene from the Y chromosome), or any structural defect of the X chromosome (46XXqi and 45X/46XXqi, 46XXr and 45X/46XXr, 46XXp and 45X/46XXp, 46XXq and 45X/46XXq, X isodicentric, translocation X—autosome or even isochromosome for the short arm of the X chromosome, Xpi). With conventional genetic analysis, the classical karyotype is detected in approximately 60% of the cases[2] and it seems to correlate with the full clinical development of the disease. The percentage of the mosaicism cases detected depends on the genetic analysis methods used. Sometimes, rarely in the cases with 45X0 karyotype, more frequently in the cases with partial deletions of an X chromosome, the nondegenerated ovarian follicles persist until puberty and determine the partial onset of the secondary sexual features.

The development of early fetal morphological assessment allowed for the description of a severe Turner phenotype, which usually causes fetal demise before midterm (the lethal Turner phenotype). Affected fetuses have very large nuchal translucency and hydrops; the ductus venosus is often absent and cardiac anomalies from the coarctation of aorta/ hypoplastic left heart spectrum are often present.

CLINICAL ASPECTS

From the point of view of the general practitioner and of the pediatrician, Turner syndrome is usually a facile diagnosis because of the very suggestive phenotype of the female patients; the characteristic physical features are rarely missing. Female patients present at puberty for the lack of onset of the secondary sexual features, primary amenorrhea, or even secondary amenorrhea (in the cases of structural defects of the X chromosome, the clinical picture is usually primary amenorrhea without Turner phenotype). However, from the obstetrician's point of view, the prenatal diagnosis of Turner syndrome and the management of the pregnancy with a Turner fetus may create problems in practice, problems that usually have to be solved in a tertiary fetal medicine center.

Early ultrasound descriptions of fetuses with Turner related to the description of fetal cystic hygroma. Malone et al. studied the prevalence, natural history, and outcome of septate cystic hygroma in the first trimester in the general obstetric population and aimed to differentiate this finding from simple increased nuchal translucency. In their study, there were 134 cases of cystic hygroma (two lost to follow-up) among 38,167 screened patients (1 in 285). Chromosomal abnormalities were diagnosed in 67 (51%), including

25 trisomy 21, 19 Turner syndrome, 13 trisomy 18, and 10 others. Major structural fetal malformations (primarily cardiac and skeletal) were diagnosed in 22 of the remaining 65 cases (34%). There were 5 cases (8%) of fetal death and 15 cases of elective pregnancy termination without evidence of abnormality. Their opinion was that first trimester cystic hygroma was a frequent finding in a general obstetric screening program. It had the strongest prenatal association with aneuploidy described to date, with significantly worse outcome compared with simple increased nuchal translucency. Most pregnancies with normal evaluation at the completion of the second trimester resulted in a healthy infant with a normal pediatric outcome.[5]

The primary defect in the formation of the lymphatic vessels is a part of a larger phenomenon of the cell migration in embryogenesis and it seems to determine many of the defects (including the cardiovascular ones[6]) that are described in the syndrome. Fetal tachycardia seems to be determined by the delay in maturation of the parasympathetic system, which results in the lack of the physiological decrease in the heart rate after 9 weeks.[7]

PATHOPHYSIOLOGY

45X0 karyotype may theoretically result from *nondisjunction in the meiosis in one of the parental gametogenetic lines*, but it is possible to practically result from a *mitosis defect*, namely the loss of a chromosome either during the germinal cell mitoses in the parental gametogenetic lines or between fertilization and the first mitotic division of the cells in the newly formed organism. It seems that these errors in the cellular division appear more frequently when one of the parental sexual chromosomes is abnormal; the chromosomal defect would determine the cellular division defect. At the first mitotic division, the phenomenon of the delay in anaphase (*anaphase lag*) may result in loss of a sexual chromosome (eventually abnormal). The defects in the ulterior divisions should lead to a genetic mosaic organism, but in those cases also the pure 45X0 karyotype may result finally through the loss of one euploid cell line, but with a probably abnormal sexual chromosome. The loss of the abnormal sexual chromosomes is a phenomenon which may appear also in the postnatal period.

The hypothesis of the mitotic error involved in the onset of Turner syndrome is sustained by clinical observations:

- Sporadic occurrence of the phenomenon, regardless of the maternal age (unlike Down syndrome or Klinefelter syndrome)
- High percentage of mosaicism cases
- Existence of monozygotic twin pregnancies with a 45X0 fetus and 46XY for the other fetus.

The percentage of the subjects identified with genetic mosaicism depends on the methods used for genetic analysis and ranges from 30 to 40% in the conventional techniques to 75% in polymerase chain reaction (PCR) amplification and in situ hybridization using specific probes (Y) techniques.[8] The extremely high rate of the in utero mortality of conceptuses with pure 45X0 karyotype led to the hypothesis that all the individuals with Turner syndrome that survive to term have mosaicism, especially as the version of the prenatal mosaicism existence with the postnatal loss of the euploid cellular lines cannot be invalidated. The idea that all the subjects with Turner syndrome who survive should have, at least initially, mosaic karyotype and is sustained by the following considerations:

- The need for existence of an euploid cellular line in the fetal membranes, where the selective imprinting of both sexual chromosomes takes place
- The existence, at birth, of a variable number of undegenerated follicles in most girls with Turner syndrome, considering that two active X chromosomes are required to maintain the gametogenetic line.

Familial cytogenetic studies showed a more frequent loss of the X chromosome with paternal origin; it seems that, in over two-thirds of the cases the paternal X chromosome is lost. It is hard to explain this phenomenon, especially considering that, although the influence of the specific imprinting of the remained X chromosome on the Turner phenotype was proved, it was not possible to reveal an advantage concerning the survival of the conceptive product that keeps the maternal—origin of X chromosome.[9] The identification and localization of the genes on X chromosome, whose haploid insufficiency leads to the phenotype in Turner syndrome ("Turner genes"), started from the idea that those genes should exist also on the chromosome Y (Ferguson–Smith). The most logical localization for these genes would be the pseudoautosomal region from the short arms of the sexual chromosomes because it is the region to participate to the crossing-over of the sexual chromosomes in the meiosis and where most of the genes are not affected by the *X-inactivation* phenomenon. The cytogenetic study of the subjects 46XYp, with the deletion of the testicular determination factor SRY, which develops as women, either with normal height or with Turner—like phenotype, depending on the additional deletions on Y chromosome, led to the identification of a 700 kb segment in the pseudoautosomal region from the end of the short arms of the sexual chromosomes, where it is found the gene whose haploid insufficiency would determine the statural hypotrophy in Turner syndrome, namely SHOX (*short-stature homeobox—gene on X chromosome*). It is a gene that encodes for a growth factor from the category of gene regulatory factors (home domain gene regulatory protein); through this growth factor, SHOX would be involved in chondrogenesis, and the lack of one of those two active copies of the gene, normally found in the cells of the body, would be (partially) responsible for the statural hypotrophy in the female patients with Turner syndrome.

SHOX is just one of the "Turner genes"; *Turner phenotype is determined by multiple factors*. Ogata and Matsuo[10] classified the phenomena that lead to its occurrence in three categories:

1. Quantitative loss or impairment of the euchromatin from extensive regions of the X chromosome (up to the absence of the entire chromosome), with global and unspecific deficiency in the development of the organism.
2. Haploid insufficiency of the growth pseudoautosomal genes, normally active on both sexual chromosomes and of the lymphogenic genes, with the appearance of the statural hypotrophy and of the "Turner marks".
3. Defective coupling of the sexual chromosomes in the prophase of the first meiosis, with loss of the gametogenetic line and gonadal dysgenesis.

Lymphogenesis defects in Turner syndrome could be due to the deficiency of a receptor for vascular endothelial derived growth factor (VEGF), namely VEGFR-3, protein of whose gene is found on X chromosome. It was also showed the deficiency of the BMX tyrosine-kinase, enzyme involved in the mediation of the VEGF effects at intracellular level, early in the embryo development, and of whose gene is also placed on the X chromosome. Macroscopically, in Turner syndrome, there is a defect in the formation of the great lymphatic vessels, which will not reach the communication with the veins in which they are supposed to flow and which, by dilatation and intrathoracic compression seems to determine the entire range of the cardiovascular defects and of the cephalic extremity defects described in the syndrome.

Gonadal dysgenesis in Turner syndrome is due to the fact that both X active chromosomes are required for the formation and maintaining of the gametogenetic line; genes from both arms of the X chromosomes are involved in the normal ovarian development. Primary germinal cells reach the gonadal ridge, but after the third month of gestation, the oocytes and the primordial follicles suffer an accelerated process of atresia, probably due to the impossibility to correctly perform the prophase of the meiosis I; therefore, the ovaries undergo a fibroconnective degeneration and they transform into gonadal streaks. The fact that the gonadal dysgenesis is caused by the accelerated atresia and not by the abnormal formation in the germinal cells was documented in the first studies about Turner syndrome and more recently studies show that, in many cases, this atresia process is not that fast to be complete at birth; almost one-third of the girls with Turner syndrome have at birth ovaries that are visible on echography, with undegenerated follicles.

Such follicles may persist until after the puberty, determining the onset of the secondary sexual features, menarche and even fertility in the female patients with Turner syndrome. Beside the interindividual variable speed of the process of follicular atresia (probably dependent on the specific of the X chromosome defect), the spontaneous onset of pregnancies in female patients with Turner syndrome may be explained by mosaicism or by the nondisjunction mitosis of the germinal 45X0 cells, with the formation of the 46XX oocytes. The women with 45X0 cellular lines have a higher rate of spontaneous abortions and of children with chromosome abnormalities than in the general population.

The consequences of the deletions to involve genetic material from X chromosome are very variable, from in utero death to normal female phenotype, with menarche and even fertility to the (eventual) installation of the secondary amenorrhea; the incidence of the mosaic karyotype with 45X0 lines in women with normal menstruation and fertility is unknown. The pattern offered for the understanding of the phenotypic consequences of the genotypic abnormalities makes Turner syndrome the subject of detailed studies.[11]

Three different mechanisms may produce triploidy:
1. Nondisjunction in meiosis I or meiosis II of spermatogenesis (sperm formation), resulting in an extra set of paternal chromosomes (diandry).
2. Nondisjunction in meiosis I or meiosis II of oogenesis (egg formation), resulting in an extra set of maternal chromosomes (digyny).
3. Double fertilization of a normal egg, resulting in an extra set of paternal chromosomes (dispermy).

Type I (diandry) triploid pregnancy presents large placenta, partial molar changes, severe symmetric growth restriction, elevated levels of maternal hCG, α-fetoprotein (AFP), inhibin A, and rarely, survives beyond the first trimester. Type II (digyny) pregnancy has a small placenta, asymmetric growth restriction, decreased levels of maternal hCG, AFP, inhibin A, and more often survives into the second trimester and eventually near term. Even if digyny is rarer, is more of interest for sonographic diagnosis.

Triploidy is lethal in utero, most of the times. Active populational screening is not justified for this condition alone, but prenatal diagnosis is of interest in individual cases. The majority of the Turner syndrome cases also end up in fetal demise. The prenatal diagnosis of the live fetuses with Turner syndrome and no major structural defects, as well as the prenatal diagnosis of the nonlethal chromosomal defects in general, is challenging from the medical and social-ethical points of view.

■ PRENATAL DIAGNOSIS

The main prenatal diagnosis methods are the ultrasound examination and serological test; these are *prenatal screening methods* for genetic conditions; the positive genetic diagnosis is made using invasive methods, amniocentesis or chorial biopsy, establishing the karyotype of the fetal cells from the sample, in the cases in which the screening indicates a high risk for chromosomal abnormalities of the fetus. Spencer et al. in one of their studies, where the first to claim that a large proportion of triploidy cases of both phenotypes could

be identified in the first trimester using nuchal translucency, maternal serum free β-hCG, and PAPP-A, while screening for trisomy 21.[12]

Echographic Screening

"First Trimester" Echography (11–14 Weeks)

The ultrasound appearance at 11–14 weeks' gestation is usually specific for both Turner syndrome and triploidy. Early studies reported that the echographic image in Turner syndrome at the end of the first trimester of gestation consists in: increased nuchal translucency **(Fig. 1)**, fetal tachycardia and early growth intrauterine restriction.[13] With the development of first trimester ultrasound, a specific "lethal" Turner phenotype has been described, consisting of: increased nuchal translucency (cystic hygroma, **Fig. 2**), absence of the ductus venosus, cardiac and renal anomalies.

Increased nuchal translucency is the most important echographic sign for all chromosomal abnormalities, between 11 and 14 weeks' gestation. Increasing nuchal translucency in fetuses with Turner syndrome is explained by the defect in the formation of the lymphatic vessels in the area of the thorax and the neck, caused by the haploid insufficiency of the lymphogenic genes in the monosomy X and which determines nuchal edema; the primary defect of the formation of the lymphatic vessels is included in a larger phenomenon of abnormalities of the cellular migration in embryogenesis.

Early studies indicated that increased nuchal translucency in the first trimester is more specific for trisomy 21, Down syndrome than for monosomy X, and Turner syndrome. In a large controlled study,[14] nuchal translucency over 5 mm was associated with 28 times increase in the incidence of Down syndrome and only nine times increase in the incidence of Turner syndrome compared to the general population. This idea was lately invalidated.

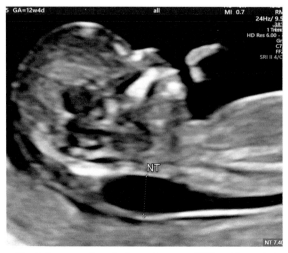

Fig. 1: Increased nuchal translucency (NT) at 12 weeks' gestational age.

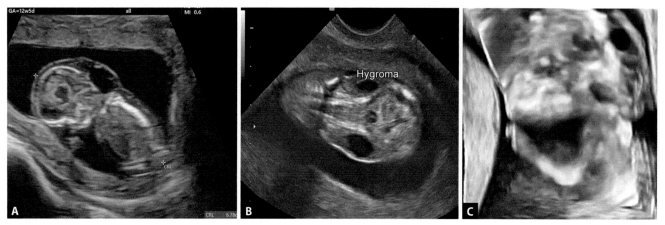

Figs. 2A to C: Two cases of cystic hygroma in Turner syndrome. (A) Increased nuchal translucency and fetal hydrops at 12 weeks' gestation; (B) Septate cystic hygroma at 12 weeks' gestational age (GA), coronal view; (C) Same case, three-dimensional (3D) view; the septum is clearly seen.

Reverse statistical analysis shows that most of the girls with monosomy X (approximately 85%) have increased nuchal translucency in trimester I, and the nuchal translucency increases to the highest values in Turner syndrome;[15,16] if in trisomy 21, the nuchal translucency increases on average with 2 mm above the normal value, in monosomy X, it increases with 7 mm above the normal value. Also, the hypoechoic nuchal image is hardly remitted in the fetuses with Turner syndrome, often persisting in the second trimester as cystic hygroma.

Attempts for an even earlier diagnosis of Turner syndrome had been made. Falcon et al. tried to determine the potential value of measuring the gestational sac volume (GSV) at 11–13^{+6} weeks of gestation in screening for chromosomal defects. The conclusion was that the measurement of the GSV at 11–13^{+6} weeks of gestation is unlikely to provide useful prediction of the major chromosomal defects. In trisomy 13 and triploidy, the small GSV may be due to early onset fetal growth restriction and reduced amniotic fluid volume. In trisomy 18, the increase in GSV is probably due to the presence of associated fetal abnormalities that interfere with fetal swallowing.[17]

Fetal tachycardia observed in the first trimester in Turner syndrome, consequence of the delay in maturation of the parasympathetic system, is not a constant finding but can be significant, even leading to functional fetal heart failure.[7]

Retardation in intrauterine growth in trimester I is moderate,[13] and, according to some studies, insignificant.[18]

Bronshtein et al. studied a population of 40,123 consecutive pregnant women at 14–16 weeks of gestation in which fetal karyotyping was performed in 9,348 cases. Turner syndrome was detected in 13 fetuses (0.03%, 1/3,086 early pregnancies). Septate cystic hygroma, severe subcutaneous edema, and hydrops were observed in all cases. A short femur was detected in 12 of 13 fetuses. A narrow aortic arch was visualized in all eight fetuses that were scanned after scanning of the aortic arch became

mandatory in that institution. They conclusioned that a reliable diagnosis of Turner syndrome by sonographic means is possible in early pregnancy.[19]

"Second Trimester" Echography (18–23 Weeks)

The fetuses with 45X0 Turner syndrome develop in the second trimester severe lymphatic abnormalities, observable on echography. The most typically sign, almost characteristic, is septate cystic hygroma, **(Figs. 3 and 4)** but clear in the rest, homogeneously hypoechoic. According to one study, from the fetuses with cystic hygroma, 75% have chromosomal abnormalities, and in over 95% of the cases the abnormality is the Turner syndrome.[20] Other echographic findings usually found in Turner syndrome in the second trimester include: lymphedema of the limbs, hydrothorax, and ascites **(Fig. 5)**. The intrauterine death is usually caused by the fetal hydrops that determines a characteristically echographic aspect, "space suit" **(Figs. 6 to 8)**.

Turner syndrome is associated also with other abnormalities visible on the echography, namely: cardiac abnormalities, especially of the left heart (coarctation of the aorta, defects of the aortic valve); renal abnormalities; skeletal dysplasia (shorten femoral bone), as well as with minor abnormalities, shared with other chromosomal defects.[20] The totality of the echographic signs in Turner syndrome in the second trimester—the "sonographic syndrome" is more suggestive than in other aneuploidies (especially in Down syndrome) **(Fig. 9)**; therefore, there are authors to sustain that the diagnosis of the Turner syndrome may be established on echography (unlike Down syndrome).[19] In case that on ultrasound we see major defects (signs), even isolated, it is recommended to analyze the fetal karyotype; the indication is valid also for severe hydrops, probably lethal, for establishing the recurrence risk (the risk for recurrence in monosomy X is theoretically absent).

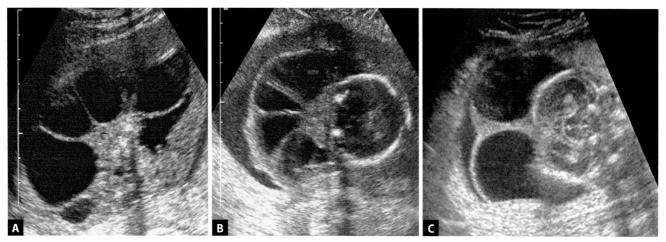

Figs. 3A to C: Multiseptated cystic hygroma in Turner Syndrome in the second trimester of gestation. (A and B) Multiseptated cystic hygroma; (C) Septate cystic hygroma at 16 weeks' gestational age (GA).
Courtesy: Professor Pelinescu D.

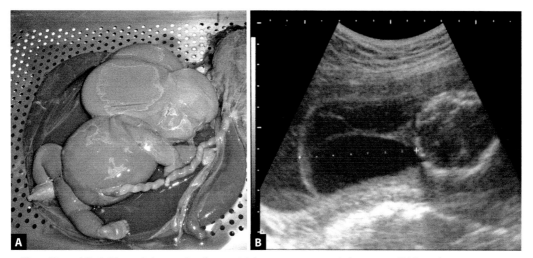

Figs. 4A and B: A 19 weeks' gestation fetus with large septate cystic hygroma. (A) Postabortum aspect; (B) Ultrasound view of the hygroma.

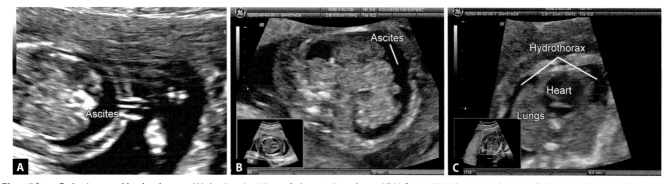

Figs. 5A to C: Ascites and hydrothorax. (A) Ascites in 15 weeks' gestational age (GA) fetus; (B) Ultrasound view of 22 weeks' fetus with ascites, notice the bowels surrounded by fluid; (C) The same case showing hydrothorax.

There is also a "sonographic syndrome" in triploidy second trimester ultrasound findings.[21,22] However, triploidy is rare in the second trimester. Besides the very high in utero mortality, the first trimester diagnosis of digynic triploidy is straightforward, based on the combination of low hormones serum levels and the characteristic appearance of the early asymmetric fetal growth restriction **(Fig. 10)**. In the second trimester, triploidy associates minor facial anomalies, facial asymmetry, low set ears, mild ventriculomegaly, multiple major structural defects of the internal organs, intrauterine growth restriction (IUGR) (asymmetric most frequently) and syndactyly (of third and fourth fingers, most frequently). Other possible ultrasound findings in triploidy are: hypertelorism and microphthalmos, micrognathia,

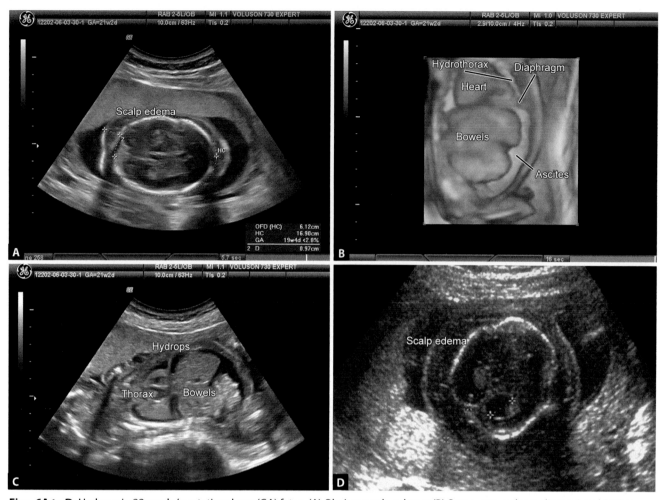

Figs. 6A to D: Hydrops in 22 weeks' gestational age (GA) fetus. (A) Obvious scalp edema; (B) Same case, a three-dimensional (3D) image showing fluid in all abdomen and thorax; (C) Same case, 2D sonography; (D) Another case, hydrops with scalp edema.

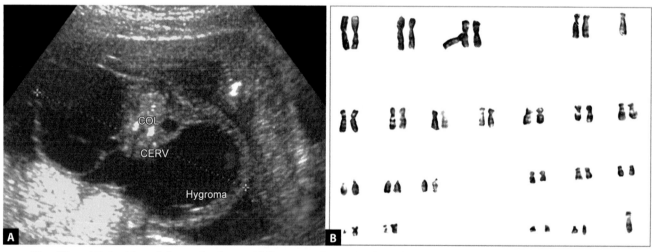

Figs. 7A and B: An 18 weeks' gestation fetus with Turner syndrome. (A) Cystic hygroma at the level of the fetal cervical spine (col. cerv. - cervical spine); (B) Turner karyotype of the case.

major facial anomalies (cleft), agenesis of corpus callosum, cardiac malformations, septal defects, single umbilical artery, omphalocele, renal anomalies **(Figs. 11 and 12 and Table 2)**.

Jauniaux et al. investigated the role of ultrasonography and maternal serum hCG in the early prenatal diagnosis of triploid pregnancies. Overall, there were 18 cases of triploidy

identified in a population of 58,862 singleton pregnancies, giving a prevalence of 1 in 3,270. Fetal defects were observed in 8 (44.4%) of these cases; these included holoprosencephaly (n = 4), exomphalos (n = 3), and posterior fossa cyst (n = 1). In six (33.3%) cases, the placenta showed molar changes. The fetal crown-rump length was below the 5th percentile

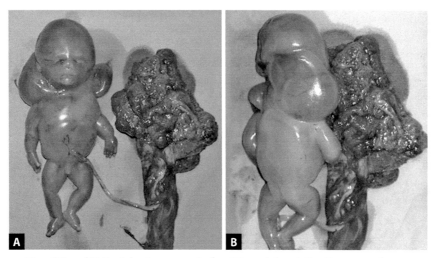

Figs. 8A and B: Postabortum aspect of an 18 weeks' gestation Turner syndrome.

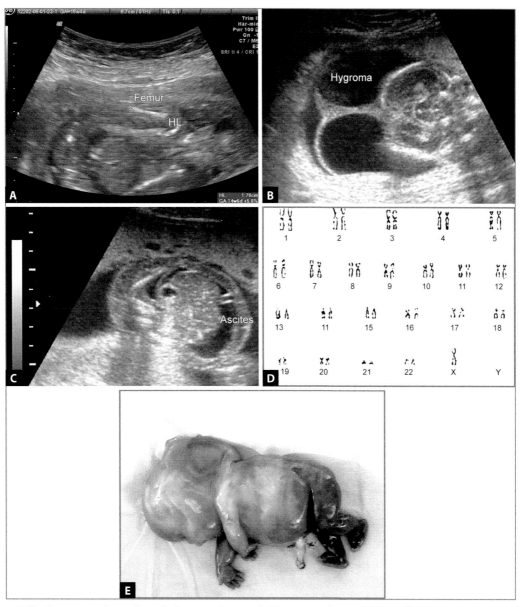

Figs. 9A to E: The "sonographic syndrome" of a case of 17 weeks' Turner syndrome. (A) Short femur (<5%); (B) Cystic hygroma; (C) Ascites; (D) Karyotype; (E) Postabortum aspect.

in 10 of the 16 (62.5%) cases for which the menstrual age was also available. Fetal nuchal translucency thickness was above the 95th percentile in 12 (66.7%) cases, and the fetal heart rate was below the 5th percentile in 4 of the 13 (30.8%) cases evaluated. The maternal hCG level was high in 11 of the 13 (84.6%) cases tested, with similar distribution of the high values in molar and nonmolar triploidies. As a conclusion, the combination of ultrasonographic examination of the fetoplacental features and measurement of the maternal serum level of hCG enables the diagnosis of most cases of triploidy at 10–14 weeks' gestation.[23]

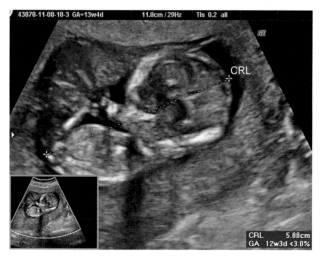

Fig. 10: Typical appearance of digynic triploidy at 13 weeks' gestational age (GA). (CRL: crown-rump length)

Specific Prenatal Diagnosis of the Turner Syndrome and Perspectives for the Direct Noninvasive Prenatal Diagnosis of the Chromosomal Defects

Positive diagnosis of monosomy X is established by determining the karyotype of the fetal cells obtained through *amniocentesis or chorial biopsy*, invasive procedures practiced in high-risk pregnancies (combined screening methods described above help that this risk to be better defined). The risk for miscarriage is 0.5% for amniocentesis in general, 5% for early amniocentesis and 0.5–2% for chorial biopsy.

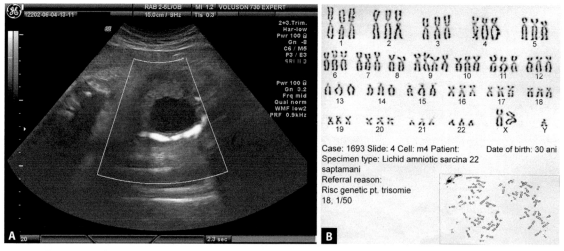

Figs. 11A and B: A case of triploidy at 22 weeks' gestation. (A) Typical aspect of a single umbilical artery; (B) Karyotype 69 XXY.

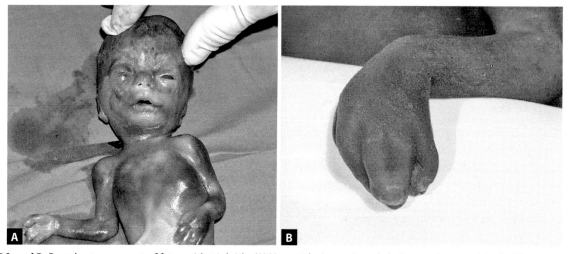

Figs. 12A and B: Postabortum aspect of fetus with triploidy. (A) Hypertelorism, microphthalmos, micrognathia, facial asymmetry, and low set ears; (B) Syndactyly of third and fourth fingers at the left upper limb.

TABLE 2: Ultrasound findings in triploidy.

	Jauniaux 1996	Rijhisingai 1997	Mittal 1998	De Vigan 2001	Combined data
No. of fetuses	70	17	20	4444	151
Increased NT/hygroma	11%	0	5%	7%	9%
Holoprosencephaly	3%	0	0	4%	3%
Ventriculomegaly	34%	23%	25%	21%	23%
Facial cleft	1%	0	0	2%	1%
Micrognathia	24%				24%
Abnormal limbs	49%		5%		38%
Abdominal wall defect	6%	12%	0	4%	5%
Central nervous system abnormality	29%	41%	45%	30%	35%
Cardiac defect	31%	6%	5%	11%	20%
Intrauterine growth restriction		71%	55%	32%	44%
Urinary tract anomaly	11%	23%	15%	7%	13%
Myelomeningocele	7%		25%		9%
Oligohydramnios	44%	59%	60%		50%
Posterior fossa anomaly	7%	12%	0		7%
>1 anomaly	100%	94%	85%	79%	92%

Source: Adapted from reference 23.

Of note, in the case of Turner syndrome, the karyotype of the cells obtained through chorial biopsy in the trimester I may be differentiated from those of the cells obtained through amniocentesis in the trimester II (real placental genetic mosaicism).

The risk involved by the invasive procedures practiced for positive diagnosis of the fetal chromosomal defects determined the search for noninvasive methods for the fetal genetic diagnosis.

Deoxyribonucleic acid (DNA) analysis of the fetal cells from maternal blood might be theoretically performed through fluorescent in situ hybridization (FISH); it is necessary to concentrate the fetal cells from maternal blood from 10^{-5} in average to at least 10^{-2}, which can be experimentally done but could not be implemented into clinical practice.

Instead, analysis of the free fetal DNA from the maternal blood to assess the risk for common aneuploidies has been available for clinical use for several years.[24] At present, the test is validated to use for trisomies 21, 18, and 13; its use for sex chromosome anomalies, including Turner syndrome, is debatable.[24]

DISCUSSION

The importance of a correct confirmed diagnosis for any child, in particular, for a family faced with a "dysmorphic" baby and planning to have further children cannot be overemphasized. Prenatal counseling and management are simplified if the genetic diagnosis is a lethal chromosomal anomaly. Triploidy is a lethal genetic condition with low risk of recurrence. Pregnancies with Turner fetus are characterized by a very high rate of in utero fetal mortality and of spontaneous abortion; >99% of the pregnancies with embryos with 45X0 karyotype have such fatal outcome. In such fetuses, defects of the lymphatic circulation in the early period and, when the gestational age allows studying the fetal morphology—cardiovascular, renal, or complex malformations are seen. Almost all fetuses diagnosed in utero with Turner syndrome have septated cystic hygroma and develop hydrops, but not all fetuses with cystic hygroma and hydrops are Turner. Occasionally, the prenatal diagnosis of a Turner karyotype is made in a fetus with no major structural anomalies; the counseling and management are challenging in such cases, as the postnatal phenotype is difficult to predict under the circumstances.

As a conclusion both triploidy and Turner syndrome must be taken into consideration if sonography reveals minor or major abnormalities in first or second trimester of pregnancy. Active screening in the general population is not justified for these conditions alone. Prenatal management of nonlethal sex chromosome anomalies, including nonlethal Turner syndrome, is challenging. Prenatal diagnosis of nonlethal Turner syndrome cases is likely to increase with the expanding use of the free fetal DNA from maternal blood analysis.[25]

REFERENCES

1. Jones KL. Triploidy syndrome and diploid/triploid mixoploidy syndrome. In: Smith's Recognizable Patterns of Human Malformation, 4th edition. Philadelphia: WB Saunders; 1988. pp. 32-3.

2. Hook EB, Warburton D. The distribution of chromosome genotypes associated with Turner's syndrome. Hum Genet. 1993;64:24-7.

3. Nielsen J, Wohlert M. Chromosome abnormalities found among 34,910 newborn children: results of a 13-year study in Denmark. Hum Genet. 1991;87:81-3.

4. Leisti JT, Raivio KO, Rapola MH, Saksela EJ, Aula PP. The phenotype of human triploidy. Birth Defects Orig Artic Ser. 1974;10:248-53.

5. Malone FD, Ball RH, Comstock CH, Saade GR, Berkowitz RL, Gross SJ, et al. First-trimester septated cystic hygroma: prevalence, natural history, and pediatric outcome. Obstet Gynecol. 2005;106(2):288-94.

6. Lacro RV, Jones KL, Benirschke K. Coarctation of aorta in Turner syndrome: a pathologic study of fetuses with nuchal cystic hygromas, hydrops fetalis and female genitalia. Pediatrics. 1988;81:445-51.

7. Hyett JA, Brizot ML, McKie AT. Cardiac gene expression of atrial natriuretic peptide and brain natriuretic peptide in trisomic fetuses. Obstet Gynecol. 1996;87:506-10.

8. Binder G, Koch A, Wajs E, Ranke MB. Nested polymerase chain reaction study of 53 cases with Turner syndrome. Clin Endocrinol Metab. 1995;80:3532-6.

9. Lorda-Sanchez I, Binkert F, Maechler M. Molecular study of 45X conceptuses: correlation with clinical findings. Am J Med Genet. 1992;42:487-90.

10. Ogata T, Matsuo N. Turner syndrome and female sex chromosome aberrations: deduction of the principal factors involved in the develpment of clinical features. Hum Genet. 1995;95:607-29.

11. Zinn AR. Growing interest in Turner syndrome. Nat Genet. 1997;16:3-4.

12. Spencer K, Liao AW, Skentou H, et al. Screening for triploidy by fetal nuchal translucency and maternal serum free beta-hCG and PAPP-A at 10-14 weeks of gestation. Prenat Diagn. 2000;20(6):495-9.

13. Sebire NJ, Snijders R, Brown R. Detection of sex chromosome abnormalities by nuchal translucency screenig at 10-14 weeks. Prenat Diagn. 1998;18:581-4.

14. Pandya PP, Kondylios A, Hilbert L, Snijders RJ, Nicolaides KH. Chromosomal defects and outcome in 1015 fetuses with increased nuchal translucency. Ultrasound Obstet Gynecol. 1995;5(1):15-9.

15. Falcon O, Wegrzyn P, Faro C, Peralta CF, Nicolaides KH. Gestational sac volume measured by three-dimensional ultrasound at 11 to 13 + 6 weeks of gestation: relation to chromosomal defects. Ultrasound Obstet Gynecol. 2005;25(6):546-50.

16. Van Vugt JMG, Van Zalen RM, Kostense PJ. First trimester nuchal translucency: a risk analysis on fetal abormality. Radiology. 1996;200:537-40.

17. Nadel A, Bromley B, Benacerraf BR. Nuchal thickening or cystic hygromas in first and early second trimester fetuses: prognosis and outcome. Obstet Gynecol. 1993;82:43-8.

18. Schemmer G, Wapner RJ, Johnson A. First-trimester growth patterns of aneuploid fetuses. Prenat Diagn. 1997;17(2):155-9.

19. Bronshtein M, Zimmer EZ, Blazer S. A characteristic cluster of fetal sonographic markers that are predictive of fetal Turner syndrome in early pregnancy. Am J Obstet Gynecol. 2003;188(4):1016-20.

20. Azar G, Snijders RJ, Gosden C, Nicolaides KH. Fetal nuchal cystic hygromata: associated malformations and chromosomal defects. Fetal Diagn Ther. 1991;6:46-57.

21. Jauniaux E, Brown R, Snijders RJ, Noble P, Nicolaides KH. Early prenatal diagnosis of triploidy. Am J Obstet Gynecol. 1997;176(3):550-4.

22. Goldberg JD, Norton ME. Genetics and Prenatal Diagnosis. In: Callen PW (Ed). Ultrasonography in Obstetrics and Gynecology, 4th edition. Philadelphia, PA: Saunders; 2000. pp. 18-38.

23. Nyberg DA, Souter VL. Chromosal abnormalities. In: Nyberg DA, McGahan JP, Pretorius DH, Pilu G (Eds). Diagnostic Imaging of Fetal Anomalies, Philadelphia, PA: Lippincott Williams & Wilkins; 2003. p. 869.

24. Gil MM, Accurti V, Santacruz B, Plana MN, Nicolaides KH. Analysis of cell-free DNA in maternal blood in screening for aneuploidies: updated meta-analysis. Ultrasound Obstet Gynecol. 2017;50(3):302-14.

25. Norton ME, Kuppermann M. Women should decide which conditions matter. Am J Obstet Gynecol. 2016;215(5):583-7.e1.

Bioethical Standards of Ultrasonographic and Invasive Prenatal Diagnosis: Practical Aspects*

Jose Maria Carrera, Bernat Serra Zantop

INTRODUCTION

In the last 30 years, a great deal of new knowledge has been acquired alongside the implementation of new technologies in the field of embryos/fetuses, geared toward developing methods for carrying out a "prenatal diagnosis" (PD) of most congenital defects (CDs) affecting embryos/fetuses.

According to various research groups working under the auspices of the World Health Organization (WHO), PD refers to "any prenatal method aimed at detecting and/or diagnosing a CD, i.e., any anomaly present at birth (although it may appear later) in relation to the morphological, structural, functional, or molecular development, which can be external or internal, steady or sporadic, hereditary or otherwise, and unique or multiple". Therefore, chromosomal impairments and malformations fall within the scope of PD, as well as any other type of disorder affecting fetal development and functionality.

In practice, a distinction should be made between "suspicion", "detection", and "diagnosis". While the first term only refers to the presence of indirect and presumptive signs of fetal impairments, detection is related to the fact of locating (by ultrasound, biochemistry, etc.) a specific impairment, and diagnosis to that of effectively identifying a determined CD.

The incidence of CD at birth ranges between 3 and 5% of newborns; 20% of all CDs are caused by a chromosomal impairment (typically trisomy), 25% are of a genetic origin, while the remaining part is attributable to the environment or has a multifactorial cause. In broad terms, in most cases where a diagnosis is recommended (the couple is ethically and legally entitled to request a diagnosis), the outcome is negative, that is to say that the fetus does not present with any diagnosable disorder.

We now have the technology at our disposal to detect and diagnose most CDs. However, even though the diagnostic ability usually stands at 100% in a range of areas, it is sometimes much more limited. From a strictly ethical point of view, such methods can be accompanied by a series of difficulties arising from the current disproportion that exists between diagnostic capacity and the actual therapeutic possibilities (insufficient at present).

This chapter concerned the ultrasonographic techniques and the *invasive tests* intended for detecting the CDs of the fetus.

In practice, these risks must be balanced against the extent of the risk subject to diagnosis and its incidence in the population under study. As a result, efforts have been made in the past few years to carry out a customized evaluation of both risks (of the test and of the possibility of detecting a defect).

Several issues account for the reason why so many ethical, social, and legal conflicts have erupted in this area, such as the complexity of the issue at stake (there are thousands of different CDs), the degree of sophistication of the technology required (which involves heavy investments by hospitals), the need to be a specialist in PD (which not all gynecologists are), the social exclusion of people suffering from a deficiency and, above all, the ideological background underlying the decision-making process.

LEGAL ISSUES

Based on the premise that any invasive PD is a "medical act", it may only be legally permitted provided that it complies with the three basic requirements described here:

1. The physician who carries out the test must *hold the appropriate qualification.*

---

*This report has been drawn up according to the recommendations of "Bioethical aspects of invasive techniques for prenatal diagnosis", which was drafted by a bioethical committee of the Spanish Society of Obstetrics and Gynecology. The author of this report piloted the redaction of those recommendations.

2. *Appropriate professional skills.* The specialist in obstetrics or gynecology must also have undergone sufficient training for carrying out such tests, which involve a degree of risk to the mother and to the fetus that lies within the normal range of risk as reported statistically.

3. *Consent of the patient.* It is a fact that the notion of "informed consent" should not solely be regarded as an ethical requirement, but also as a legal requisite.

In some countries, ultrasonographic examination may be performed (either in whole or in part) by nonmedical staff. However, the specialized sonographer responsible for the examination has to issue a diagnosis, which he/she must also sign.

■ GENERAL ETHICAL PRINCIPLES

There is a general consensus over the following principles:

- All pregnant women (and their partners) are entitled to have access to objective information about the CD risk and the possibilities of PD.
- The information about current PD methods must include the indications related to such methods, as well as any specific risks and alternative options available.
- The physician should not attempt to impose his own views on patients; on the contrary, he should inform them of any existing aspect and option.
- All PD methods should be carried out according to *lex artis* (sufficient experience, appropriate technology, and suitable environment). In any other case, the patient should be referred to another level of care where the requirements are met.
- The results of the explorations must be kept secret, and access to such results must be restricted.
- The physician's task does not end once diagnosis has been completed or, where appropriate, following termination of pregnancy. In fact, the physician must endeavor at all times to provide relevant genetic counseling to the couple to help them deciding between the options available.
- The physician must abide by any decision that the couple may take within the framework of the legislation in force at the time.
- The ethical dilemmas normally arise at five different stages which are all linked to PD, namely: (1) Upon disclosing the *information,* (2) Upon communicating the *indication,* (3) Upon *carrying out the indication,* (4) Upon *communicating the diagnosis* and finally, (5) Upon any *subsequent decision making.*

We will now set out to analyze the accepted practice, inappropriate practice, and recommendations in view of such potentially conflictive situations with regard to each of the stages mentioned above.

■ INFORMATION

Accepted Practice

- All preconception and pregnancy consultations should include information about the individual risks to the couple (or to each member of the couple) regarding the risk of conceiving a child with CD, as well as the existing means of prevention and the possibilities of PD.
- As a rule, the information given should be adapted to the age and the personal and family history of the couple.
- The preconception risk is chiefly assessed according to the age of the couple, their personal history (such as the fact of having another child affected by CD, balanced translocation in parents, etc.), their family history (affected first-degree relatives), and their environment.
- The risk during pregnancy should be calculated (risk index) according to the above factors and, specially for the most frequent trisomies (21, 18, and 13), to the results of the *screening* tests, especially the *biochemical screening* and *ultrasound screening* (nuchal sonolucency and other ultrasonographic signs).
- It should be stressed that the definitive diagnosis regarding the presence or absence of chromosomal disorders in the fetus is carried out by means of an invasive test designed to determine its karyotype, chromosomal microarray, or even exome or genome.
- Therefore, the information should include a list of the various methods available in terms of detection (anamnesis, biochemical, and ultrasound *screening*) and PD (invasive tests), together with a detailed explanation of what method is advisable in each particular case.

In any case, the content of the information should be clear, comprehensive, easily understandable, and consistent with the patient's personal characteristics (idiosyncrasy, culture, etc.).

Inappropriate Practice

The following should be avoided:

- Failing to inform the patient about CD risks and of the PD tests available for detecting such risks/conditions, whether on ideological grounds (such as for religious reasons, etc.) or simply because of professional negligence.
- Providing biased information (such as underestimating CD risks or overestimating the risks linked to the tests).
- Providing partial or incomplete information on the actual possibilities of each test (what does it do and what does it not do).

Recommendations with Regard to Potentially Conflictive Situations

If the couple expressly states their refusal to resort to PD methods, the physician must respect their choice, provided that he has previously made sure that it is based on a free and informed decision. This, however, should not stop the physician from requesting the patients to sign a "nonconsent" statement.

- Any medical information about the genetic disease of a patient is absolutely confidential and cannot be disclosed to any member of the family without the patient's explicit consent. However, the physician should advise the affected couple to inform those members of the family that play a crucial role in ensuring that the PD is carried out appropriately.

■ INDICATIONS

Accepted Practice

The fact of indicating a particular test (for *detection* and/or *diagnosis* purposes) depends basically on the age and on the history of the pregnant patient.

- Both the number and the chronology of the ultrasonographic examinations to be performed are determined to the indication and outcome of each case. For ethical reasons, a policy of excessive number of examinations should be avoided. In general, the protocols and/or recommendations of the scientific societies must be complied with.
- If the pregnant patient is a *low anamnesis risk* individual for chromosomal defects, combined biochemical and/or ultrasonographic screening for evaluating the *risk index* is recommended.
- If the pregnant patient is considered a high-risk individual, by means of a previous screening procedure or by being either parent a carrier of an alteration that can be transmitted to the offspring, an invasive test will be indicated. The choice of a specific method (amniocentesis or chorionic villus sampling) is made on the basis of the indication, the gestational age at which the decision is taken, and the experience of the physician.

Inappropriate Practice

- Indicating a method (ultrasonography, invasive test, etc.) which is not the most suitable due to personal limitations (little experience, if any) or to the resources of the medical facilities (single-member private medical care, low standards, etc.).
- Indicating invasive tests without any specific indication (unethical policy regarding indications). The reasons for this are multiple: they may be related to economic motives (especially in the private medical sector), incomplete information given to the patient (inappropriate balance of risks/benefits), erroneous indications (such as an indication due to teratogens), or a masked study, etc.
- Failing to recommend invasive tests in cases where they should be indicated. The *threshold point* should

not be modified on the sole grounds of the physician's opinions (in which case inaccurate information would be provided).

- Unduly delaying (negligence, ideological convictions, etc.) the diagnosis until the legal time limit for abortion has been reached, thus increasing the level of risks in connection with late abortion.

Recommendations with Regard to Potentially Conflictive Situations

- The indication of *maternal anxiety* will only apply where, after providing accurate information to the patient, the state of anxiety persists. If the anxiety suffered is severe, the intervention of a specialist might be required.
- As a rule, PD invasive tests should not be carried out unless strictly medical indications are made to that effect. Except in the case of genital diseases, any request for such a test, which is aimed at knowing the sex of the fetus, should be rejected, especially if there is a strong suspicion that the patient might request an abortion depending on the results of the tests. Choosing the sex of a fetus infringes the principle of equality between genders.
- Only in exceptional cases (judiciary order, severe pathological situations, etc.) will a request for a prenatal paternity test be satisfied.
- If a test is required as a result of a correct medical indication, it must be carried out even if the couple states that they will only use the results for information purposes, and that under no circumstances will they decide to terminate the pregnancy. The couple is entitled to be informed of their situation, regardless of what decision they make afterward.

■ IMPLEMENTATION (PERFORMING THE TESTS)

Accepted Practice

- The operator (sonographer or sonographist) should be sufficiently qualified and experienced to obtain as much information as possible from the ultrasonographic examination. The technique must be performed with an appropriate level of care. The standards of ultrasonographic safety must be observed in all cases.
- The ultrasonographic examination must be carried out in an appropriate environment (with privacy, peace of mind, reduced family pressure, etc.). Under the supervision of a suitable technical team and appropriate method. The overall structure of the care center should provide the necessary time and resources while respecting the dignity of patients all times.
- Invasive PD, given the specific risks it involves, can only be carried out by skilled professionals working within a suitable technological infrastructure and medical

environment. In fact, most hospitals have a prenatal diagnosis section or unit.

- The decision to use a particular method must be made on the basis of the objective characteristics of each case and not solely on the basis of the technical experience of the physician. A series of semiobjective criteria (number of tests carried out, etc.) are now available for assessing the physician's experience.
- If the physician does not have the required experience and/or if the appropriate technology is not available, the patient should be referred to a prenatal diagnosis centre with proven experience. Such a referral should be decided on the basis of health considerations, and not on economic grounds.
- Before carrying out the test, the physician should have a conversation with the couple to assure that they know the reason for performing the test, the possible risks involved, and the precautions that should be taken.
- Complying with the appropriate procedure in terms of *informed consent*.
- The professional who performs the invasive procedure must ensure adequate identification of the sample obtained and must clearly state in the request to the laboratory that will process the sample the reason for the study and the test(s) that are requested.

Inappropriate Practice

The following should be avoided:
- Carrying out the test without the necessary experience, as this could increase the level of risk.
- Carrying out the test in a negligent manner or with little diligence (incomplete asepsis, etc.).
- Failing to take the steps required to ensure the safety and confidentiality of the testing and of the ensuing results (promiscuity between patients, verbal information given in public, mistakes, interchanging results, backing up the information in an inappropriate way, etc.).

Recommendations with Regard to Potentially Conflictive Situations

- It is absolutely right for a care center to carry out invasive PD even when it cannot provide patients with legal abortion facilities afterward (such as religious hospitals or hospitals whose practitioners have declared their conscientious objection to abortion), provided that such a restriction has been previously notified to the couple.
- Invasive PD must only be performed in those hospitals, whether public or private, that have the appropriate equipment to ensure maximum safety for the patient and the fetus. Accordingly, the staff must be trained to carry out the tests and resolve any problem that may arise in the process.

■ COMMUNICATING THE DIAGNOSIS

Accepted Practice

- In addition to being duly notified in writing, the diagnosis (normal and pathological) must be communicated verbally to the patient, in person, by a member of the medical staff.
- It is desirable that the person responsible for informing the patient of the diagnosis be the obstetrician in charge of the case, since the latter knows all the aspects of the case, including the idiosyncrasy of the patients. Therefore, the practitioner should be adequately trained in this area of specialism and, if this is not the case, he should seek the assistance of the specialist most skilled in this field.
- The information should be communicated in a way that can be easily understood by the couple, particularly in the case of a pathological diagnosis. In other words, the information should take their personal circumstances into account whilst being explained in plain language.
- In some cases, the prognosis and the options available should not be confirmed until all necessary additional screenings have been carried out.
- Where necessary, special psychological or psychiatric support should be provided, including social services assistance in some cases, in addition to the assistance and emotional support given by the attending physician.
- In any case, the focus should be on ensuring that the patients are treated by the same member of staff throughout their stay in hospital (to avoid mistakes and any possible disagreement), while allowing them to have a second opinion (from a list of physicians or centers).

Inappropriate Practice

The following should be avoided:
- Untimely communication of the diagnosis by unqualified staff, or by members of staff who do not know the particulars of the case in question
- Communicating the information via third parties or by any other indirect means, thereby increasing the chances of a misunderstanding while jeopardizing the confidentiality of the diagnosis
- Communicating the diagnosis with too much haste, without previously analyzing and examining the case (delicate situations), a situation which is likely to give rise to errors in terms of diagnosis
- Failing to provide the appropriate psychological support, thus increasing the chance of *chronic grief*.

Recommendations with Regard to Potentially Conflictive Situations

- Wherever possible, it is recommended that the specialist (sonologist, geneticist, etc.) avoid making any additional diagnosis-related decision (such as carrying out an invasive test following the suspicion of aneuploidy upon ultrasound examination) and/or any therapeutic decision without the opinion and approval of the treating obstetrician. Such decision-making is only possible in cases where, in view of the hospital structure and of the urgency of the case, there is a need to avoid excessive waste of time.

- It is desirable that the obstetrician in charge of the patient's care be informed as soon as possible of any pathological diagnosis, so that he can inform the patient of the results, in person and in due time. However, if this is not possible (due to the structure of the hospital, the pressure exerted by the patient, etc.), it is perfectly right for the geneticist or the specialist physician to provide such information to the patient.
- The results of the PD must be treated as confidential, just like the rest of the hospital records. Furthermore, each care center and practitioner must take any step necessary to restrict access to this information to the authorized staff only.

■ DECISION-MAKING FOLLOWING DIAGNOSIS

Accepted Practice

- Before issuing any diagnosis and suggesting alternative options to the couple with a view to helping them make their decision, all the different possibilities available for reaching a consistent diagnosis and for identifying the strategy to be followed must be explored.
- The case must be examined by all the specialists involved (geneticist, sonologist, obstetrician, neonatologist, etc.), where possible, within the framework of a *Hospital Committee of Congenital Defects.* The aim is to examine the results of the tests carried out while evaluating the risks and advantages of any decision and option.
- It is needless to say that the information provided to the couple regarding the issues mentioned above must be easily understandable, clear, complete, and suited to their personal circumstances. This information is designed to help the couple decide freely and in accordance with their needs and beliefs.
- The information will be provided within the scope of the *genetic advice,* or of the *reproductive health advice* and, as such, must include relevant information about the reproductive health outlook for the couple (possibilities and options). The couple should be reminded of the need to carry out a necropsy study in case of fetal death or legal abortion to confirm the PD and follow-up the case in an appropriate manner.
- After explaining the diagnosis, prognosis and available options, the physician must, within the limits of the

law, fully respect the decisions made by the patient (or the couple). If the hospital or its practitioners have duly stated their conscientious objection, the case must be referred to another hospital or practitioner who has not declared any conscientious objection. In all cases, the patients should be able to seek a second opinion.

- The psychological assistance provided to patients should be aimed at supporting their final decision.

Inappropriate Practice

The following should be avoided:

- Unduly delaying the decision as to whether to terminate pregnancy, thereby giving rise to an increase in the risk of complications, given that late abortion (in particular, illegal abortion) is more dangerous
- Giving one-sided advice that pinpoints one single option (legal abortion), without discussing any other alternatives with the couple
- Causing the patient to opt for termination on the basis of mere conjecture (absence of any relevant prenatal study) or for trivial reasons (such as an alleged exposure to teratogens)
- Failing to recommend legal termination in cases of severe fetal pathology, while underestimating the problems caused to the child in the future
- Providing inaccurate or negligent information regarding the outcome and prospects of the necropsy study and of the *reproductive health advice* (such as "the harm has already been done" or "there is nothing we can do to avoid it")
- Carrying out legal termination of pregnancy without taking the samples necessary for carrying out a subsequent study of the product (necropsy and cytogenetic study). Such practices will make it impossible to confirm the PD or provide adequate counseling to the couple.

Recommendations with Regard to Potentially Conflictive Situations

- The information provided regarding any possible options must not be based on the ideology and/or religious beliefs of the physician or indeed on those of the patient or couple. If the patient wishes to obtain information about specific religious criteria, she must be asked to request it from the relevant authorities (priests, etc.). Ultimately, it is the patient's sense of right and wrong that will determine any subsequent moral decision. Accordingly, the patient's principles should be respected at all times, and no attempt whatsoever should be made to manipulate the patient whether directly or indirectly.

3D and 4D Ultrasound for Congenital Fetal Anomalies

Sonal Panchal

■ INTRODUCTION

Invention of three-dimensional (3D) and four-dimensional (4D) ultrasound (US) has brought an immense revolution in fetal imaging. Three-dimensional US helps to see the fetus in perspective, appreciate depth, and thus allows better demonstration of limb and facial defects of the fetus that are diagnosed or suspected on two-dimensional (2D) US. Four-dimensional US is a real-time 3D. Speedy 3D reconstruction can produce real-time 3D images and this is 4D US. Four-dimensional US allows not only to demonstrate structural abnormalities but also allows to study abnormalities of movements that may be because of flexion or extension deformities of the limbs or even because of major neurological abnormalities. Apart from this because of better spatial resolution and multiplanar imaging, abnormalities of fetal internal organs and related anatomy are also better demonstrated.

Tips for volume ultrasound for second- and third-trimester fetus:

- Use convex volume probe.
- Use volume angle large enough to include the whole structure of interest.
- Acquisition can be done with multiplanar or render mode though it is better to acquire with optimally selected render mode preset.
- Using curved render line is often required for fetal volume imaging.
- Rendering for internal structures is done with surface texture, in combination with maximum or minimum transparent mode.
- Rendering for limbs and facial defects, is best done with surface smooth and gradient modes in combination or by HD live mode. Changing light direction does help in better demonstration of subtle abnormalities. Silhouette mode may be added as and when required especially for anechoic structures and bones. Fluid interface is absolutely essential for surface rendering.

- Inversion mode rendering or sonographic automated volume count (AVC) general may be used for assessment of fluid-filled structures/lesions (hydrocephalus, hydronephrosis, duodenal atresia, etc.).
  - However for better understanding of related anatomy, tomographic ultrasound imaging (TUI) with or without volume contrast imaging (VCI) is used.
  - For better understanding of anatomy align the sectional planes in anatomical identifiable orthogonal planes before interpretation.
  - Spatial temporal image correlation (STIC) is an excellent tool for assessment of fetal heart.
  - Generally "up–down" render direction is used but for STIC volumes and 3D power Doppler "front-back" render direction is used. However, render direction may be changed as per requirement.
  - VOCAL may be used for volume calculation of fetal organs or lesions (e.g., lung volume in diaphragmatic hernia, renal volume in dysplastic kidneys, etc.).
  - Angiomode or glass body mode is especially useful when vascular abnormalities are suspected.
  - Omniview is widely used for assessment of fetal spine, limbs, corpus callosum, etc.

■ 3D–4D US APPLICATIONS FOR CONGENITAL FETAL ANOMALIES

Systematic study of the fetus with 3D–4D US must always be preceded by a detailed and systematic assessment of the fetus by 2D US. A high-quality 2D US is absolutely essential for a high-class 3D US image.

Facial Abnormalities

Volume US is the only modality that actually allows to study the fetal face. Surface smooth in a combination with gradient light is the rendering mode to be used to demonstrate the fetal face. HD live is a better render mode **(Figs. 1A and B)**.

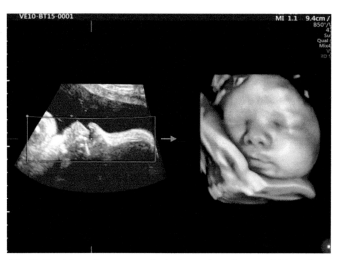

Fig. 2: Fetal front face on render is seen when the acquisition plane shows fetal face profile, when up–down render mode is selected.

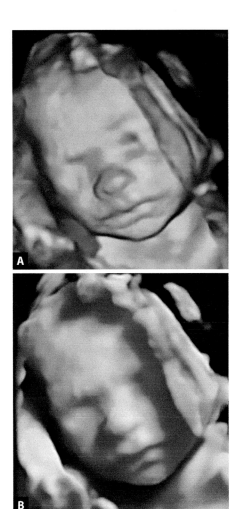

Figs. 1A and B: (A) Fetal face rendered in surface mode; (B) The same face as in (A) is rendered in HD live mode.

Scanning the face profile and using up–down viewing direction is the most common way of demonstrating the fetal face. Though the fetus actively moves in the second trimester, 4D instead of 3D is better used.

To get a proper position pressing mother's abdomen repeatedly, turning mother to one or another side, or reexamining after a few minutes would help when fetus is not in a favorable position to see the face. The absolute essential is fluid interface.

Best time to see the fetal face is between 23 and 30 weeks but proper fetal position is essential. In 90% of cases, correct and reproducible face images can be produced in second trimester. However, this reduces to only 30% after 34 weeks due to the obligatory position that the fetus has to attain with its growing size. Fetal limbs overlap on fetal face to accommodate its growing size in relatively small intrauterine space.

When volume of the face is acquired and rendered to demonstrate facial abnormalities suspected on 2D US, front of the face is required and in that case on 2D US a profile view of the fetus is required **(Fig. 2)**. But when fetal face is to be rendered photographic purpose only, whatever may be the position of the fetus seen on 2D US, face can be rendered, the only requirement is that there should be an adequate fluid interface **(Figs. 3A and B)**.

Three-dimensional US has an important role in diagnosis of facial cleft, micrognathia, nasal abnormalities, ear abnormalities, including low set ears, and eye abnormalities **(Figs. 4A and B)**. Merz et al. have reported well-defined facial images as early as ninth week of pregnancy **(Fig. 5)**.[1] Defects of the orbits like hypertelorism, hypotelorism, single orbit, microphthalmia, commonly a part of genetic syndromes, may be suspected by 2D US, but the confirmation and demonstration are not possible without the use of volume US.

Cleft lip is suspected on 2D US as a cut in the upper lip **(Figs. 6A and B)**. It may be central, unilateral, or bilateral. Surface rendering and HD live are the best modes to demonstrate the defect. Rotten and Levaillant have proved that 3D–4D is superior to 2D US for diagnosis of facial clefts.[2] Rendering for the palate can also be done with flipped face technique **(Fig. 7)**.[3] Three-dimensional US can also pick up isolated soft palate defects as shown in studies by Pilu et al.[4] Another technique to detect the cleft palate is the 3D "reverse face" view **(Figs. 8A and B)**.[5] After acquiring the face volume, the viewing direction is changed to back instead of front, to see the facial bones from inside the skull. Maxilla and palate can be reliably studied as early as 11 weeks.

Though cleft lip is very well demonstrated on surface rendering **(Fig. 9)**, cleft palate needs studying the multiplanar planes. Cleft palate can be diagnosed by TUI in axial plane, just caudal to the orbital plane **(Fig. 10)**.[6] TUI in coronal plane is also useful for demonstration of the connecting passage between the oral and nasal cavity in cleft palate **(Fig. 11)**. Diagnosis of cleft lip and palate is almost 100%, including the cleft of soft palate also.[2,4,7] Omniview with VCI is suggested by Benacerraf et al.[8] Omniview is used with three polylines **(Figs. 12A and B)**.

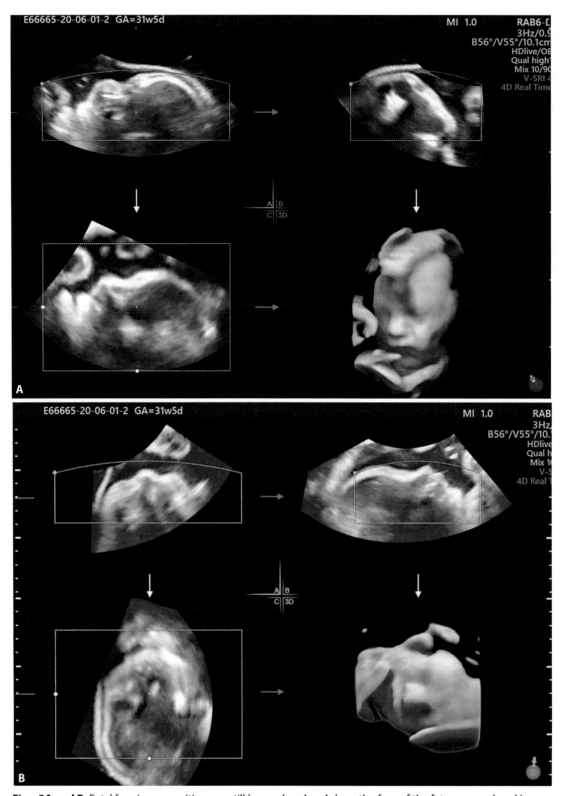

Figs. 3A and B: Fetal face in any position can still be rendered and show the face of the fetus on rendered image, though not the front of the face.

A rare condition where the cleft of the lip extends up to the medial angle of the eye **(Fig. 13)**, can be diagnosed by volume US only as it is not easy to document the facial extension on 2D US. Generalized information of the facial bony defects available on 3D multiplanar mode or TUI helps decide the surgical approach. Cleft lip with volume US is best diagnosed between 20 and 24 weeks.

Early diagnosis of median cleft syndrome is possible in which the frontal bones and nasal bones are largely separated with hypertelorism, flat nasal bridge, rudimentary nostrils,

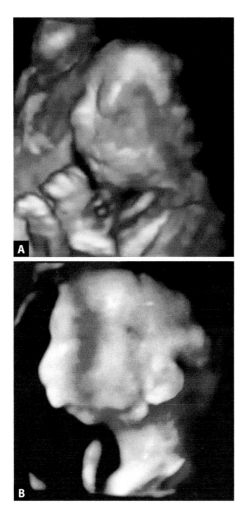

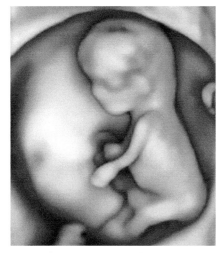

Figs. 4A and B: (A) Rendered image of fetal profile showing flat nasal bridge and micrognathia; (B) Rendered image of fetal profile showing micrognathia and low set ears.

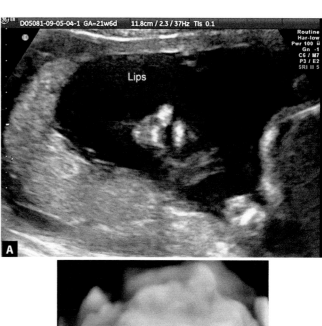

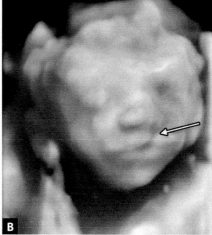

Figs. 6A and B: (A) B-mode ultrasound image of fetal lips in coronal plane with break in the upper lip shadow-cleft lip; (B) 3D ultrasound HD live rendered image of fetal face with cleft lip.

those without protuberant premaxillary segment. This protuberance is more evident in second trimester and may appear like a beak, and is more apparent than the cleft itself. Risk of chromosomal abnormalities is higher when there is a *cleft lip and palate* and higher when it is *bilateral or median* (15–30%).

Micrognathia/Retrognathia

Micrognathia is diffuse smallness of mandible whereas retrognathia is reduced anteroposterior (AP) extent of mandible. The two conditions may often coexist. But mandibular abnormalities often do not become evident till 24 weeks.

Three-dimensional US shows precise alignment of orthogonal planes in which accurate measurements can be made and allows creation of rendered casts of the mandibular bone. Micrognathia is diagnosed subjectively by rendered 3D image of fetal face **(Fig. 14)** on face profile or objectively by measurement of inferior facial angle[10] and jaw index: AP diameter of mandible/biparietal diameter (BPD) (<0.23 is micrognathia) **(Figs. 15A and B)**.[11,12]

Fig. 5: HD live rendered 3D ultrasound image of the 1st trimester fetus.

and other facial abnormalities.[9] Median clefts may also be associated with holoprosencephaly, nasal abnormalities, and other midline defects.

Bilateral cleft lip and palate can be further categorized as those having protuberant premaxillary segment and

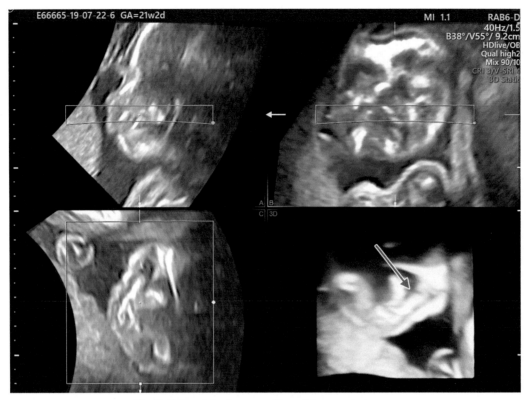

Fig. 7: Cleft palate shown on flipped face rendering.

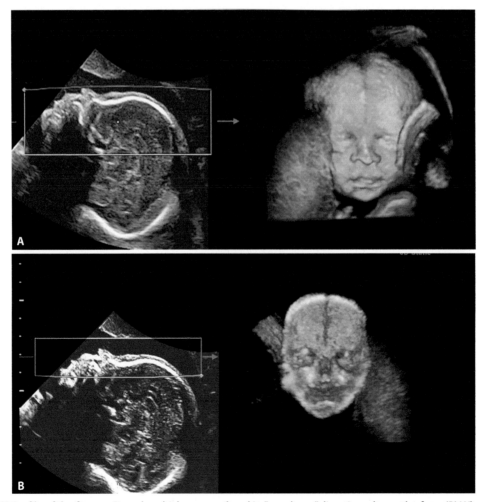

Figs. 8A and B: (A) Profile of the face on B mode, which was rendered in "up–down" direction, shows the face; (B) When render direction was reversed, it shows the bony face for the assessment of the cleft palate—reverse face view.

Micrognathia is known to be associated with trisomy 13 and 18. It is also a component of Treacher Collins syndrome, Neu–Laxova syndrome, Pena–Shokeir syndrome, and multiple pterygium syndrome.

Ear Abnormalities

Size, morphology, and placement of the ear are important for diagnosis of chromosomal abnormalities. 70% of trisomy 21 babies have helix-lobe lengths more than two standard deviation from mean. Detection of ear appendices may be a marker of renal malformation. Size and shape of the ear may sometimes be assessed on 2D US, but position of the ear can only be assessed by volume US **(Figs. 16A and B)**. Therefore

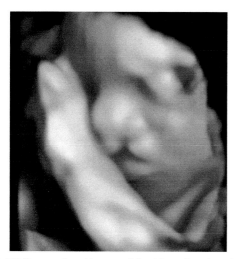

Fig. 9: HD live rendered image of fetal face showing cleft lip.

low placed ears, an important marker for trisomy 21 can only be demonstrated by volume US.

Abnormal profiles like frontal bossing can also be better demonstrated on volume US.

Nasal bone is usually seen on the mid-sagittal plane. But coronal plane-retronasal triangle view is also used to confirm both the nasal bones. Using 3D US with maximum mode rendering has been proved to be more reliable between 18 and 33 weeks of gestational age for diagnosis of absence or hypoplasia of the nasal bones **(Fig. 17)**.[13] If the gap between the two nasal bones is >0.6 mm, it indicates absent nasal bone at 12 weeks scan.

Flat nasal bridge, an important sign for aneuploidy, though can be diagnosed on B-mode US, it may be more easily understandable for the non-scan person by 3D US **(Fig. 18)**.

Orbital Abnormalities

Sepulveda et al. have documented diagnosis of congenital dacryocystocele by 3D US.[14] Though hypertelorism and hypotelorism are diagnosed on 2D US, on a transorbital axial plane, 3D US may make the demonstration of these lesions more understandable to a lay person. Same holds true for microphthalmia, anophthalmia, and congenital cataract.

Three-dimensional US also has a role in diagnosis of rare fetal tumors including palatal teratoma, epulis, hemangiomas of face and neck, epignathus, etc. It helps in assessment of the extension of the tumor and if at all involvement of the airway.

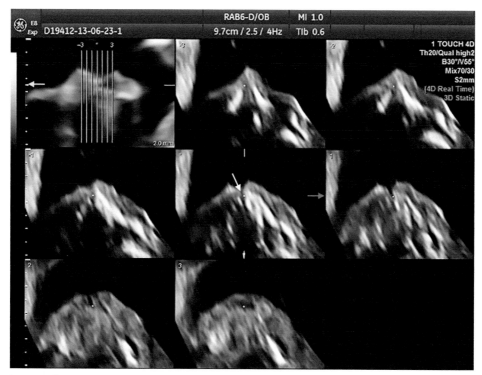

Fig. 10: The same fetus as in Figure 9, on axial plane tomographic ultrasound imaging, shows the cleft in the palate.

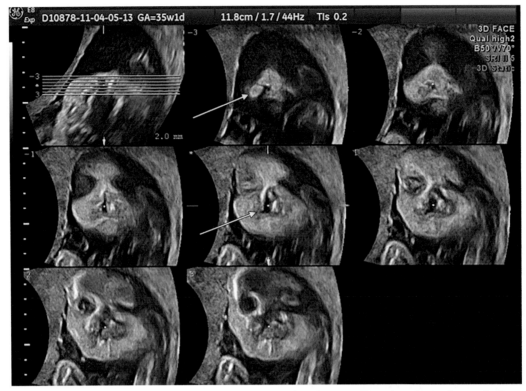

Fig. 11: The same fetus as in Figure 9, on coronal plane tomographic ultrasound imaging, shows the gap in the maxilla, the gap extending toward the nasal cavity.

Apart from the defects or anatomical variations, only volume US can show the fetal expressions that represent the fetal behavior and neurological development of the fetus.

The *expressions* recorded so far are:
- Yawning **(Fig. 19)**
- Smiling **(Fig. 20)**
- Swallowing
- Sucking
- Blinking **(Figs. 21A and B)**
- Grimacing **(Fig. 22)**
- Mouthing **(Fig. 23A)**
- Tongue expulsion **(Fig. 23B)**

Lot more about this is discussed in the chapter 8 of this book.

Cranial Abnormalities

Skull bones and sutures can be visualized by 3D US[15] **(Fig. 24)**, which is difficult with 2D US due to natural curve of the skull. Maximum transparency mode is used for this. Excessive diastases of the sutures can be seen in cranium bifidum occultum and premature closure can diagnose craniostenosis and microcephaly early.[16]

Volume US shows fontanelle very clearly **(Fig. 25)**. Paladini et al. have documented that the size of anterior fontanelle increases as gestational age increases but in relation to fetal head volume its size decreases with advancing gestational age. The anterior fontanelle is larger in trisomy 21.[17]

Features of fetal head dysmorphism like flattening or prominence of occipital bones or frontal bones, and altered facial angles—superior or inferior can be diagnosed by volume US on facial profile views. Small meningoceles that are easily overlooked by 2D US, would be clearly demonstrated by volume US **(Fig. 26)**.

Central Nervous System

In late second and third trimesters, if fetus is in cephalic presentation, transvaginal approach can be a better approach to study fetal brain. Placenta and thick skull bones may be obstructing the vision on transabdominal approach. Gentle pressure on the fetal head with steady hand while acquiring the volume of the head can avoid bone shadowing and help better visualization of the brain. When transvaginal route is used, the fontanelle which is open is used as acoustic window **(Fig. 27)**. Once the fetal brain volume is acquired, it is then possible to navigate in the stored volume. By multiplanar display, the brain anatomy can be studied in detail. Development of brain in second trimester has three developmental landmarks:
1. Development of lateral ventricle into frontal, occipital, and temporal horns
2. Development of corpus callosum
3. Development of cerebellum and its vermis.

Whenever any abnormality of the fetal brain is suspected on B-mode US due to simple signs like mild ventriculomegaly

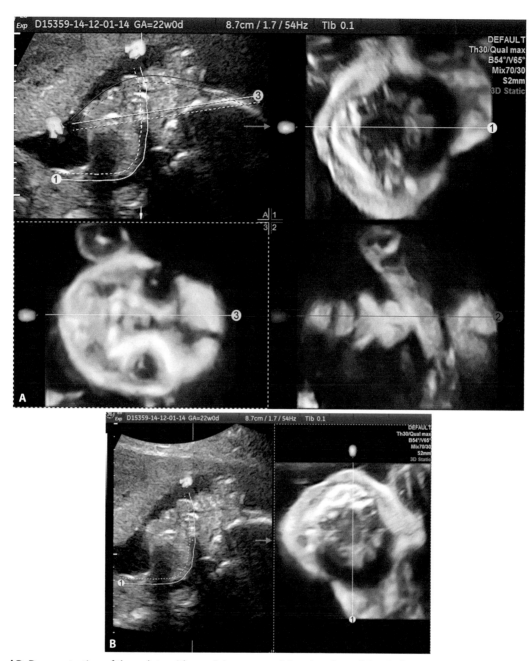

Figs. 12A and B: Demonstration of the palate with omniview on omniview 1 and omniview 3. Omniview 2 shows coronal plane of lips.

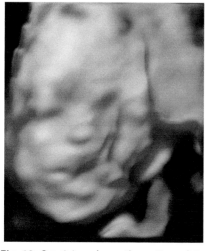

Fig. 13: Omniview shows the entire palate.

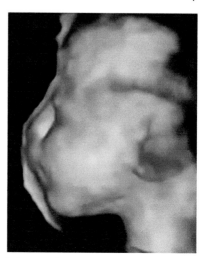

Fig. 14: HD live rendered image of fetal face with facial cleft extending to medial angle of the eye.

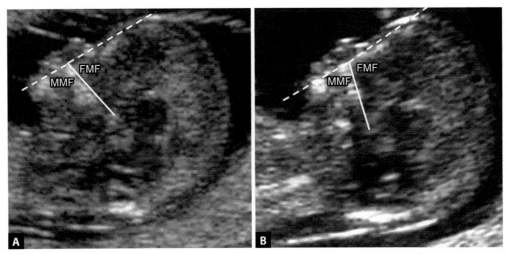

Figs. 15A and B: Mid-sagittal view of the fetal face demonstrating the measurement of the frontomaxillary facial (FMF) angle and the mandibulomaxillary facial (MMF) angle in (A) a chromosomally normal fetus; (B) A fetus with trisomy 18.

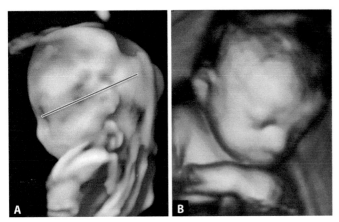

Figs. 16A and B: (A) Normal position of the ear on rendered image of fetal head; (B) Low placed ear on rendered image of fetal head.

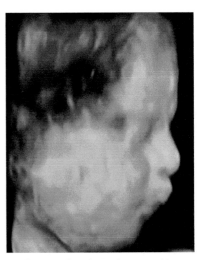

Fig. 18: Surface rendered 3D ultrasound image of fetal face in profile shows flat nasal bridge and retrognathia.

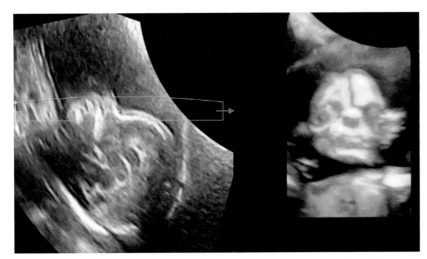

Fig. 17: Maximum mode of fetal face to show maxillary triangle and nasal bones.

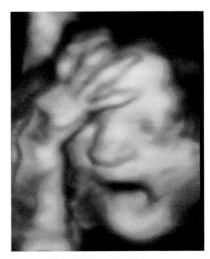

Fig. 19: Yawning fetus.

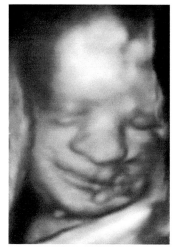

Fig. 20: Smiling fetus.

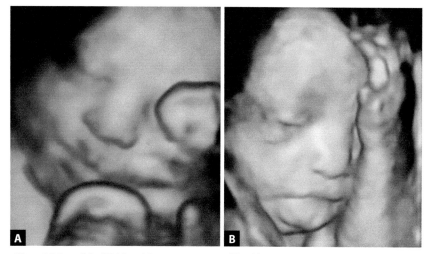

Figs. 23A and B: (A) Mouthing movement of fetal lips; (B) Fetus protruding tongue.

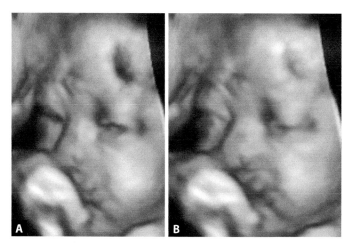

Figs. 21A and B: Opening and closing of eyes of the fetus.

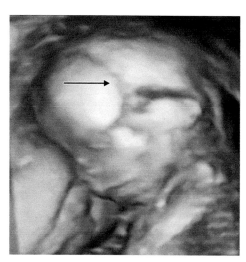

Fig. 24: Cranial sutures (arrow) seen on surface rendered 3D ultrasound image of fetal head.

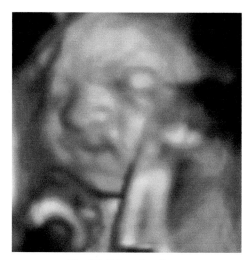

Fig. 22: Grimacing fetus.

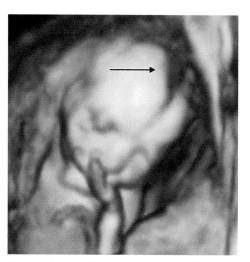

Fig. 25: Anterior fontanelle (arrow) seen on surface rendered 3D ultrasound image of fetal head.

to major abnormalities like hydrocephalus or midline shift, a detailed neurosonogram is required. Using TUI in all the three orthogonal planes, all the coronal, sagittal, and axial sections required for a detailed neurosonogram can be achieved by one single sweep of the fetal head. This consists of **(Figs. 28A to C)**:

- *Three axial planes*:
  1. Transventricular
  2. Transthalamic
  3. Transcerebellar

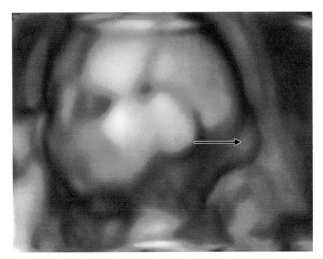

Fig. 26: Small occipital meningocele (arrow) seen on surface rendered 3D ultrasound image of fetal head.

- *Four coronal planes*:
  1. Transfrontal plane (frontal 2 plane)
  2. Transcaudate plane (midcoronal 1 plane)
  3. Transthalamic plane (midcoronal 2 plane)
  4. Transcerebellar plane (occipital 1 and 2 plane)
- *Three sagittal planes*:
  1. Mid-sagittal
  2. Two parasagittal sections

VOCAL may be used for volume calculation of dilated ventricles and intracranial lesions. Volume contrast imaging in coronal plane depicts the midline structures like corpus callosum, brain stem, cerebellar vermis, and optic chiasma.

Agenesis of corpus callosum and cerebellar vermian hypoplasias—Dandy–Walker syndrome can be demonstrated using VCI C in axial or coronal plane **(Figs. 29A and B)**. Transvaginal transfontanelle 3D US has been preferred for confirmation of corpus callosum in some studies.[18] Volume acquisition if is done from sagittal plane corpus callosum appears echolucent but where as if acquisition is acquired in axial plane corpus callosum appears echogenic.[19] Normal corpus callosum and cerebellar vermis with ventriculomegaly is most likely due to aqueduct stenosis. In case of mild ventriculomegaly, it is essential to confirm the status of corpus callosum and cerebellar vermis. Ventriculomegaly can be quantitatively evaluated and clearly delineated using inversion mode for rendering and also by sono AVC general **(Figs. 30A and B)**.

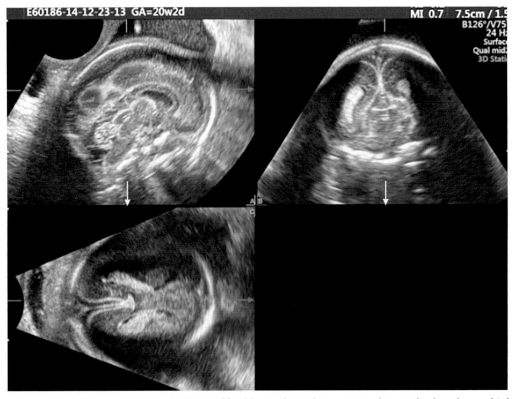

Fig. 27: Three-dimensional ultrasound acquired volume of fetal brain, through transvaginal route displayed as multiplanar images.

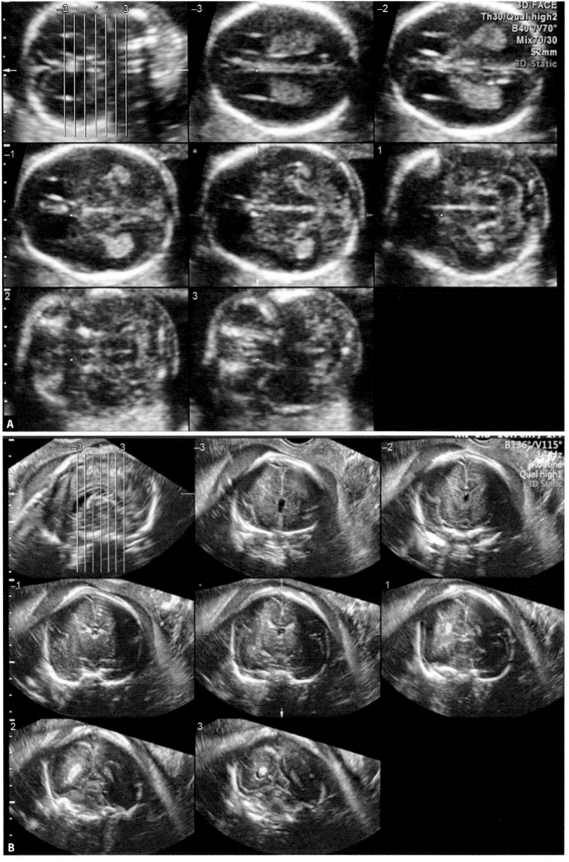

Figs. 28A and B

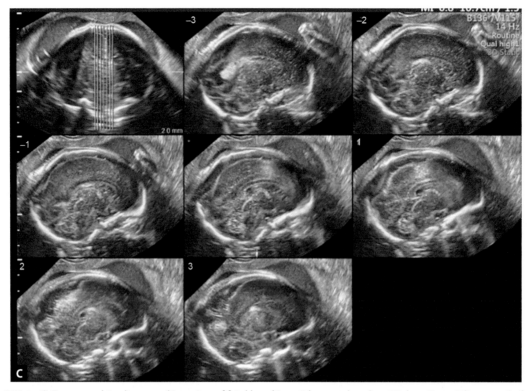

Figs. 28A to C: Tomographic ultrasound imaging of fetal head in axial coronal and sagittal sections: Ultrasound of sections of detailed neurosonogram.

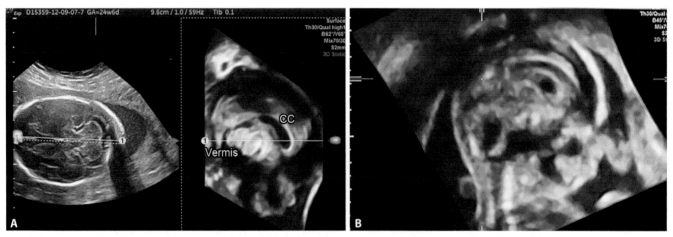

Figs. 29A and B: (A) Omniview used on transcerebellar axial plane with omniview line passing through midline (falx) showing mid-sagittal plane with corpus callosum, midbrain, pons, and cerebellar vermis; (B) Omniview showing absent vermis (Dandy–Walker syndrome).

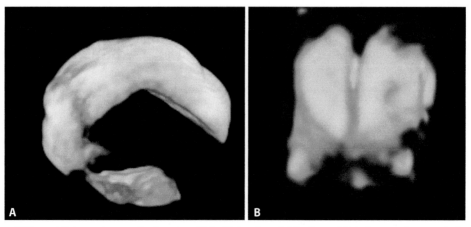

Figs. 30A and B: Inversion mode showing dilated lateral ventricles in sagittal plane and coronal plane.

Paladini and Volpe[20] have suggested measuring tentorovermian angle, tentoroclivus angle, clivovermian angle, etc. to diagnose vermian abnormalities **(Fig. 31)**. Tentoroclivus and clivovermian angle both can demonstrate the upward displacement of vermis in fetuses with Dandy–Walker variant. The normal tentoroclivus angle is 4 ± 4.2 and normal clivovermian angle is 47.8 ± 7.3 **(Fig. 32)**. This study concludes that 3D US is the modality of choice to demonstrate the key features important for diagnosis of posterior fossa lesions like the upward displacement of the tentorium, the counter-clockwise rotation, and the significant hypoplasia of the cerebellar vermis.[20]

Skull base development can be assessed by measurement of anterior skull base length and posterior cranial fossa length and skull base angle.[21] Brain growth leads to higher increment in posterior cranial fossa length leading to 6° flexion in the skull base angle.[21] Craniofacial variability index (CVI) can assist in fetal facial anatomy to study craniofacial development.[22] Sections of the skull required for all these measurements can be all achieved and measured by TUI and multiplanar mode. This technique has proved to be almost as sensitive as computed tomography (CT) scan or magnetic resonance imaging (MRI) for study of brain lesions. Three-dimensional US may be applied to every central nervous system (CNS) abnormality diagnosed with traditional 2D technique and may offer further information useful for correct diagnosis. It can delineate the exact nature and anatomic level of anomaly.

Three-dimensional power Doppler also delineates the cerebral vasculature and its abnormalities **(Fig. 33)**. Several workers have proved the role of 3D power Doppler for demonstration of vein of Galen aneurysm and have also claimed the technique to be comparable with MRI.[23] Though power Doppler does show the vascular architecture in detail, especially with transvaginal approach, 3D power Doppler may add to the information.

Study of *fetal motorial and behavioral pattern* is essential for complete evaluation or functional integrity of fetal CNS. Only 4D US allows the evaluation of fetal motorial and behavioral patterns. With 4D US it is possible to better define the degree of normality and pathology of fetal neurological functions in utero and to find out which fetuses are at risk of bad neurological outcome. Kurjak A et al. have described patterns of neurodevelopmental behavior during the three trimesters of pregnancy using 4D US.[24] The changes in the motorial pattern expresses the evolution of the maturative process of CNS during intrauterine life. These fetal behavior and movements can help diagnosis of abnormal motoric development **(Figs. 34A to C)**. Delayed motoric development is seen in fetuses of diabetic mothers. Infolding of the thumb in the fist of the fetus is typically described as neurological thumb being a sign **(Fig. 35)** of some neurological deficit. Fetuses with arthrogryposis show early disturbances in motoric development with absent limb movement and joint contractures **(Figs. 36A and B)**. Fetal functional neurology has been discussed in detail in chapter 8 of this book.

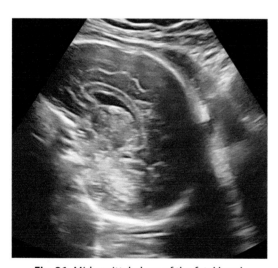

Fig. 31: Mid-sagittal plane of the fetal head.

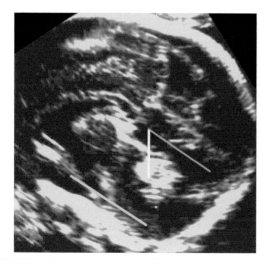

Fig. 32: Mid-sagittal plane of the fetal head showing measurement of tentoroclivus and clivovermian angle.

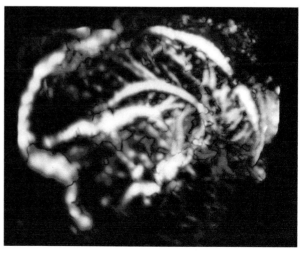

Fig. 33: Cerebral vasculature seen on 3D power Doppler angiomode.

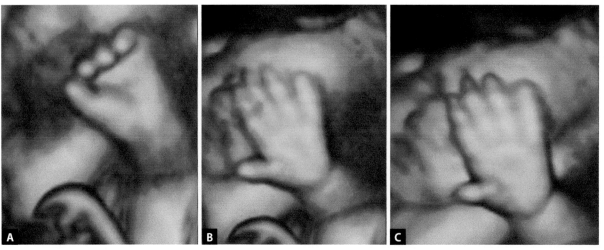

Figs. 34A to C: Movements of hand documented by series of images.

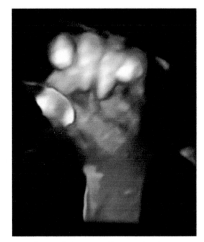

Fig. 35: Neurological thumb (thumb folded inside the fist).

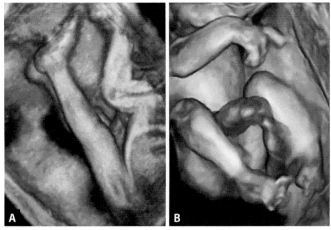

Figs. 36A and B: (A) Persistent extension deformity of lower limbs seen on 3D ultrasound surface rendered image; (B) Multiple joint abnormalities of upper and lower limbs seen on 3D ultrasound surface rendered image.

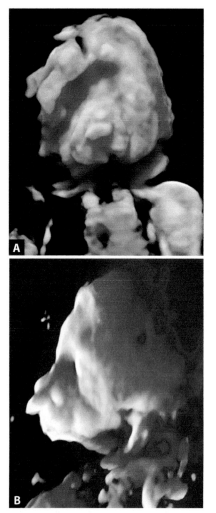

Figs. 37A and B: Coronal and sagittal plane HD live rendered images of major facial fetal abnormality.

Neck Abnormalities

Chiefly cystic hygroma and thyroid goiter are the two most common lesions seen in the fetal neck. Though these can be diagnosed on B-mode US, 3D can be used for better demonstration of the same.[25,26]

Apart from these, various studies have shown that 3D US has been used for diagnosis of trisomy 18 and for diagnosis of rare abnormalities of the face like Treacher Collins syndrome, cebocephaly, otocephaly, etc. **(Figs. 37A and B)**.

Spinal Abnormalities

Evaluation of the CNS cannot be called complete without evaluation of the spine. Evaluation of spine in sagittal, coronal, and axial all three planes is essential to diagnose spinal abnormalities correctly. All the three views cannot be achieved in one fetal position on 2D US. Three-dimensional US saves examination time and clearly can show all the three views at a time on multiplanar mode along with the overlying skin surface by using maximum mode transparent rendering and surface rendering **(Fig. 38A)**. Using 4D VCI C can also show coronal view even when on 2D US only axial section is seen **(Figs. 38B and C)**. Spinal column abnormalities like spinal canal defects, hemivertebrae, diastematomyelia, can all be well demonstrated by 3D US **(Figs. 39A to D)**.

Using Magicut and 3D rotation, it is also possible to see each vertebra separately on transverse section **(Fig. 40A)** and to define the extent of lesion especially in cases of open spinal canal defects. In case of lesions like teratomas or spinal canal defects, meningomyeloceles **(Figs. 40B and C)**, 3D US allows to exactly define the number of involved vertebrae. Volume US has almost 100% sensitivity and very high specificity for diagnosis of spinal abnormalities. Longitudinal scan of the fetus is used with maximum mode to evaluate the thoracic cage, clavicle, and scapulae **(Fig. 41)**. HD live is an even better mode to evaluate the spine. The settings for this are important. To render the bones on HD live usually zero threshold and high silhouette is used.

Chest

Multiplanar mode and TUI allows to study the spatial relationship between lungs, heart, oesophagus, and diaphragm **(Figs. 42A to C)**.[27] Trachea and oesophagus morphology can be studied **(Fig. 43)**. Thus helping to diagnose tracheoesophageal fistulae early and decide the type in utero. It is important to mention here that tracheoesophageal fistula is searched for on 2D US only in high-risk cases or in those fetuses in whom stomach is persistently small or not seen. Randomly seeing for the oesophagus and trachea for every scan is not done. Moreover, it is also important to note here that not all patients with tracheoesophageal fistula will show small or absent stomach shadow.

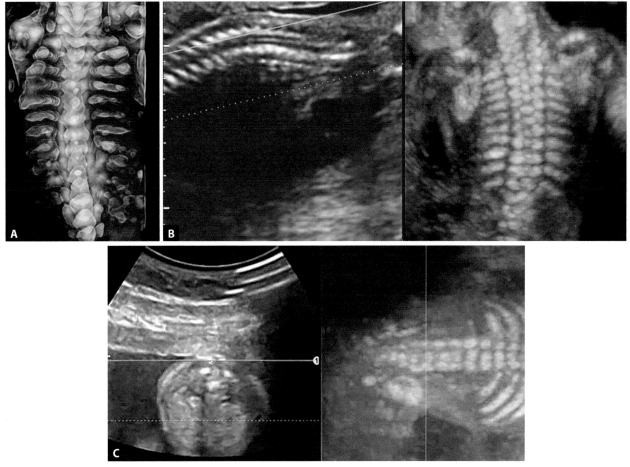

Figs. 38A to C: (A) 3D ultrasound HD live silhouette rendered image of normal spine; (B) Omniview is used on sagittal section of trunk to image the spine in coronal plane using VCI C; (C) Omniview is used on axial section of trunk to image the spine in coronal plane.

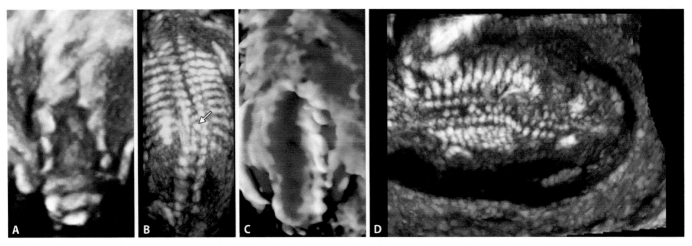

Figs. 39A to D: (A) Large open spinal canal defect of the lumbar spine rendered by 3D ultrasound with combination of surface and maximum mode; (B) Hemivertebra in lower thoracic spine rendered by 3D ultrasound with combination of surface and maximum mode; (C) Large open spinal canal defect with a large myelomeningocele rendered on HD live; (D) Multiple vertebral abnormalities rendered on maximum mode.

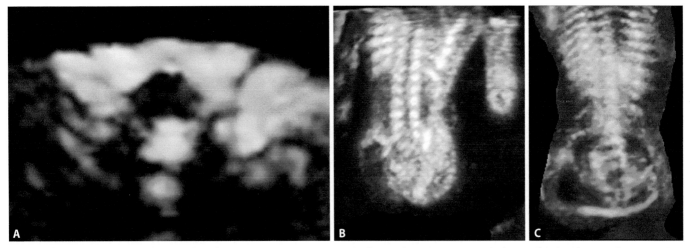

Figs. 40A to C: (A) Single vertebra rendered in transverse section using rendering the spine in coronal plane, selecting the vertebra, scooping it out by Magicut, and then *x* rotation; (B) Coronal plane of spine rendered in maximum mode showing absence of the sacral spine with soft-tissue mass lesion—sacrococcygeal teratoma; (C) Coronal plane of spine rendered in maximum mode showing widening of the sacral spine with a round echolucent lesion—sacral meningocele.

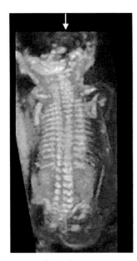

Fig. 41: Longitudinal scan of the fetus is used with maximum mode to evaluate the thoracic cage, clavicle, and scapulae.

Diaphragmatic hernia can be easily diagnosed by 2D US. Three-dimensional US with VOCAL and 3D–4D multiplanar mode is useful for assessment of fetal lung volume, which is the prognosis deciding parameter in cases of diaphragmatic hernia and pulmonary hypoplasia also.

Studies have evaluated the potential of 3D power Doppler to predict neonatal outcome and pulmonary arterial hypertension in fetuses with congenital diaphragmatic hernia and have found that severity of pulmonary arterial hypertension was associated with progressive reduction in prenatal vascular indices.[28,29] Pulmonary hypoplasia may also be due to oligohydramnios due to any cause, premature rupture of membranes, chylothorax, etc. and it may be the deciding factor for prognosis. Lung volume assessment as mentioned earlier can help predict the prognosis in these cases too. To calculate the lung volume, 3D volume of the

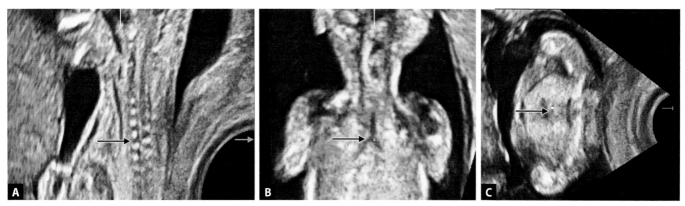

Figs. 42A to C: Multiplanar images of the fetal thorax, explaining the spatial relation of thoracic anatomy. Arrow showing tracheal bifurcation at the reference dot.

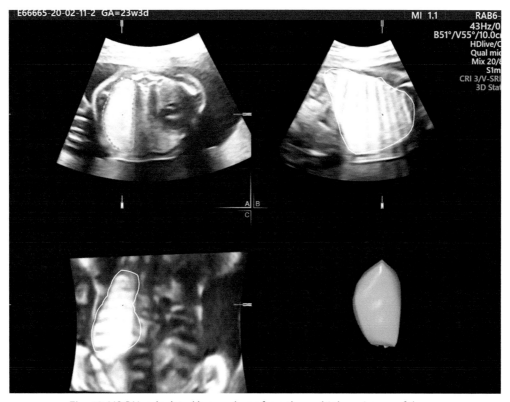

Fig. 43: VOCAL calculated lung volume from the multiplanar image of thorax.

thorax is acquired in axial plane including the entire thorax, volume angle about 50–60° depending on the gestational age. Lung volume assessment is also helpful in cases with congenital cystic adenomatoid malformation of the lung **(Fig. 43)**. Select either lung, one after the other and use VOCAL to calculate the volume. Though sequestration of the lung and cystic adenomatoid malformation of the lung are diagnosed on B-mode US, 3D power Doppler may give more confident diagnosis by identification of the vessels **(Fig. 44)**.

Abdomen

Using transparent mode and multiplanar mode, the abdominal organs can be very well identified with definition of all tissue planes. Three-dimensional US is an effective tool for diagnosis of gastrointestinal malformations and gives

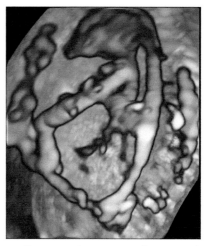

Fig. 44: Three-dimensional power Doppler image showing fetal trunk vasculature.

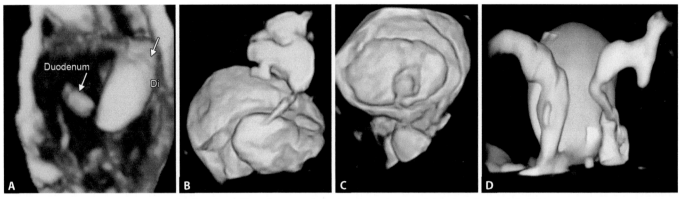

Figs. 45A to D: (A) Inversion mode showing dilated stomach and pylorus (case of duodenal atresia); (B) Inversion mode rendering of hydronephrosis; (C) Inversion mode rendering of the distended urinary bladder with ureterocele inside the bladder; (D) Bilateral hydronephrosis and hydroureter shown in inversion mode rendering.

additional information over 2D US for pediatric surgeons for surgical planning and for counseling with parents. Inversion mode helps to define cystic lesions and can be best used to confirm the diagnosis of pyloric stenosis, duodenal atresia, posterior urethral valves, obstructive uropathy, etc. **(Figs. 45A to D)**. All abdominal masses may be better evaluated by multiplanar mode for their origin and extension.

Hydronephrosis, hydroureter, and even the bladder abnormalities including posterior urethral valve can be well demonstrated by 3D US **(Fig. 45D)**. Congenital renal tumors—nephroblastoma—and their extent can be assessed by 3D US TUI, and 3D power Doppler also helps to assess the extent of the lesion. VOCAL may be used to calculate the tumor volume, volume of dilated pelvicalyceal system, distended bladder, and these can be of help for comparison for follow up of these lesions and to prognosticate them. Surface rendering allows clear visualization of genitals and thus can be a helpful tool to demonstrate the abnormalities of the genitals that may be of major importance for the family. Hypospadias is seen as "tulip sign"[22] and clitoral hypertrophy can be diagnosed in third trimester.

Anterior abdominal wall defects are usually diagnosed on 2D US but are well demonstrated on volume US. Three-dimensional with power Doppler is very useful to differentiate the bowel containing from the liver containing omphalocele. Use of 3D multiplanar display is more accurate than the use of 2D US for measuring the size of omphalocele. Omphalocele and gastroschisis can be confidently differentiated by 3D US.

Three-dimensional US with VOCAL can be used to calculate the liver volume as for the lungs. Liver volume has been considered as a parameter that correlates with fetal growth retardation.[30] Study of the abdominal vasculature is facilitated by 3D power Doppler.

Limb Abnormalities

Though limb abnormalities are fairly well demonstrated on 2D US, 3D US produces a more understandable picture

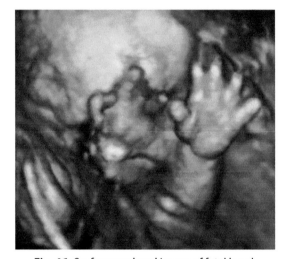

Fig. 46: Surface rendered image of fetal hand.

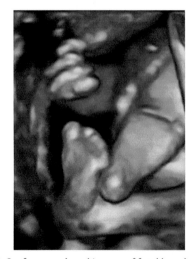

Fig. 47: Surface rendered image of fetal hand and foot.

for patient explanation. Accurate analysis of majority of bony structures can be done by using maximum mode rendering of 3D US or omniview, though in general limb abnormalities can also be demonstrated well by surface mode **(Figs. 46 and 47)**. 3D-4D US enables detailed examination of fingers and toes with almost 100% certainty

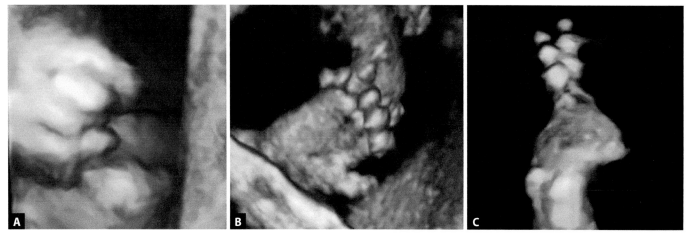

Figs. 48A to C: Surface rendered image of (A) Overriding of fingers; (B) Polydactyly; (C) Radial aplasia.

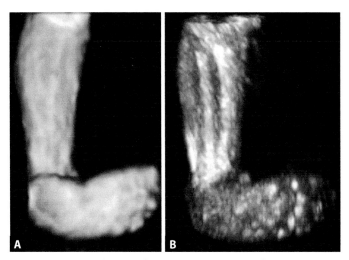

Figs. 49A and B: Clubfoot rendered on (A) Surface mode;
(B) Maximum mode after Magicut.

of detecting agenesis and extra digits **(Figs. 48A to C)**. Motor abnormalities and abnormal attitude of fingers, toes or hands, and legs like clubfeet **(Figs. 49A and B)**, overriding of fingers, flexion/extension deformities, the joints as in arthrogryposis, or thumb in the fist may be manifestations of chromosomal or neurological abnormality. Clubfeet can also be ruled out or demonstrated with omniview when rendering is difficult due to fetal position or reduced amniotic fluid amount.

Placenta

It is known that pregnancy-induced hypertension occurs only after at least 70% of the placental vasculature is obliterated. Three-dimensional power Doppler with angiomode of the placental vasculature may show obliteration of the placental vessels and pruning effect and help to predict pregnancy-induced hypertension much earlier **(Figs. 50A and B)**. Morbidly adherent placenta, though is diagnosed by B-mode US, 3D power Doppler helps to assess the extent of vascularity and thus confirm the penetration of the placenta **(Figs. 50C and D)**.

Normal cord vessels can be visualized on color Doppler and 3D added to this gives more real life and clear image **(Fig. 51A)**.

Cord abnormalities like hypercoiling **(Fig. 51B)**, abnormal cord insertion also can be confirmed with 3D and Doppler. Cord round the neck, true knot in cord can be more confidently diagnosed by 3D Doppler **(Figs. 52A and B)**.

Benacerraf et al.[31] have described a novel use of 3D US in offline fetal evaluation. According to their study, five volume sweeps should be taken of every fetus, and they are examined offline. This method has proved to be successful in detailed evaluation of fetal anatomy and very sensitive for diagnosing fetal anomalies. These sweeps are axial section of fetal head, axial section of fetal thorax, axial section of fetal abdomen, longitudinal sweep of lower limbs, and longitudinal section of head.

■ 3D–4D FOR FETAL ECHOCARDIOGRAPHY

Cardiac evaluations have been made less time consuming and much easier with advancing technology. New 4D US technology with STIC can be used for offline 4D cardiac evaluation. It is one of the best teaching and learning tools especially in cases with cardiac abnormalities. After optimizing the 2D image, a single sweep is taken from the upper abdomen to the upper chest in 7.5–15 seconds. Hundreds of images of the heart during different phases of cardiac cycle are captured and stored. The computer depending on its calculated heart rate divides these images into systolic and diastolic phase and synchronizes one after the other in correct sequence of events and then plays the entire clip of the cardiac cycle continuously as a volume. This can be seen in all three planes like any other volume imaging—X, Y, Z (sagittal, axial, and coronal) **(Fig. 53)** and can be run as a continuous cardiac cycle. This acquisition and display can also be done with color or power Doppler **(Fig. 54)**. Volume of the heart can be acquired in with heart on 2D seen as four-chamber heart view. Before acquisition, it must be confirmed that you have selected the fetal cardiac preset that has more bright grey map and high contrast. If the

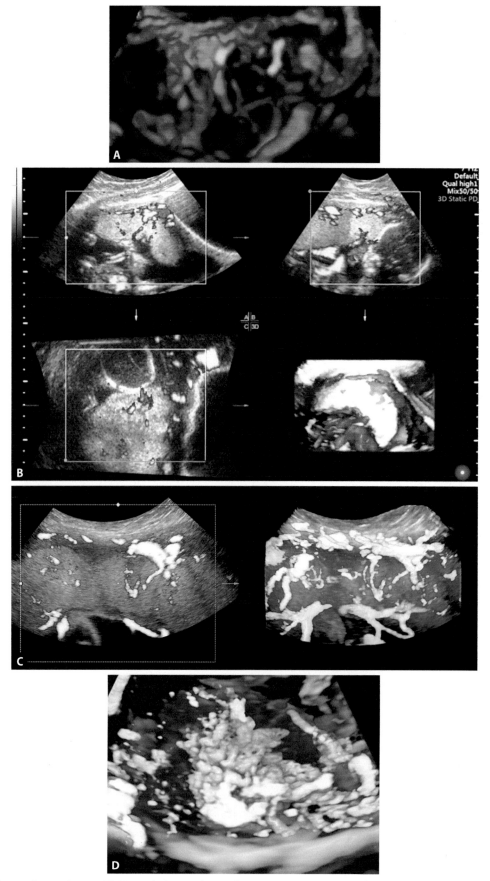

Figs. 50A to D: Placental vasculature. (A) Normal placental vasculature on 3D power Doppler; (B) 3D power Doppler multiplanar and rendered image showing scanty placental vascularity with pruning of vessels; (C) 3D HD flow showing normal placental vasculature; (D) Placental increta with placental vasculature extending till uterine serosa.

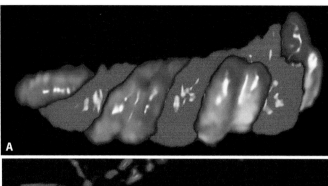

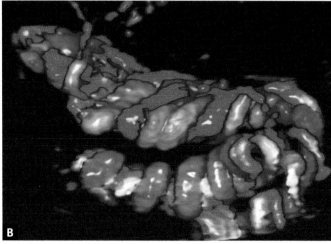

Figs. 51A and B: (A) Normal cord on 3D power Doppler with Magicut; (B) Hypercoiling of cord.

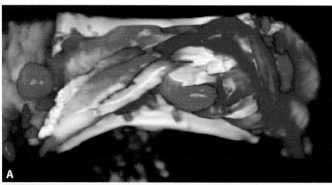

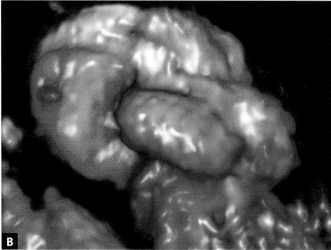

Figs. 52A and B: (A) Two loops of cord round the neck; (B) True knot in the cord. Both images are rendered in 3D power Doppler with Magicut.

volume is to be acquired with color Doppler, the color settings in the cardiac preset present have high pulse repetition frequency (PRF) and high wall motion filter. The color gains should be set such that they fill up the cardiac chambers completely and do not spill out. The best possible volume quality is selected according to the fetal movements. However, it is best to wait for the fetus to calm down before STIC volume is acquired. Fetal movements can lead to significant distortions in the image. The volume angle selected is between 20 and 35° depending on the gestational age so that the volume contains upper thorax to upper abdomen. Stomach should be seen in the lower most section and it should extend just beyond the three vessel trachea view. Once the volume is acquired, usually z rotation is used to achieve an apical four-chamber view. The x and y rotations may be used to correct any errors in the four-chamber section. Once that image is perfect, then the analysis is started. Analysis is started with the reference point on the crux of the heart. Rendering is usually done in front-back or back-front direction. The render box size and position are adjusted according to what structure is to be rendered. However, usually front-back render direction is selected.

Walking through these sections gives all the planes required for complete cardiac evaluation, like four-chamber view, left ventricular outflow tract view, right ventricular outflow tract view, three-vessel view, short-axis view, aortic-arch view, ductus-arch view, etc. These views can be seen simultaneously by using TUI with 3D or 4D **(Fig. 55)**. The image can also be seen as live 3D by various rendering modes.

Inversion mode of rendering can be a useful tool to demonstrate small septal defects difficult to image otherwise and also for demonstration of outflow tracts and great vessels **(Fig. 56A)**. HD live and glass body mode is used for valvular defects, outflow tract defects, and septal defects. Angiomode **(Fig. 56B)** is especially useful for the study of the arch views and relationship of great vessels and study of their branches or vascular abnormalities. Rendering from different directions can give all those views of the heart that were never possible by any other modality; for example, basic view or surgical view of the heart **(Fig. 56C)**, which shows relationship of all the four valves, is very informative for outflow tract relationship, inflow tract abnormalities, and important for surgeons. For this view, the render direction selected is up–down. Individual valves can be studied by omniview or rendering.

Volume computer aided display (VCAD) can be more useful for beginners. When working with this, the essential views of the heart are only a button touch away. No manual rotations or walking through are necessary. Volume of the heart is acquired as usual. The A plane is manipulated (rotation and zoom–unzoom) to match the predrawn four-chamber heart diagram of the heart **(Fig. 57)**. The predrawn diagram is placed on A image that is showing four-chamber

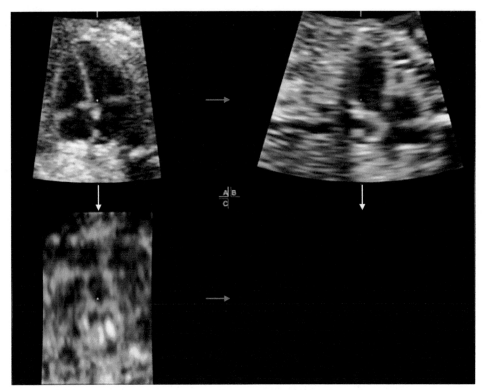

Fig. 53: Multiplanar display of the spatial temporal image correlation—acquired volume of fetal heart.

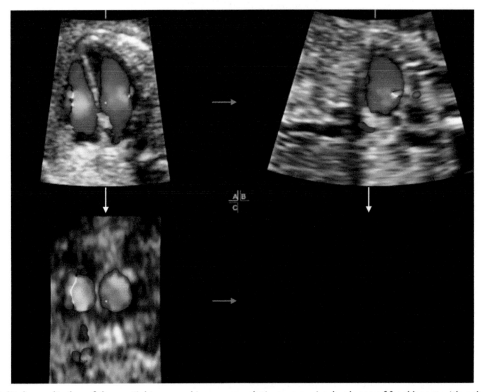

Fig. 54: Multiplanar display of the spatial temporal image correlation—acquired volume of fetal heart with color Doppler.

view of the heart and then various sections required are automatically achieved by only a button touch. This makes cardiac evaluation much quicker both online and offline. Using rendering, the heart is reconstructed in four-chamber view and then is cut by a line from apex to base, closely placed near the septum, and then rotating it shows the interventricular septum en face. This view is excellent for demonstration of location and extent of ventricular septal defect (VSD). In cases of cardiac tumors or also for study of the chordae tendinae, the viewing line is placed parallel

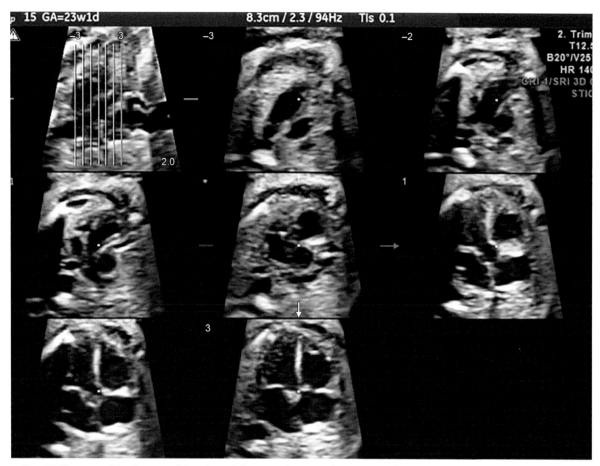

Fig. 55: Tomographic ultrasound imaging of the spatial temporal image correlation—acquired volume of fetal heart.

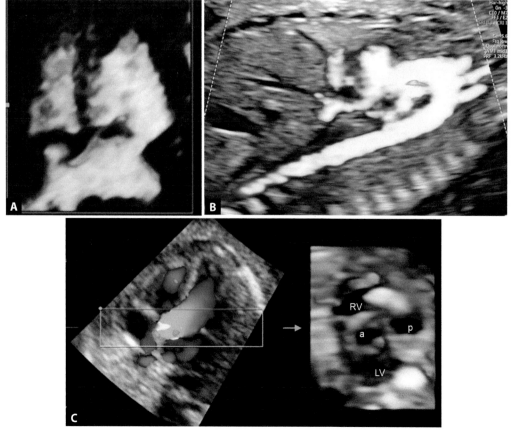

Figs. 56A to C: Inversion mode rendering of the heart.

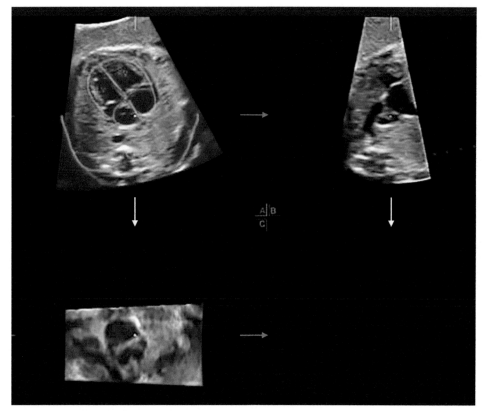

Fig. 57: Volume computer aided display used on spatial temporal image correlation—acquired volume of the heart.

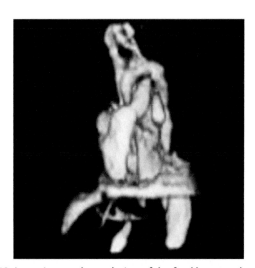

Fig. 58: Inversion mode rendering of the fetal heart and outflow tracts with the two arches in coronal plane.

to interventricular septum in the ventricle of interest. Relationship of the two arches can be best studied when the volume is acquired in sagittal plane of the fetus and the viewing line is placed cephalic to the arches, either on inversion mode or on angiomode **(Fig. 58)**. A few of these are narrated here for the reader's interest but there can be lot of innovations in this.

Omniview also can be used to save time and also for some difficult-to-get image planes. It is chiefly used on outflow tracts or three-vessel or three-vessel trachea view.

To establish the identity of a particular vessel, especially in cases of suspected abnormities, omniview may be used to see the long axis of the vessel or its relationship to surrounding structures.

Conjoined Twins

In conjoined twins, practicability and the consequent morbidity of the fetuses after separation depend on the degree of codivision of organs and vascular structures. Therefore, detailed and accurate anatomic and vascular map is fundamental for evaluation of joined organs in conjoined fetuses is of fundamental importance to decide the line of treatment. Moreover defects like orofacial cleft, diaphragmatic hernia, imperforate anus, and neural tube defects are also common. Bega et al. have reported that combining multiplanar display and surface rendering can assess these fetuses fairly reliably, as early as 10 weeks.[32] Three-dimensional US can be of great help in classifying more accurately the type of conjoined twins and color Doppler may be of further help **(Fig. 59)**.

■ LIMITATIONS OF 3D–4D ULTRASOUND

As for 2D US maternal obesity, maternal scar, maternal movements, excessive fetal movements and air, calcifications or bones that come in way of sound propagation are obstacles for 3D US also. Oligohydramnios does not permit sufficient

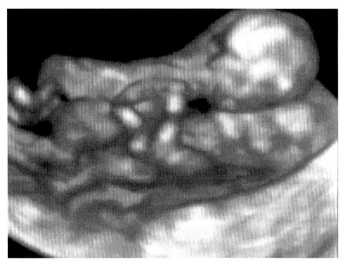

Fig. 59: Surface rendered image of thoracopagus conjoined twins.

fluid interface that is an absolute essential for surface rendering and so is not a favorable factor for reconstruction and surface rendering.

CONCLUSION

Volume US is a very valuable tool for diagnosis and demonstration of fetal abnormalities in spite of these limitations. Volume US gives better accuracy with a shorter examination time. Three-dimensional orientation and multiplanar imaging gives unlimited tomograms, with only limited probe manipulation and minimizes the fetal exposure to US.

REFERENCES

1. Merz E, Weber G, Bahlmann F, Miric-Tesanic D. Application of transvaginal and abdominal three-dimensional ultrasound for detection or exclusion of fetal malformations of fetal face. Ultrasound Obstet Gynecol. 1997;9:237-43.
2. Rotten D, Levaillant JM. Two- and three-dimensional sonographic assessment of the fetal face. 2. Analysis of cleft lip, alveolus and palate. Ultrasound Obstet Gynecol. 2004;24(4):402-11.
3. Platt LD, Devore GR, Pretorius DH. Improving cleft palate/cleft lip antenatal diagnosis by three-dimensional sonography: the "flipped face" view. J Ultrasound Med. 2006;25(11):1423-30.
4. Pilu G, Segata M. A novel technique for visualization of the normal and cleft fetal secondary palate: angled insonation and three-dimensional ultrasound. Ultrasound Obstet Gynecol. 2007;29(2):166-9.
5. Campbell S, Lees C, Moscoso G, Hall P. Ultrasound antenatal diagnosis of cleft palate by a new technique: the 3D "reverse face" view. Ultrasound Obstet Gynecol. 2005;25(1):12-8.
6. McGahan MC, Ramos GA, Landry C, Wolfson T, Sowell BB, D'Agostini D, et al. Multislice display of the fetal face using three-dimensional ultrasonography. J Ultrasound Med. 2008;27(11):1573-81.
7. Kurjak A, Azumendi G, Andonotopo W, Salihagic-Kadic A. Three- and four-dimensional ultrasonography for the structural and functional evaluation of the fetal face. Am J Obstet Gynecol. 2007;196(1):16-28.
8. Benacerraf BR, Sadow PM, Barnewolt CE, Estroff JA, Benson C. Cleft of the secondary palate without cleft lip diagnosed with three-dimensional ultrasound and magnetic resonance imaging in fetus with Fryns' syndrome. Ultrasound Obstet Gynecol. 2006;27(5):566-70.
9. Sleurs E, Goncalves LF, Jhonson A, Espinoza J, Devers P, Chaiworapongsa T, et al. First-trimester three-dimensional ultrasonic findings in a fetus with frontonasal malformation. J Matern Fetal Neonatal Med. 2004;16(3):187-97.
10. Rotten D, Levaillant JM, Martinez H, le Pointe HD, Vicaut E. The fetal mandible: a 2D and 3D sonographic approach to the diagnosis of retrognathia and micrognathia. Ultrasound Obstet Gynecol. 2002;19(2):122-30.
11. Paladini D, Morra T, Teodoro A, Lamberti A, Tremolaterra F, Martinelli P. Objective diagnosis of micrognathia in the fetus: the jaw index. Obstet Gynecol. 1999;93(3):382-6.
12. Borenstein M, Perisco N, Strobl I, Sonek J, Nicolaides KH. Frontomaxillary and mandibulomaxillary facial angles at 11 + 0 to 13 + 6 weeks in fetuses with trisomy 18. Ultrasound Obstet Gynecol. 2007;30(7):928-33.
13. Benoitt B, Chaoui R. Three-dimensional ultrasound with maximal mode rendering: a novel technique for the diagnosis of bilateral or unilateral absence or hypoplasia of nasal bones in second-trimester screening for Down syndrome. Ultrasound Obstet Gynecol. 2005;25(1):19-24.
14. Sepulveda W, Wojakowski AB, Elias D, Otano L, Gutierrez J. Congenital dacrocystocoele: prenatal 2- and three-dimensional sonographic findings. J Ultrasound Med. 2005;24(2):225-30.
15. Krakow D, Santulli T, Platt LD. Use of three-dimensional ultrasonography in differentiating craniosynostosis from severe fetal molding. J Ultrasound Med. 2001;20:427-31.
16. Dikkeboom CM, Roelfsema NM, Van Adrichem LNA, Wladimiroff JW. The role of three-dimensional ultrasound in visualizing the fetal cranial sutures and fontanels during the second half of pregnancy. Ultrasound Obstet Gynecol. 2004;24(4):412-6.
17. Paladini D, Vassallo M, Sglavo G, Pastore G, Lapadula C, Nappi C. Normal and abnormal development of the fetal anterior fontanelle: a three-dimensional ultrasound study. Ultrasound Obstet Gynecol. 2008;32(6):755-61.
18. Timor-Tristch IE, Monteagudo A, Mayberry P. Three-dimensional ultrasound evaluation of the fetal brain: the three horn view. Ultrasound Obstet Gynecol. 2000;16(4):302-6.
19. Plasencia W, Dagklis T, Borenstein M, Csapo B, Nicolaides KH. Assessment of corpus callosum at 20-24 weeks' gestation by three-dimensional ultrasound examination. Ultrasound Obstet Gynecol. 2007;30(2):169-72.
20. Paladini D, Volpe P. Posterior fossa and vermian morphometry in the characterization of fetal cerebellar abnormalities: a perspective three-dimensional ultrasound study. Ultrasound Obstet Gynecol. 2006;27(5):482-9.
21. Roelfsema NM, Grijseels EWM, Hop WCJ, Wladimiroff JW. Three-dimensional sonography of prenatal skull base development. Ultrasound Obstet Gynecol. 2007;29(4):372-7.
22. Roelf NM, Hop WCJ, van Adrichem LNA, Wladimiroff JW. Craniofacial variability index in utero: a three-dimensional ultrasound study. Ultrasound Obstet Gynecol. 2007;29(3):258-64.

23. Ruano R, Benachi A, Aubry MC, Brunelle F, Dumez Y, Dommergues M. Perinatal three-dimensional color power Doppler ultrasonography of vein of Galen aneurysms. J Ultrasound Med. 2003;22(12):1357-62.

24. Kurjak A, Pooh RK, Merce LT, Carrera JM, Slihagic-Kadic A, Andonotopo W. Structural and functional early human development assessed by three-dimensional and four-dimensional sonography. Fertil Steril. 2005;84(5):1285-99.

25. Bonilla-Musoles F, Raga F, Villalobos A, Blanes J, Osborne NG. First-trimester neck abnormalities: three-dimensional evaluation. J Ultrasound Med. 1998;17(7):419-25.

26. Nath CA, Oyelese Y, Yeo L, Chavez M, Kontopoulos EV, Giannaina G, et al. Three-dimensional sonography in the evaluation and management of fetal goiter. Ultrasound Obstet Gynecol. 2005;25(3):312-4.

27. Gerards FA, Twisk JW, Bakker M, Barkhof F, van Vugt JM. Fetal lung volume: three-dimensional ultrasonography compared with magnetic resonance imaging. Ultrasound Obstet Gynecol. 2007;29(5):533-6.

28. Spaggiari E, Strinneman JJ, Sonigo P, Khen-Dunlop N, De Saint Blanquat L, Ville Y. Prenatal prediction of pulmonary arterial hypertension in congenital diaphragmatic hernia. Ultrasound Obstet Gynecol. 2015;45(5): 572-7.

29. Harting MT. Congenital diaphragmatic hernia-associated pulmonary hypertension. Semin Peadiatr Surg. 2017; 26(3):147-53.

30. Kuno A, Hayashi Y, Akiyama M, Yamashiro C, Tanaka H, Yanagihara T, et al. Three-dimensional sonographic measurement of liver volume in small for gestational age fetus. J Ultrasound Med. 2002;21:361-6.

31. Benacerraf BR, Bromley B, Shipp TS. Can 3D volume sets alone be used to detect fetal malformations? ISUOG. 2006.

32. Bega G, Wapner R, Lev-Toaff A, Kuhlman K. Diagnosis of conjoined twins at 10 weeks using three-dimensional ultrasound: a case report. Ultrasound Obstet Gynecol. 2000;388-90.

Fetal Face Malformations in Ultrasound

Marek Pietryga, Kinga Toboła-Wróbel, Rafał Iciek, Jacek Brązert

■ INTRODUCTION

Interruption of normal embryologic growth and differentiation of the face and skull results in a wide variety of craniofacial abnormalities. Thanks to the development of ultrasound techniques, it is possible to assess and recognize abnormalities of craniofacial structure at an early stage of development. The aim of this chapter is to present possibilities of prenatal diagnosis in recent times based on own data.

Fetal cranial abnormalities are observed as isolated face changes and as coexisting and accompanying other developmental defects in genetic and nongenetic syndromes. Facial abnormalities associated with malformation syndromes are easier to recognize than isolated defects, which are particularly difficult to recognize in cases of oligohydramnios and uterine defects (forced placement in these cases). Therefore, a very important element of prenatal diagnosis is the correct assessment of the fetal face at the right time—around the 20th week of pregnancy. It should be noted that the increasingly better resolution of ultrasound machines results in the fact, that craniofacial imaging is in some cases possible from 12th to 17th week of pregnancy.

The first facial defects (cleft lip and palate) were visualized prenatally in the 1980s. Currently, ultrasound diagnostics of craniofacial defects allow the diagnosis of 50–90% malformations.[1-4] In developmental defect sets, detection can reach 100%, while in isolated defects only about 50%, although this percentage has doubled in the last 20 years.[1,5,6]

■ EMBRYOLOGY

Branchial arches appear around 4–5th week of embryological development, and the fourth branchial arch with a bunch of mesenchymal tissue is separated by the palate. At the turn of 4th/5th week, the stomodeum is formed in the central part of the face and surrounded by the first pair of branchial arches. Each arch consists of an ectoderm, endoderm, and "neural crest cells" that help in the development of the facial skeleton.

The mesodermal tissue of the arches forms the muscular parts of the face and neck.[2] The first bronchial arch gives rise to facial formation and to the growth of the jaw. Facial formation occurs at the 5th week of pregnancy **(Figs. 1 and 2)**.

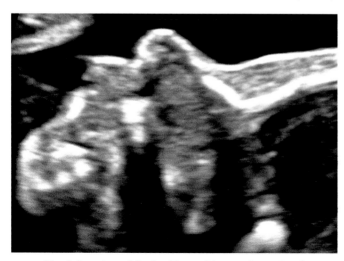

Fig. 1: Imaging of the fetal face with two-dimensional (2D) ultrasound.

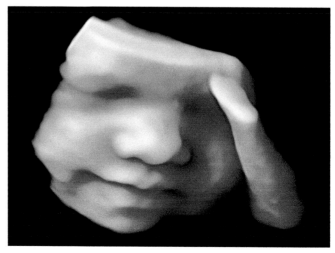

Fig. 2: Imaging of the fetal face with three-dimensional (3D) ultrasound.

The nasal plate forms the nasal cavity, and the surrounding crests form the frontal nasal eminence, at which time the mandible eminence is also formed. Between 5th and 8th week of pregnancy, the maxillary tuberosity increases, closing the sulcus between the nasal and maxillary eminences. The upper lip is formed by the fusion of maxillary tuberosity with middle nasal eminence. Mandibular protrusion forms the lower lip, cheek, and jaw.[2]

The nose is formed from five eminences:[2]

- Frontal haughtiness of the face (bridge of the nose)
- Two middle nasal eminences (comb, tip, and central part of the lip)
- Two lateral nasal eminences (nose wings).

A very important stage of development is the time of merging the two medial nasal eminences, the combination of which forms the middle segment of the jaw and partly the upper lip, teeth, anterior palate, and primary palate **(Fig. 3)**.[1-4,7] Joints of jaw eminences with middle nasal is a key element of forming lips and palate.

The total lack or partial combination of these eminences results in one-sided or two-sided cleft of lip and palate at 6 weeks of pregnancy. Cleft lateral appears between the lateral incisors and the canine, lengthwise upper lip in the middle position. Central (middle) lip strain is caused by the incomplete union of the two medial nasal eminences.

This disadvantage is associated with heavy multiorgan defects, especially with holoprosencephalia.

Irregularities that are primarily related to the first branchial arch as a result of failure of cell migration to this bow, we can observe as Treacher Collins Syndrome (TCS) (mandibulofacial dysostosis) and Pierre Robin syndrome.[1] These cells also take part in the formation of the aorta, pulmonary arteries, and their abnormality might cause congenital heart disease[1] **(Fig. 3)**.

Standard craniofacial ultrasound imaging in two-dimensional (2D) projection should be performed during the second prenatal examination between 18 and 22nd week of pregnancy, in three basic planes **(Fig. 4)**:[1,2,5,6,8]

1. *Coronal/frontal plane*
2. *Sagittal plane*
3. *Transverse plane*

In addition, we can use Doppler study:

In the coronal plane we assess: nostrils, nasal column, alveolus, nasal septum, hard palate, and the vomer (most important ones in the evaluation of the integrity of facial anatomy) **(Fig. 4A)**

In the sagittal plane we assess: forehead, profile, nasal bones and nasal column, upper lip with philtrum/medical cleft, secondary palate, tongue, lower lip, and chin (at the height of the forehead) (useful in the assessment of the normality of the profile) **(Figs. 4B and C)**.

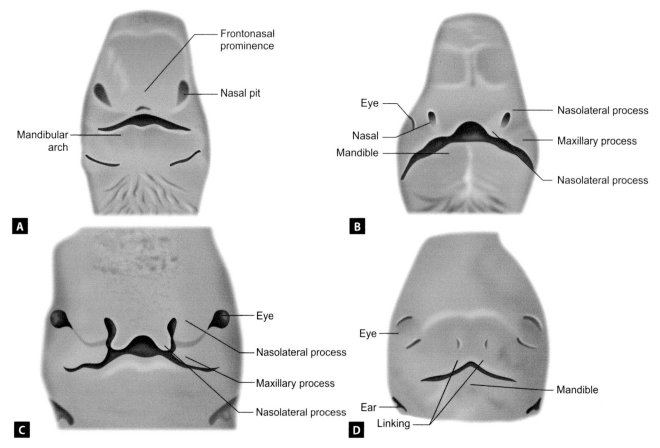

Figs. 3A to D: Craniofacial development.

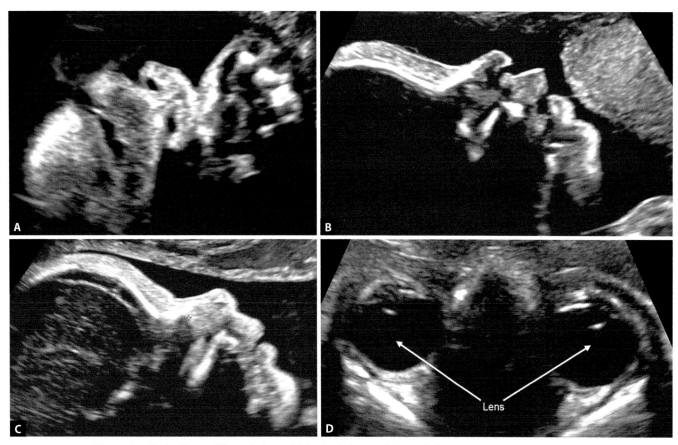

Figs. 4A to D: (A) Coronal/frontal plane; (B) Sagittal plane; (C) Sagittal plane; (D) Transverse/axial plane.

In the transverse (axial) plane, we assess: orbits—interorbital and biorbital distance, nasal septum, upper lip, jaw with compounded teeth, hard palate, tongue, and V-shaped mandible (easily reveals both orbits) **(Fig. 4D)**

In the craniofacial imaging, we can perform the following measurements:[9]

- Lip width
- Interbuccal frenum distance (chick to chick diameter)
- Mandible
- Tongue
- Eye sockets (inter- and biorbital distances)
- Nose.

We carry out these measurements in cases of malformations, diagnostic doubts, but not in routine ultrasound examination.

In assessing the continuity of the upper lip and palate, proper imaging is very important.

In order to get a clear picture of the lips, we cannot press the probe, but sometimes move it away. On the other hand, if we want to assess the alveolar arch—the "image of the seagull"—in the case of cleft palate, we will see a hypoechoic fissure in the arch behind the incisor teeth. Then we have to move the probe in the same position, toward the head[5] **(Fig. 5)**.

In extreme facial edema, we observe distortion of the facial contours in frontal and axial planes. Deformations are

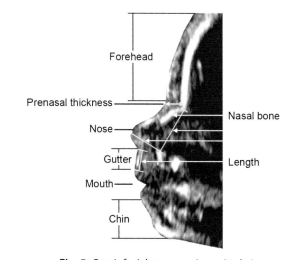

Fig. 5: Craniofacial structure in sagittal view.

so intense that it is impossible to highlight the nose, lips, or eyelids **(Figs. 6 and 7)**.

In other cases, the changes are insignificant, for example, a slight degree of nasal bone hypoplasia and dilatation of the anterior tissue in trisomy 21.

◼ NOSE IMAGING

Nose imaging is performed in the sagittal and coronary planes.

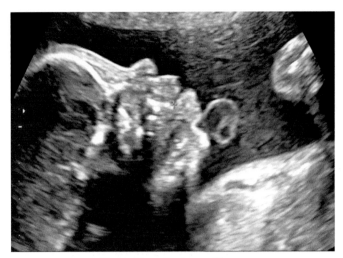

Fig. 6: Hypoplastic nasal bone.

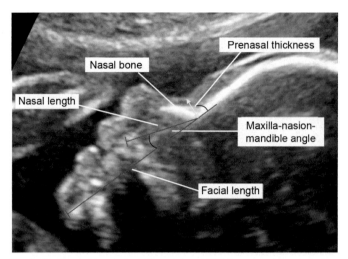

Fig. 8: Fetal nasal bone two-dimensional (2D) imaging. Measurement of prenasal thickness as a marker of trisomy 21 in the second trimester of pregnancy and maxilla–nasion–mandible (MNM) angle.

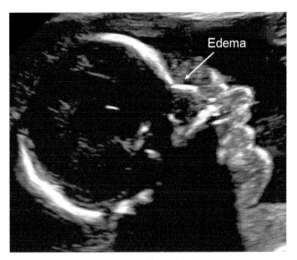

Fig. 7: Face profile and edema.

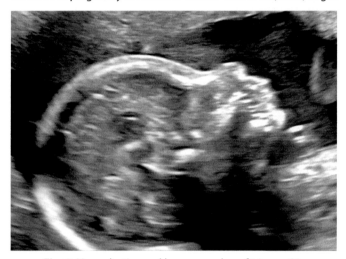

Fig. 9: Hypoplastic nasal bone—marker of trisomy 21.

Nasal abnormalities are mainly associated with chromosomal abnormalities (hypoplasia or lack of nasal bone in trisomy 21, triploidy, or tetrasomy). In the second trimester of pregnancy, the trisomy 21 marker is also frontal thickening—prenasal thickness. Maxilla–nasion–mandible (MNM) angle measurement is also very important **(Fig. 8)**.

We can also observe a flat and small nose in other malformation syndromes:
- Binder syndrome
- Aarskog syndrome
- Raine syndrome
- Brachmann-de Lange syndrome
- Pierre Robin syndrome and after exposure to valproic acid during epilepsy treatment **(Figs. 9 to 14)**.[15,16]

▪ IMAGING OF THE LIPS AND PALATE

Imaging of the lips is performed in the coronary plane, showing: the tip of the nose, nostrils, upper and lower lip, chin, and tongue. By moving the probe toward the head, we can see the alveolar arch, tooth buds, and palate **(Figs. 15 to 21)**.

The most common facial cranial defect that we can diagnose prenatally with ultrasound is cleft lip and palate.

Imaging of the lip and palate is performed in 2D ultrasonography according to standards. However, if we have the option of additional three-dimensional (3D) imaging, it is also helpful. Sensitivity of the test 2D and 3D in the diagnosis of cleft are similar, although in some cases 3D examination is more sensitive. However, these differences are small, between 2 and 5%[10] **(Figs. 22 and 23)**.

▪ TECHNICAL DIFFICULTIES IN THREE-DIMENSIONAL IMAGING

The condition for 3D imaging is the correct position of the fetus and the right amount of amniotic fluid.

Imaging difficulties can be caused by **(Fig. 24)**:[5,8]
- Oligohydramnios/insufficient amniotic fluid over the fetus's face

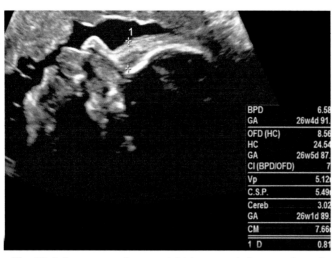

Fig. 10: Enlargement of prenasal thickness and absence of nasal bone—markers of trisomy 21.

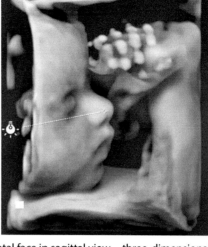

Fig. 13: Fetal face in sagittal view—three-dimensional (3D) view.

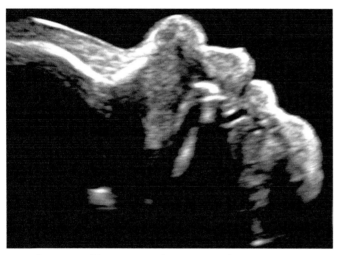

Fig. 11: Fetal face in sagittal view—two-dimensional (2D).

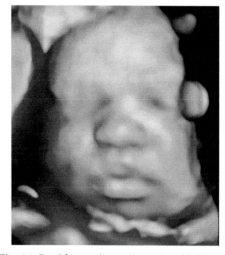

Fig. 14: Fetal face—three-dimensional (3D) view.

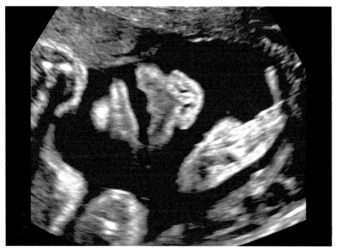

Fig. 12: Fetal mouth imaging—two-dimensional (2D) view.

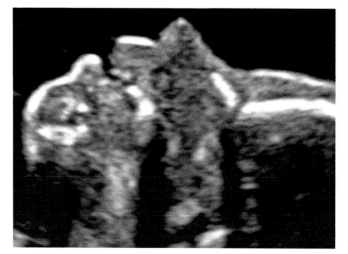

Fig. 15: Sagittal view of the fetal face.

- "Low-reaching" head or other unfavorable positioning of the fetus
- Umbilical cord loops above the fetus's face
- Fetal hands covering the face.

In 3D imaging, we use the rendering function as well. To select individual elements of face we can also use the magic-cut function.

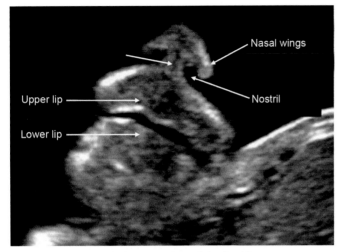

Fig. 16: Coronary view of the fetal face.

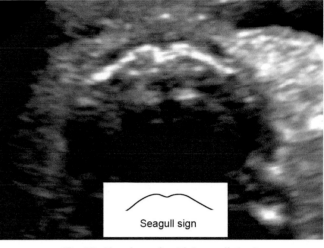

Fig. 19: Alveolar arch with "seagull sign".

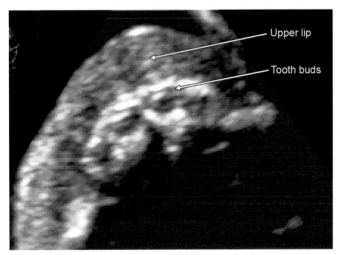

Fig. 17: Axial view of the fetal face.

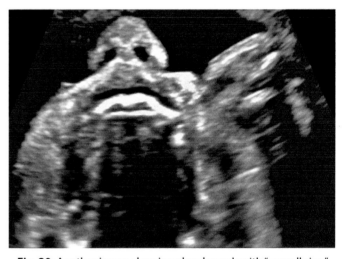

Fig. 20: Another image showing alveolar arch with "seagull sign".

■ EYE SOCKET IMAGING

The measurements of the distance between the eye sockets are associated with the concepts of hypo- and hypertelorism. To recognize them we should measure the interocular and binocular distances **(Fig. 26)**. After 20th week of pregnancy we can visualize: a transparent, round lens in the eye socket, muscle fibers, optic nerve, and yolk artery[11] **(Figs. 27 to 29)**.

Hypertelorism

- Aneuploidic syndrome (TR 21,13, 45X)
- *Nonaneuploidic syndrome*:
  - Aarskog syndrome
  - Apert syndrome
  - Crouzon syndrome
  - DiGeorge syndrome
  - Ehlers–Danlos syndrome
  - Frontonasal dysplasia
  - Greig syndrome
  - Gorlin syndrome
  - LEOPARD syndrome

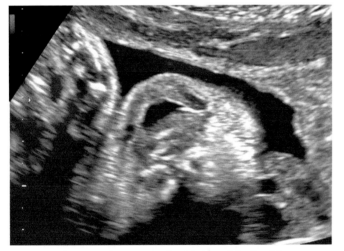

Fig. 18: Another image of axial view of the fetal face.

The latest improvement in 3D technique is 3D-HD imaging. The image obtained in this projection reflects natural colors and is very similar to visualization in fetoscopy. Changing the "light" setting during the examination may turn out to be a new direction in 3D research **(Fig. 25)**.

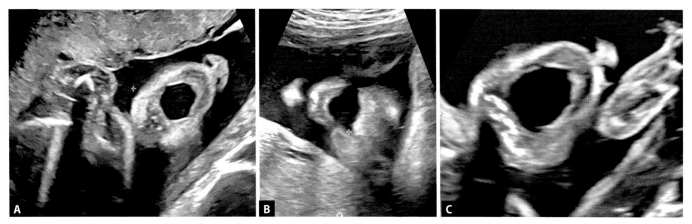

Figs. 21A to C: Fetus mouth imaging at 27 weeks of pregnancy.

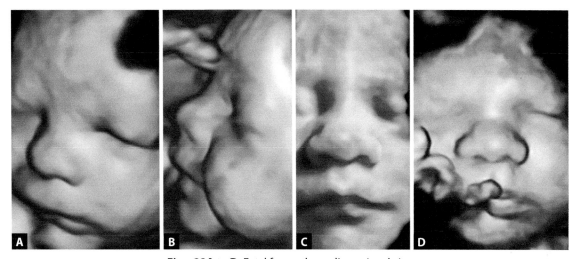

Figs. 22A to D: Fetal face—three-dimensional view.

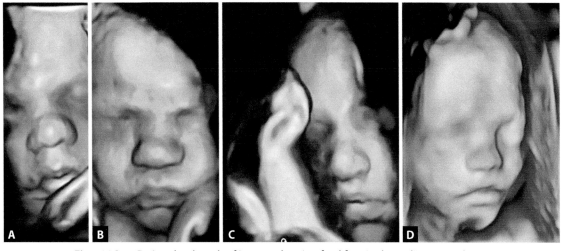

Figs. 23A to D: Another bunch of images showing fetal face in three-dimensional view.

- Loeys–Dietz syndrome (LDS)
- Mucopolysaccharidoses
- Morquio syndrome
- Neu–Laxova syndrome (NLS)
- Noonan syndrome
- Saethre-Chotzen syndrome
- Sotos syndrome
- Weaver syndrome
- Wolf-Hirschhorn syndrome

In cases of eyeball reduction or lack thereof, we can recognize microphthalmia (small eyes) or anophthalmia (no eyeball). Microphthalmia is observed in Fraser's syndrome (associated with mental retardation—prenatal diagnosis is very difficult), and in some cases it is a "genetic

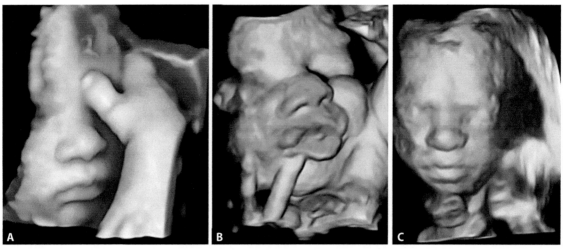

Figs. 24A to C: Difficulties in three-dimensional (3D) fetal face imaging.

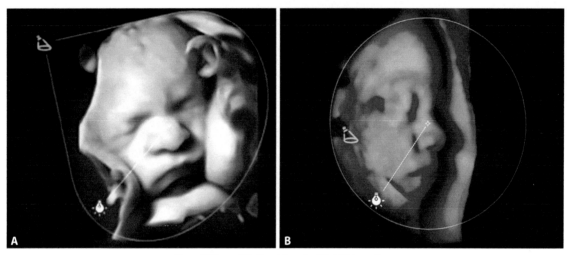

Figs. 25A and B: Fetal face in 3D-HD imaging.

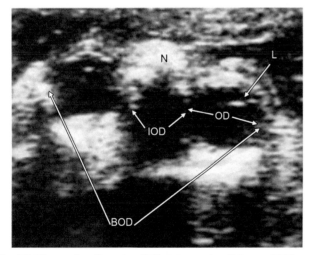

Fig. 26: The ocular diameter (OD), interocular distance (IOD), and binocular distance (BOD) are demonstrated in this scan. The lens (L) is visible in the eye. (N: nasal process)

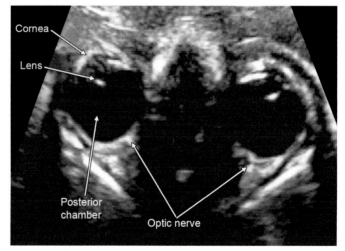

Fig. 27: Orbit and lens ultrasound imaging of the eye.

beauty" that occurs in the family, without changes in the brain.

Orbital imaging and visualization of the lenses in the eyeball provide opportunities in the diagnosis of congenital cataracts from 14th week of pregnancy. Congenital cataracts are also associated with chromosomal aberrations, mainly with trisomy 13, and may also be a symptom of cytomegalovirus (CMV) infection, rubella, and toxoplasmosis.[1-3]

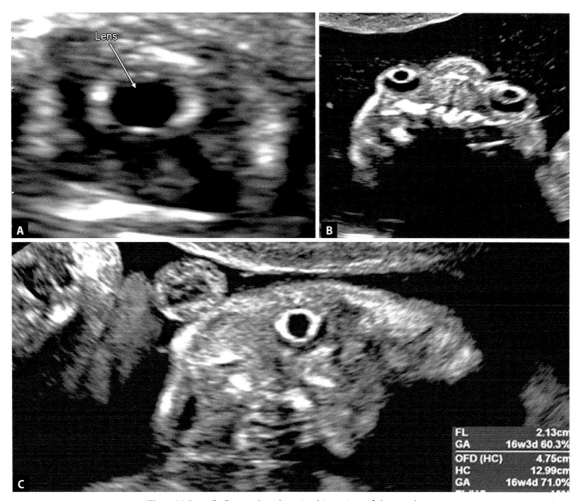

Figs. 28A to C: Coronal and sagittal imaging of the eye lens.

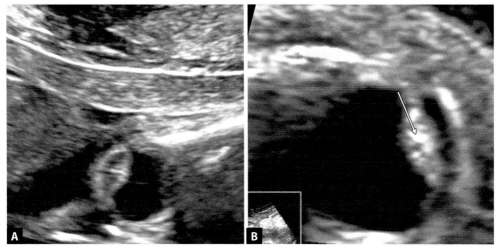

Figs. 29A and B: Congenital cataract with hyperechogenic lens—sagittal view.

Due to the very rare occurrence, prenatal diagnosis as an isolated defect is very difficult **(Figs. 30 and 32)**. Cataracts can be caused by:

- Idiopathic (~50%)
- Hereditary, e.g.:
  - Down syndrome
  - Trisomy 13
  - Lowe syndrome
- Marfan syndrome
- Arthrogryposis
- Cerebro-oculo-facio-skeletal (COFS) syndrome
- Roberts syndrome
- Chondrodysplasia
- Neu–Laxova syndrome
- Smith–Lemli–Opitz syndrome
- Branchio-oculo-facial syndrome

- Infection, e.g., rubella, varicella zoster virus (VZV), CMV, herpes simplex virus (HSV), and toxoplasmosis
- Metabolic, e.g., galactokinase deficiency, and homocystinuria.

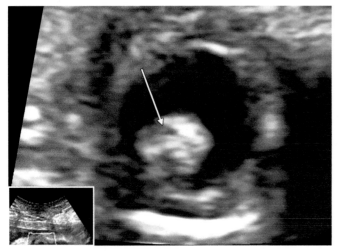

Fig. 30: Congenital cataract in coronal view.

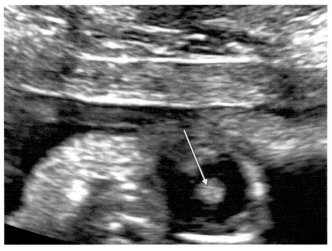

Fig. 31: Congenital cataract in coronal view.

Tear Bag Cyst (Dacryocystocele)

Dacryocystocele: It is a rare variant of a relatively common congenital nasolacrimal duct obstruction, accounting for only 0.1% of infants with congenital nasolacrimal duct obstruction[11] **(Fig. 33)**.

■ IMAGING OF THE LANGUAGE

The language can be represented by an axial and sagittal plane.

Macroglossia (enlargement of the tongue) may be caused by a wide variety of congenital and acquired conditions.

The most common causes are: Beckwith–Wiedemann syndrome and chromosomal aberration: mainly in Down syndrome.

However, the ultrasound recognition of the enlarged tongue over time is not entirely true. Partially sticking out or not, the hiding tongue we see during the ultrasound is not always associated with its enlargement. In the case of Beckwith–Wiedemans syndrome, the enlargement of the tongue is true because the lips are too small to hide it freely. In cases of chromosomal aberrations, these magnification is not always associated with the lip line and the exposure beyond the lip line is associated with hypotonia **(Figs. 34 and 35)**.[1-4,9] In such cases we can also observe a flattening and reduction of the auricle.

■ HAIR

In ultrasound imaging, the deposition of mineral syntaxes in amniotic fluid on the hair of the fetus is shown as a hyperechoic layer. This layer can be imaged from the 30th week of pregnancy (best visible after the 34th week of pregnancy), and in some cases even after the 20th week of pregnancy **(Fig. 36)**.

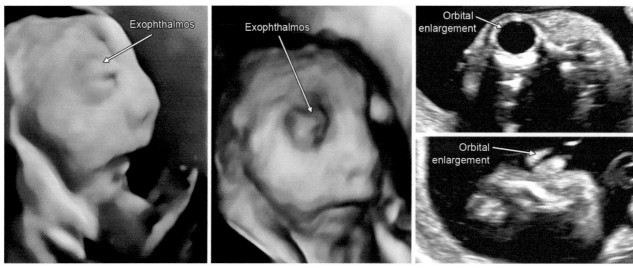

Fig. 32: Exophthalmos and orbital enlargement—2D and 3D.

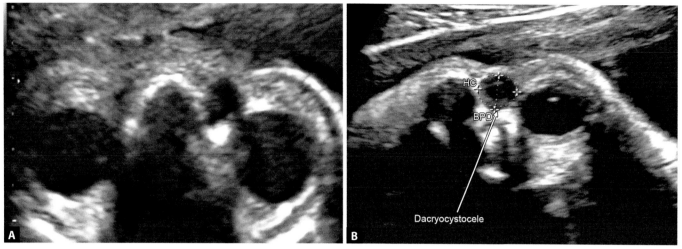

Figs. 33A and B: Dacryocystocele. (BPD: biparietal diameter)

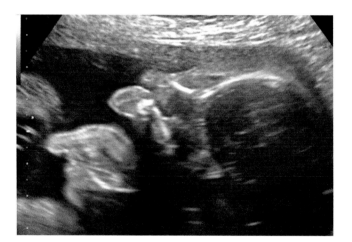

Fig. 34: Macroglossia—two-dimensional (2D) imaging.

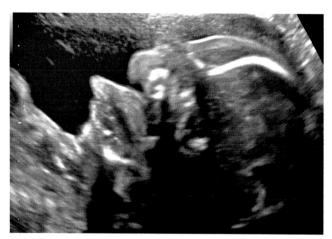

Fig. 35: Another image of macroglossia in two-dimensional (2D) imaging.

CLEFT LIP AND PALATE

The first classifications of lip and palate clefts in ultrasonography were published in 1995 by Nyberg.[3] This classification did not differentiate between alveolar cleft and hard palate cleft.

In recent years, prenatal detection of lip cleft and palate cleft in the low-risk population reaches 23–58%, and the detection of isolated cleft without lip cleft is close to zero. In high-risk pregnancies, the detection rate for lip cleft is 80–90% and for cleft palate, once lip cleft is detected, the detection rate is up to 97% **(Fig. 37)**.

In fetuses with cleft lips and palates, other developmental defects accompany about 50–60%, most often with chromosomal aberrations, heart defects, foot deformities, and additional toes. The risk of cleft occurrence in the fetus, when one of the parents has this defect, increases by about 5%, while for both parents it increases to about 60% **(Figs. 38 to 41)**.

Common Forms of Cleft Lip and Palate

- *Group I:*[4,9,12]
  - *Upper lip clefts:*
    - Subcutaneous-submucosal (unilateral)
    - Partial (middle)
    - Total (two-sided)
- *Group II:*
  - *Clefts of the upper lip and alveolar process:*
    - Subcutaneous-subcutaneous (unilateral)
    - Partial (middle)
    - Total - to the ashesal opening (two-sided)
- *Group III:*
  - *Clefts of the palate:*
    - Submucosal
    - Partial soft
    - Total soft
    - Total soft and partial hard
    - Total hard and soft (to the incisive foramen)

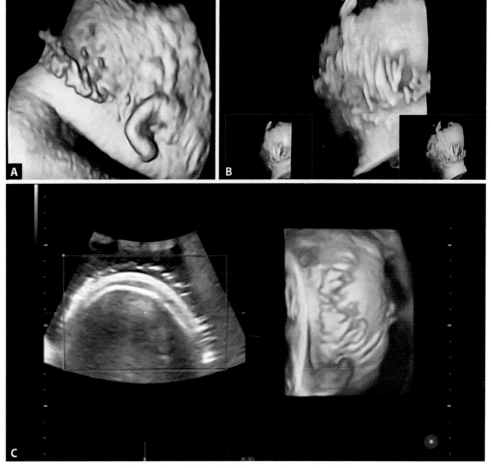

Figs. 36A to C: Fetal hair in two-dimensional view.

- *Group IV:*
  - *Clefts of the upper lip, alveolar process, and the palate:*
    - Unilateral
    - Bilateral
- *Group V:*
  - Combination clefts.

Group I—Lip Cleft: Hidden, Partial, and Total (Cheiloschisis: Oculta, Partialis, and Totalis)

Depending on the severity of the developmental defect, the continuity of tissues within the skin, the circular muscle of the mouth and mucous membrane is interrupted. In one-sided form, the cleft line runs laterally from the midline of the body. A cleft includes part or all of the height of the lip. There is also subcutaneous-subcutaneous-mucosal cleft, the so-called hidden cleft, which only affects the circular muscle of the mouth. Lip cleft causes disorders in its normal anatomical system. The activity of the lip is impaired. In a double-sided lip cleft, a discontinuation occurs on both sides of the gutter. As a result, the upper lip is divided into three parts. The middle part contains the prolabium and the two lateral sections of the lip.

In the sagittal plane, the assimilated labial red is visible beyond the lip line (most often in connection with the nose, no possibility of imaging the correct post in case of bilateral clefts) and the nose is flattened. In the coronary plane, there is a visible loss of lip continuity. In the axial plane, there is a visible loss of lip continuity, the emphasis of the labial red and flattened nostrils with wings of normal anatomy.

In the axial plane, a visible cleavage covering the peritoneal bone (the protrusion of the peritoneal bone with red lips) or reaching it with a displacement of the jaw plane. In the coronary plane, there is no continuity of the alveolar arch.

In the sagittal and parasagittal planes, there is no continuity of the hard palate and hyperechoic vomer.

In the axial plane, the most common is the lack of continuity in the bilateral cleft and the hyperechoic vomer. In the coronary plane, a visible cleft with uneven palate surfaces and a blade supported on the damaged part—a one-sided cleft, and in the case of a two-sided cleft, there is no possibility of imaging the hard palate—a vomer without visible support.

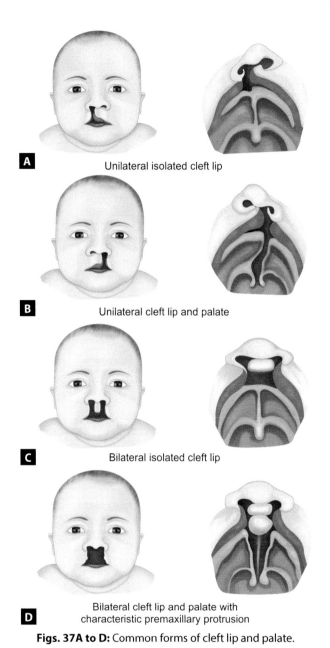

Figs. 37A to D: Common forms of cleft lip and palate.

A — Unilateral isolated cleft lip

B — Unilateral cleft lip and palate

C — Bilateral isolated cleft lip

D — Bilateral cleft lip and palate with characteristic premaxillary protrusion

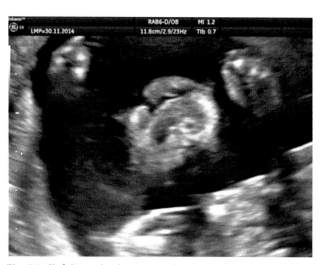

Fig. 39: Cleft lip and palate—two-dimensional ultrasonography.

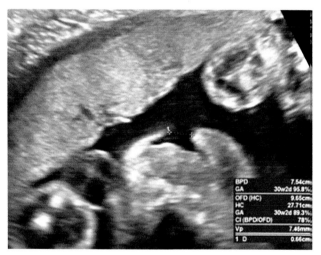

Fig. 40: Cleft lip and palate—two-dimensional ultrasonography.

Group II—Lip and Alveolar Cleft: Hidden, Partialis, and Totalis (Cheiloschisis: Oculta, Partialis, and Totalis)

In this form, the lip and alveolar process are split into the incisive foramen. This group of clefts is characterized by significant displacement of the lip and alveolar process. In one-sided forms, part of the lip from the prolabium and part of the alveolar process of a larger section containing the peritoneal bone are displaced forward and upwards in a healthy direction. A defective jaw and vomer arrangement, which supports the skeleton of the nose, leads to a significant disturbance in its shape.

In one-sided forms, part of the lip from the prolabium and part of the alveolar process of a larger section containing the peritoneal bone are displaced forward and upward in a healthy direction. A defective jaw and blade arrangement, which supports the skeleton of the nose, leads to a significant disturbance in its shape.

In the bilateral clefts, the peritoneal bone and the prolabium are protruded forward. There is a significant functional and esthetic disturbance of the face.

Fig. 38: Cleft lip and palate—two-dimensional ultrasonography.

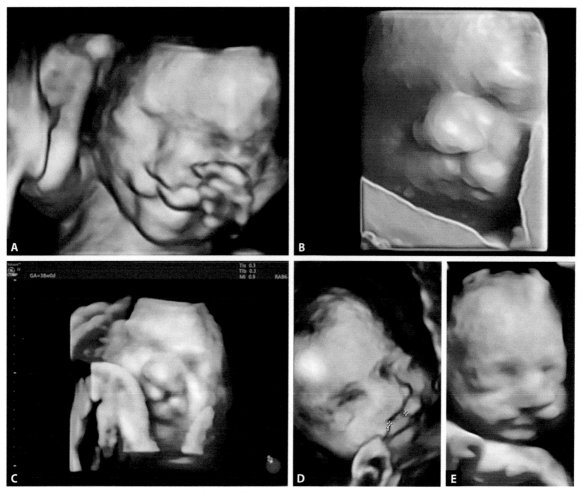

Figs. 41A to E: Cleft lip and palate—three-dimensional ultrasonography.

Group III—Hard and Soft Palate Cleft: Hidden, Partial, and Total (Uranostaphyloschisis: Oculta, Partialis, and Totalis)

In palate cleft, there is a lack of continuity of tissues within the oral cavity mucosa and nasal mucosa and a discontinuity of bone that reaches to the incisive foramen. In the hidden form of a cleft, only the continuity of the palate muscles is broken.

Group IV—Lip, Alveolar Process, and Palate Cleft (Cheilognathouranostaphyloschisis)

In the unilateral forms of clefts of the upper lip, alveolar process and palate, the anatomical continuity of the tissues within the upper lip, nasal fundus, alveolar process, and palate is broken, dividing the lip and jaw into two unequal parts. The larger section includes the lateral side of the lip, the prolabium with a philtrum and Cupid's bow, the alveolar process with the peritoneal bone and the palate connected in the line of the palatal suture with the vomer. The smaller section contains the remaining lip, alveolar process, and palate.

Anatomical abnormalities in this form of cleft are characterized primarily by a cleft gap whose width varies from 0.3 to 3 cm and displacement of the lip, alveolar process, and palate in relation to three spatial planes. The larger section of the lip within the prolabium is displaced upward and forward together with the bone base. There is a significant vertical shortening of the lip, and the lip philtrum runs obliquely. The outline of Cupid's bow is distorted.

■ FACE AND NECK TUMORS

We can also diagnose lesions that occur very rarely, e.g., changes in the interorbital region—a tumor arising from the ethmoid bone **(Fig. 42)** and changes in the neck (thyroid goiter, lymphatic angioma) **(Fig. 43)** as well as changes in the lips [epulis or edema of the incisive bone—**(Fig. 44)**].

- *Facial tumors:*
  - *Mouth:*
    - Sarcoma, gingival granuloma, and Neumann's tumor (epulis)
    - Oropharyngeal teratoma (epignathus)
  - *Nasal cavity:*
    - Teratoma
  - *Cheek and soft tissues:*
    - Hemangioma
    - Rhabdomyosarcoma

- Cerebral hernia (encephalocele)
- Lymphangioma and vascular hamartoma
- *Neck tumors:*
  - Teratoma
  - Goiter

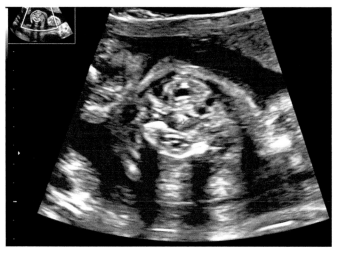

Fig. 42: Tumor arising from the ethmoid bone.

- Lymphangiomas
- Hemangiomas.

MANDIBULAR RETRACTION (MICROGNATHIA)

Micrognathia, or mandibular retraction, is a result of mandibular hypoplasia occurring between 6 and 7 weeks of pregnancy. Isolated micrognathia is rare and is associated with family, constitutional factors. In most cases, it is associated with other malformations and chromosomal aberrations. Usually we recognize micrognathia between 18 and 22th week of gestation but in some cases, there is a possibility of imaging it in the first trimester **(Figs. 45 to 49)**.[5,6,13]

- *Syndromes with micrognathia:*
  - Achondrogenesis
  - Amniotic band syndrome (ABS)
  - Atelosteogenesis
  - Campomelic dysplasia
  - Carpenter's syndrome
  - Cornelia de Lange Syndrome (CdLS)

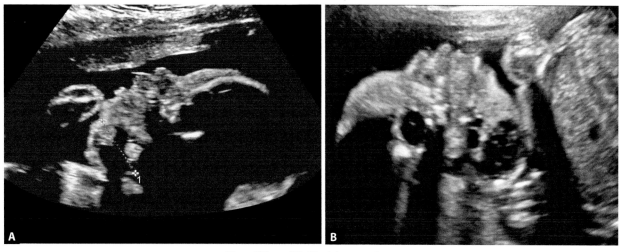

Figs. 43A and B: Neck hemangioma.

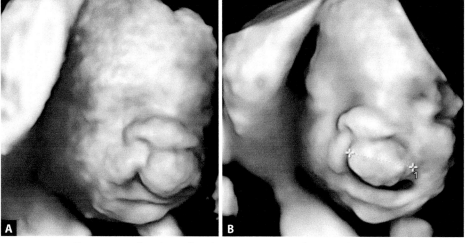

Figs. 44A and B: Craniofacial tumor—growing from the fetus's lips.

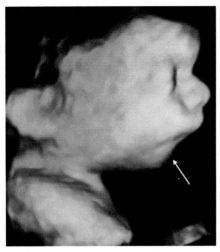

Fig. 45: Micrognathia—three-dimensional view.

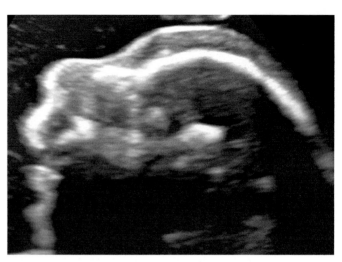

Fig. 48: Micrognathia—two-dimensional view.

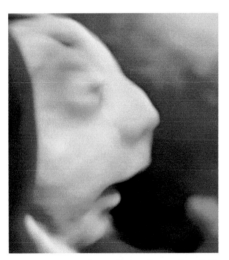

Fig. 46: Micrognathia—three-dimensional view.

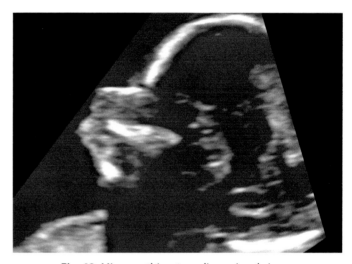

Fig. 49: Micrognathia—two-dimensional view.

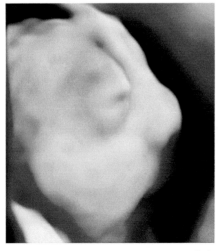

Fig. 47: Micrognathia—three-dimensional view.

- Crouzon syndrome
- Jacobsen syndrome (11q terminal deletion disorder)
- Wolf-Hirschhorn syndrome
- Fryns syndrome
- Goldenhar syndrome (GS)
- Joubert syndrome
- Meckel–Gruber syndrome
- Nager syndrome
- Neu-Laxova syndrome
- Mohr syndrome
- CHARGE team (coloboma, heart anomaly, anal atresia, retardation, and genital and ear anomalies)
- Pena-Shokeir syndrome
- Pierre Robin syndrome
- Roberts syndrome
- Seckel syndrome
- Shprintzen syndrome

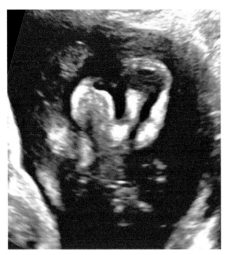

Fig. 50: Healthy fetal ears.

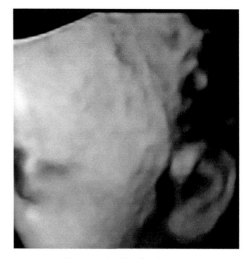

Fig. 52: Healthy fetal ears.

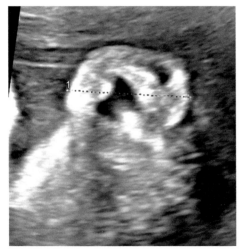

Fig. 51: Healthy fetal ears.

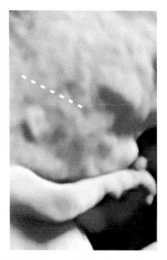

Fig. 53: Hypoplastic—low set ears.

- Smith–Lemli–Opitz syndrome
- Thrombocytopenia
- Treacher Collins syndrome
- Triploidy
- Trisomy 10
- Trisomy 18
- Trisomy 9
- *Pierre Robin syndrome is characterized by the triad of symptoms:*
  - Palate cleft
  - Micrognathia
  - Glossoptosis
- *Differential diagnosis:* trisomy 13, 18, otocephalia.
- *Otocephalia:*
  - Abnormal development of the auricles, very low ears set forward
  - Always associated with micrognathia or agnathia
  - Absence of the mandible
  - Hypo- or hypertelorism

- Central eye
- Proboscis
- Holoprosencephalia
- Cephalocele
- Tracheoesophageal fistula
- Heart defects
- Situs inversus
- Kidney malformations
- Adrenal hypoplasia
- Single umbilical artery (SUA)
- Rib defects.

■ IMAGING THE EAR

The ear grows linearly with gestational age, its length is one-third of the biparietal diameter (BPD). It has been shown that reduced size (<0.8), flattened shape and low-set ears correlate with trisomy 21—75–98% **(Figs. 50 to 55)**.[5,8,14]

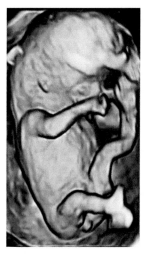

Fig. 54: Hypoplastic—low set ears.

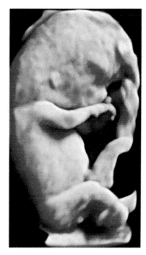

Fig. 55: Hypoplastic—low set ears.

■ REFERENCES

1. Nyberg DA, McGahan JP, Pretorius DH, Pilu G. Diagnostic Imaging of Fetal Anomalies. Philadelphia: Lippincott, Williams and Wilkins; 2003. pp. 335-80.
2. Callen PW. Ultrasonography in Obstetrics and Gynecology. Philadelphia: Saunders Elsevier; 2008. pp. 392-418.
3. Nyberg DA, Sickler GH, Hegge FN, Kramer DJ, Kropp RJ. Fetal cleft lip with and without cleft palate: US classification and correlation with outcome. Radiology. 1995;195:677-84.
4. Maarse W, Bergé SJ, Pistorius L, van Barneveld T, Kon M, Breugem C, et al. Diagnostic accuracy of transabdominal ultrasound in detecting prenatal cleft lip and palate: a systematic review. Ultrasound Obstet Gynecol. 2010;35: 495-502.
5. Pietryga M. Ultrasonografia w ginekologii i położnictwie. Wydawnictwo Exemplum. 2020 ISBN: 9788362690473.
6. Kurjak A, Azumendi G, Andonotopo W, Salihagic-Kadic A. Three- and four-dimensional ultrasonography for the structural and functional evaluation of the fetal face. Am J Obstet Gynecol. 2007;196(1):16-28.
7. Maarse W, Pistorius LR, van Eeten WK. Prenatal ultrasound screening for orofacial clefts. Ultrasound Obstet Gynecol. 2011;38:434-9.
8. Mak ASL, Leung KY. Prenatal ultrasonography of craniofacial abnormalities. Ultrasonography. 2019;38(1):13-24.
9. Yoon A, Pham B, Dipple K. Genetic screening in patients with craniofacial malformations. J Pediatr Genet. 2016;(4):220-4.
10. Goldstein I, Tamir A, Weiner Z. Dimensions of the fetal facial profile in normal pregnancy. Ultrasound Obstet Gynecol. 2010;35:191-4.
11. Vilaplana F, Muiños SJ, Nadal J, et al. Stickler syndrome. Epidemiology of retinal detachment. Arch Soc Esp Oftalmol. 2015;90:264-8.
12. Tessier P. Classification of rare craniofacial clefts. J Maxillofac Surg. 1976;4(2):69-92.
13. Sepulveda W, Wong AE, Viñals F. Absent mandibular gap in the retronasal triangle view: a clue to the diagnosis of micrognathia in the first trimester. Ultrasound Obstet Gynecol. 2012;39:152-6.
14. Haratz K, Viñals F, Lev D. Fetal optic nerve sheath measurement as a non-invasive tool for assessment of increased intracranial pressure. Ultrasound Obstet Gynecol. 2011;38:646-51.
15. Maymon R, Levinsohn-Tavor O, Cuckle H, Tovbin Y, Dreazen E, Wiener Y, et al. Second trimester ultrasound prenasal thickness combined with nasal bone length: a new method of Down syndrome screening. Prenat Diagn. 2005;25:906-11.
16. Krysta L. Chirurgia szczękowo-twarzowa. Warszawa PZWL; 1993: 360-406.

Three-dimensional Reconstruction of Normal Fetal Heart and Congenital Heart Disease

Toshiyuki Hata, Aya Koyanagi, Riko Takayoshi, Takahito Miyake, Kenji Kanenishi

■ INTRODUCTION

There have been numerous studies on three-dimensional (3D)/four-dimensional (4D) reconstruction of the normal fetal heart and congenital heart disease (CHD) using real-time 3D ultrasound,[1-3] B-flow,[4] HDlive,[5,6] HDlive silhouette,[7] inversion mode,[8,9] and color Doppler.[10,11] However, the image quality and resolution of these techniques were unsatisfactory.

HDlive Flow utilizes an adjustable light source to create lighting and shadowing effects to increase depth perception in 3D/4D color/power Doppler.[12,13] The use of HDlive Flow to increase the resolution of 3D/4D color/power Doppler leads to a significant improvement compared with previous 3D/4D techniques for reconstruction of the fetal heart, facilitating clear visualization of the normal fetal heart and CHD.[13-15] HDlive Flow silhouette is the further advanced technology to present vitreous-like clarity of fetal cardiovascular blood flow, and has the ability to preserve and delineate the outline and borders of blood flow, while showing its core as semitransparent.[13] Therefore, it is possible to obtain holographic images of cardiovascular blood flow, being its most unique feature.[13,16,17] In the last 5 years, numerous studies on HDlive Flow (silhouette) with spatiotemporal image correlation (STIC) for evaluation of the normal fetal heart and CHD have been published.[12-29]

In this chapter, we present the latest state-of-the-art HDlive Flow (silhouette) with STIC of the normal fetal heart and CHD. We also discuss the present and future applicability of this novel technique to evaluate the normal fetal cardiac structure and diagnose CHD.

■ NORMAL FETAL HEART

With the frontal view, the spatial relationships among the right atrium with superior vena cava and inferior vena cava can be realized **(Fig. 1)**. The target of the frontal view is to

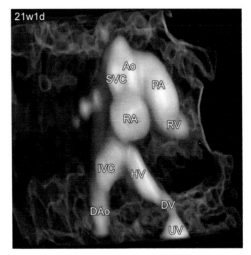

Fig. 1: Frontal view with HDlive Flow of a normal fetal heart at 21 weeks and 1 day of gestation.
(Ao: aorta; DAo: descending aorta; DV: ductus venosus; HV: hepatic vein; IVC: inferior vena cava; PA: pulmonary artery; RA: right atrium; RV: right ventricle; SVC: superior vena cava; UV: umbilical vein)

assess the inflow view of the right atrium (both superior vena cava and inferior vena cava to the right atrium). With the spatial three-vessel view, the relationships and course of the outflow tracts (crisscross arrangements of the pulmonary artery and aorta) and superior vena cava can be evaluated **(Figs. 2 and 3)**. The panoramic view demonstrates spatial relationships among the cardiac chambers and vessels, facilitating visualization of the relationships and course of the out- and inflow tracts **(Fig. 4)**. The panoramic view is a left, oblique, and lateral view, and we can clearly identify the ductal arch and descending aorta. With the posterior view, the vertical descending aorta is evident, and the right atrium with superior and inferior vena cava can be identified **(Fig. 5)**. With the right lateral view, the aortic arch and descending aorta, superior vena cava, and inferior vena cava can be clearly realized **(Figs. 6 and 7)**. This view is unique for evaluating the aortic arch.

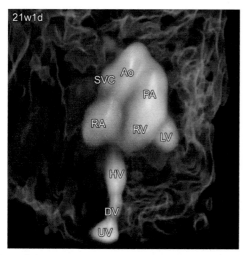

Fig. 2: Spatial three-vessel view with HDlive Flow of a normal fetal heart at 21 weeks and 1 day of gestation.
(Ao: aorta; DV: ductus venosus; HV: hepatic vessel; LV: left ventricle; PA: pulmonary artery; RA: right atrium; RV: right ventricle; SVC: superior vena cava; UV: umbilical vein)

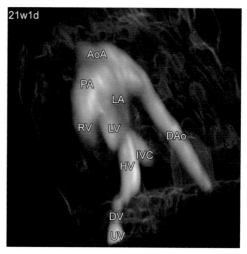

Fig. 4: Panoramic view with HDlive Flow of a normal fetal heart at 21 weeks and 1 day of gestation.
(AoA: aortic arch; DAo: descending aorta; DV: ductus venosus; HV: hepatic vein; IVC: inferior vena cava; LA: left atrium; LV: left ventricle; PA: pulmonary artery; RV: right ventricle; UV: umbilical vein)

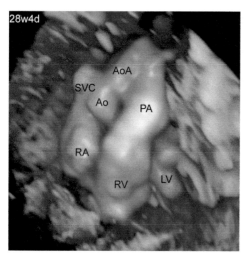

Fig. 3: Spatial three-vessel view with HDlive Flow of a normal fetal heart at 28 weeks and 4 days of gestation.
(Ao: aorta; AoA: aortic arch; LV: left ventricle; PA: pulmonary artery; RA: right atrium; RV: right ventricle; SVC: superior vena cava)

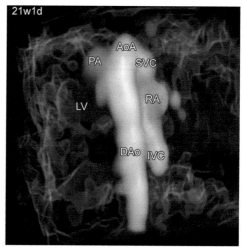

Fig. 5: Posterior view with HDlive Flow of a normal fetal heart at 21 weeks and 1 day of gestation.
(AoA: aortic arch; DAo: descending aorta; IVC: inferior vena cava; LV: left ventricle; PA: pulmonary artery; RA: right atrium; SVC: superior vena cava)

■ CONGENITAL HEART DISEASE

HDlive Flow (silhouette) with STIC facilitates an easier way to demonstrate spatial relationships among fetal cardiac chambers, great arteries, and veins. This technique also shows the size differences of great vessels, so we can easily understand complicated cardiac structures of CHD. HDlive Flow (silhouette) with STIC may be an adjunctive technology to conventional fetal echocardiography for the prenatal diagnosis of CHD. However, there may be a limitation regarding the use of HDlive Flow (silhouette) to diagnose some CHDs.

Right Aortic Arch[14,20,21]

Color Doppler showed the aortic arch on the right side of the trachea with ductus arteriosus on the left side of the trachea, connected by a vascular ring (Kommerell's diverticulum)

behind the trachea **(Fig. 8)**. Spatial three-vessel and right lateral views clearly depicted the typical vascular ring around the trachea at the level of the upper mediastinum **(Figs. 9 and 10)**.[21]

Ventricular Septal Defect

Ventricular septal defect (VSD) can be easily diagnosed using conventional color Doppler **(Fig. 11A)**. HDlive Flow may not provide any additional information for the diagnosis of VSD **(Fig. 11B)**.

Left Ventricular Diverticulum[16]

HDlive Flow revealed a hypoplastic right ventricle, left ventricular diverticulum, and left-sided single umbilical artery **(Fig. 12)**.

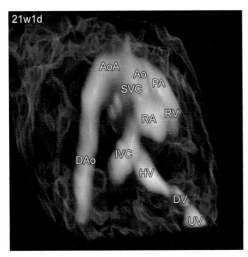

Fig. 6: Right lateral view with HDlive Flow of a normal fetal heart at 21 weeks and 1 day of gestation.
(Ao: aorta; AoA: aortic arch; DAo: descending aorta; DV: ductus venosus; HV: hepatic vein; IVC: inferior vena cava; RA: right atrium; RV: right ventricle; SVC: superior vena cava; UV: umbilical vein)

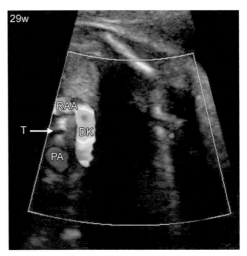

Fig. 8: Color Doppler image at 29 weeks of gestation in a case of right aortic arch (RAA). Three-vessel trachea view shows the vascular ring around the trachea (T) formed by the pulmonary artery (PA), RAA, and diverticulum of Kommerell (DK).

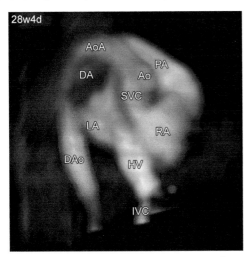

Fig. 7: Right lateral view with HDlive Flow silhouette of a normal fetal heart at 28 weeks and 4 days of gestation.
(Ao: aorta; AoA: aortic arch; DA: ductus arteriosus; DAo: descending aorta; HV: hepatic vein; IVC: inferior vena cava; LA: left atrium; PA: pulmonary artery; RA: right atrium; SVC: superior vena cava)

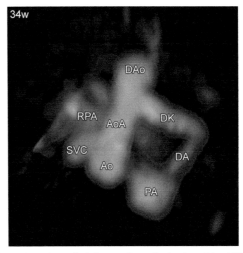

Fig. 9: Superior view of right aortic arch depicted by HDlive Flow silhouette at 34 weeks of gestation.
(Ao: aorta; AoA: aortic arch; DA: ductus arteriosus; DAo: descending aorta; DK: diverticulum of Kommerell; PA: pulmonary artery; RPA: right pulmonary artery; SVC: superior vena cava)
Source: Reprinted with permission from Jaypee Brothers Medical Publishers (P) Ltd.[21]

Pulmonary Stenosis with Poststenotic Dilatation[13]

Conventional color Doppler depicted the size differences of the aorta and pulmonary artery, and aliasing of pulmonary stenosis (PS) flow **(Fig. 13)**. A panoramic view using HDlive Flow clearly showed a large main pulmonary artery due to poststenotic dilatation **(Fig. 14)**. This technique also demonstrated the size differences of the aorta and pulmonary artery.

Hypoplastic Left Heart Syndrome[13]

Two-dimensional (2D) sonography clearly showed a diminutive left ventricle **(Fig. 15)**. A significant size difference could be identified on a spatial three-vessel

view between the pulmonary artery and aorta **(Fig. 16)**. With a panoramic view, a very small ascending aorta and tear-drop-shaped heart were noted **(Fig. 17)**. A difference in size between the aortic arch and descending aorta could also be demonstrated. Lighting and shadowing effects could create an angiographic image due to increased depth perception **(Fig. 17)**.

Transposition of Great Arteries[13,28]

Color Doppler showed the parallel arrangement of great arteries **(Fig. 18)**.[28] HDlive Flow clearly demonstrated an aorta leaving the right ventricle and a pulmonary artery leaving the left ventricle in parallel **(Figs. 19 to 21)**.[28]

In another case, HDlive Flow clearly showed the spatial parallel arrangement of the aorta left from the right ventricle and the pulmonary artery left from the left ventricle **(Figs. 22 to 24)**. With a spatial three-vessel view, the order of pulmonary artery, aorta, and superior vena cava from left to right was evident **(Fig. 22)**. With a superior view, the entire running of the aortic arch and left and right pulmonary arteries could be noted **(Fig. 23)**. With a panoramic view, the aortic arch and neck vessels could be clearly identified **(Fig. 24)**.

Double Outlet Right Ventricle[27]

Color Doppler showed a small pulmonary artery, and the parallel arrangement of great arteries **(Fig. 25)**.[27] HDlive Flow clearly demonstrated a large aorta and small pulmonary artery leaving the right ventricle in parallel **(Fig. 26)**.[27]

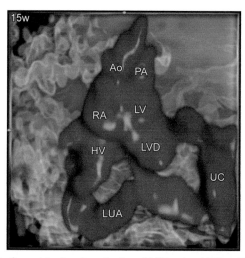

Fig. 12: Left ventricular diverticulum (LVD) using HDlive Flow at 15 weeks of gestation.
(Ao: aorta; HV: hepatic vein; LUA: left umbilical artery; LV: left ventricle; PA: pulmonary artery; RA: right atrium; UC: umbilical cord)

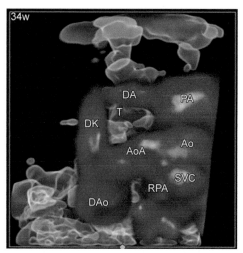

Fig. 10: Right lateral view of right aortic arch depicted by HDlive Flow at 34 weeks of gestation.
(Ao: aorta; AoA: aortic arch; DA: ductus arteriosus; DAo: descending aorta; DK: diverticulum of Kommerell; PA: pulmonary artery; RPA: right pulmonary artery; SVC: superior vena cava; T: trachea)

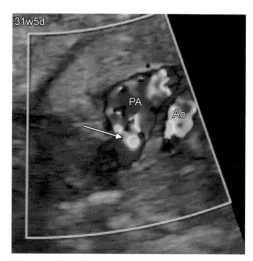

Fig. 13: Color Doppler of pulmonary stenosis (PS) with poststenotic dilatation at 31 weeks and 5 days of gestation. The size differences of the aorta (Ao) and pulmonary artery (PA), and aliasing of PS flow (arrow) can be clearly noted.

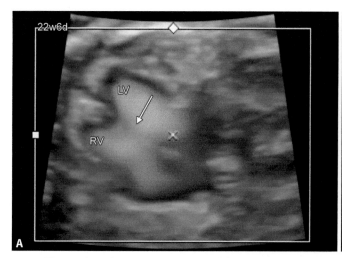

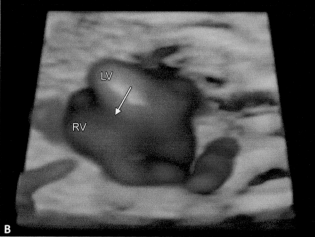

Figs. 11A and B: Ventricular septal defect (arrows) at 22 weeks and 6 days of gestation. (A) Color Doppler; (B) HDlive Flow.
(LV: left ventricle; RV: right ventricle)

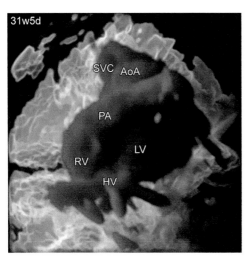

Fig. 14: A markedly large main pulmonary artery (PA) due to poststenotic dilatation is clearly demonstrated using HDlive Flow. (AoA: aortic arch; HV: hepatic vein; LV: left ventricle; RV: right ventricle; SVC: superior vena cava)

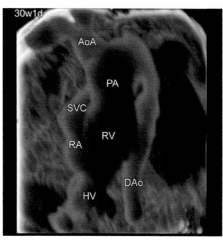

Fig. 17: Panoramic view with HDlive Flow of hypoplastic left heart syndrome at 30 weeks and 1 day of gestation. The size differences between the aortic arch (AoA) and pulmonary artery (PA) is evident. (DAo: descending aorta; HV: hepatic vein; RA: right atrium; RV: right ventricle; SVC: superior vena cava)

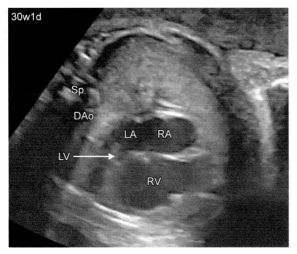

Fig. 15: Four-chamber view of hypoplastic left heart syndrome. (DAo: descending aorta; LA: left atrium; LV: left ventricle; RA: right atrium; RV: right ventricle; Sp: spine)

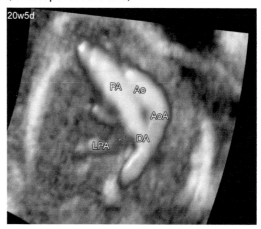

Fig. 18: Parallel arrangement of great arteries in a case of transposition of great arteries at 20 weeks and 5 days of gestation using color Doppler. (Ao: aorta; AoA: aortic arch; DA: ductus arteriosus; LPA: left pulmonary artery; PA: pulmonary artery)
Source: Reprinted with permission from Jaypee Brothers Medical Publishers (P) Ltd.[28]

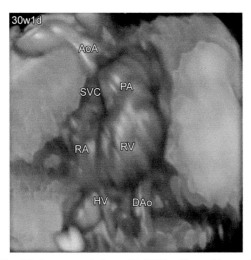

Fig. 16: Spatial three-vessel view with HDlive Flow of hypoplastic left heart syndrome at 30 weeks and 1 day of gestation. The size differences between the aortic arch (AoA) and pulmonary artery (PA) is evident. (DAo: descending aorta; HV: hepatic vein; RA: right atrium; RV: right ventricle; SVC: superior vena cava)

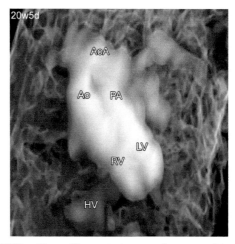

Fig. 19: HDlive Flow silhouette image of transposition of great arteries at 20 weeks and 5 days of gestation. Parallel arrangement of great arteries is clearly recognized. (Ao: aorta; AoA: aortic arch; HV: hepatic vein; LV: left ventricle; PA: pulmonary artery; RV: right ventricle)

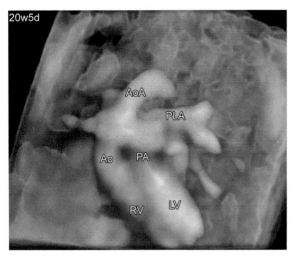

Fig. 20: HDlive Flow image of transposition of great arteries (spatial three-vessel view) at 20 weeks and 5 days of gestation. Parallel arrangement of great arteries is clearly recognized.
(Ao: aorta; AoA: aortic arch; LPA: left pulmonary artery; LV: left ventricle; PA: pulmonary artery; RV: right ventricle)

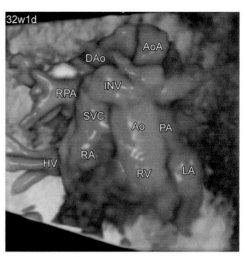

Fig. 22: Spatial three-vessel view with HDlive Flow of the transposition of great arteries at 32 weeks and 1 day of gestation. The spatial parallel arrangement of the aorta (Ao) left of the right ventricle (RV) and pulmonary artery (PA) left of the left ventricle (LV) can be clearly identified.
(AoA: aortic arch; DAo: descending aorta; HV: hepatic vein; INV: innominate vein; RA: right atrium; RPA: right pulmonary artery; SVC: superior vena cava)

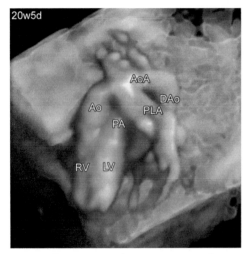

Fig. 21: HDlive Flow image of transposition of great arteries (panoramic view) at 20 weeks and 5 days of gestation. Parallel arrangement of great arteries is clearly recognized.
(Ao: aorta; AoA: aortic arch; DAo: descending aorta; LPA: left pulmonary artery; LV: left ventricle; PA: pulmonary artery; RV: right ventricle)
Source: Reprinted with permission from Jaypee Brothers Medical Publishers (P) Ltd.[28]

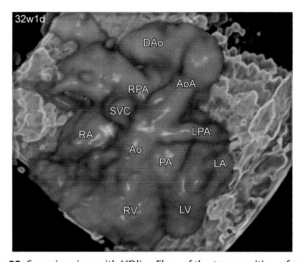

Fig. 23: Superior view with HDlive Flow of the transposition of great arteries at 32 weeks and 1 day of gestation. The spatial parallel arrangement of the aorta (Ao) left of the right ventricle (RV) and pulmonary artery (PA) left of the left ventricle (LV) is evident.
(AoA: aortic arch; DAo: descending aorta; LA: left atrium; LPA: left pulmonary artery; RA: right atrium; RPA: right pulmonary artery; SVC: superior vena cava)

Truncus Arteriosus[18]

Two-dimensional sonography revealed the presence of VSD with a single trunk **(Fig. 27)**. With a spatial three-vessel view, HDlive Flow clearly showed truncus arteriosus (TA) straddling both ventricles and giving rise to the aorta and pulmonary artery **(Fig. 28)**. With a superior view, the left and right pulmonary arteries, aortic arch, and descending aorta could also be distinguished using HDlive Flow silhouette **(Fig. 29)**.

In another case, color Doppler demonstrated VSD and a single trunk with the left pulmonary artery **(Fig. 30)**. With a superior view using HDlive Flow silhouette, TA straddling both ventricles and giving rise to the aorta and left and right pulmonary arteries could be clearly identified **(Fig. 31)**.

Persistent Left Superior Vena Cava[20]

With a three-vessel view using 2D sonography, persistent left superior vena cava (PLSVC) was noted on the left side of

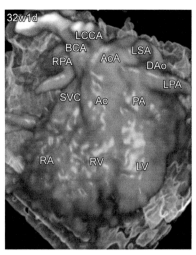

Fig. 24: Panoramic view with HDlive Flow of the transposition of great arteries at 32 weeks and 1 day of gestation.
(Ao: aorta; AoA: aortic arch; BCA: brachiocephalic artery; DAo: descending aorta; LCCA: left common carotid artery; LPA: left pulmonary artery; LSA: left subclavian artery; LV: left ventricle; PA: pulmonary artery; RA: right atrium; RV: right ventricle; RPA: right pulmonary artery; SVC: superior vena cava)

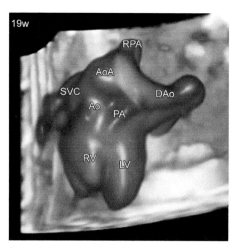

Fig. 26: HDlive Flow image of double outlet right ventricle (spatial three-vessel view) at 19 weeks of gestation. Parallel arrangement of great arteries is clearly recognized.
(Ao: aorta; AoA: aortic arch; DAo: descending artery; LV: left ventricle; PA: pulmonary artery; RPA: right pulmonary artery; RV: right ventricle; SVC: superior vena cava)
Source: Reprinted with permission from Jaypee Brothers Medical Publishers (P) Ltd.[27]

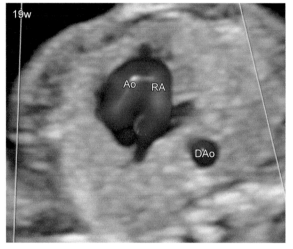

Fig. 25: Parallel arrangement of great arteries in a case of double outlet right ventricle at 19 weeks of gestation using color Doppler.
(Ao: aorta; DAo: descending aorta; PA: pulmonary artery)
Source: Reprinted with permission from Jaypee Brothers Medical Publishers (P) Ltd.[27]

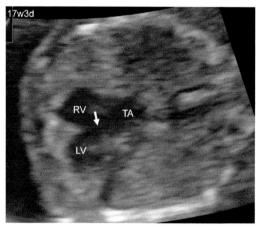

Fig. 27: Two-dimensional sonographic image of truncus arteriosus (TA) at 17 weeks and 3 days of gestation. Arrow indicates a large ventricular defect.
(LV: left ventricle; RV: right ventricle)

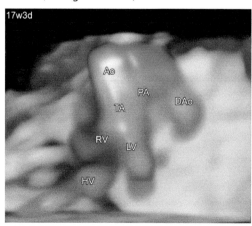

the pulmonary artery **(Fig. 32)**. With a four-chamber view, PLSVC was identified in the left atrium **(Fig. 33)**. The spatial three-vessel and panoramic views clearly demonstrated PLSVC on the left side of the pulmonary artery **(Figs. 34 and 35)**.[20]

Persistent Left Superior Vena Cava with an Absent Right Superior Vena Cava[26]

Two-dimensional sonography and color Doppler revealed a blood vessel on the left side of the pulmonary artery and absence of the superior vena cava with a three-vessel tracheal view **(Figs. 36 and 37)**. Panoramic and right lateral

Fig. 28: Spatial three-vessel view using HDlive Flow of truncus arteriosus (TA) straddling both ventricles and giving rise to the aorta (Ao) and pulmonary artery (PA) at 17 weeks and 3 days of gestation.
(DAo: descending aorta; HV: hepatic vein; LV: left ventricle; RV: right ventricle)

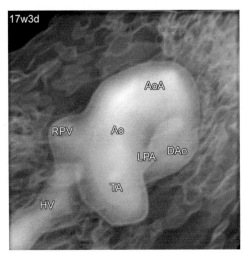

Fig. 29: Superior view of truncus arteriosus (TA) at 17 weeks and 3 days of gestation. The right (RPA) and left (LPA) pulmonary arteries, aortic arch (AoA), as well as descending aorta (DAo) were also distinguished using HDlive Flow silhouette.
(Ao: aorta; HV: hepatic vein)

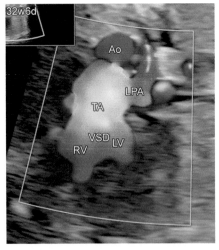

Fig. 30: Color Doppler image of truncus arteriosus (TA) at 32 weeks and 6 days of gestation.
(Ao: aorta; LPA: left pulmonary artery; LV: left ventricle; RV: right ventricle; VSD: ventricular septal defect)

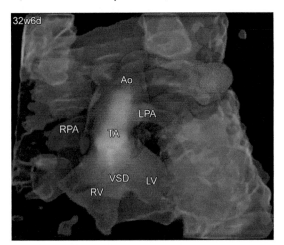

Fig. 31: HDlive Flow silhouette image of truncus arteriosus (TA) at 32 weeks and 6 days of gestation.
(Ao: aorta; LPA: left pulmonary artery; LV: left ventricle; RPA: right pulmonary artery; RV: right ventricle; VSD: ventricular septal defect)

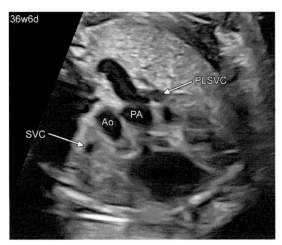

Fig. 32: Three-vessel view of persistent left superior vena cava (PLSVC) at 36 weeks and 6 days of gestation.
(Ao: aorta; PA: pulmonary artery; SVC: superior vena cava)

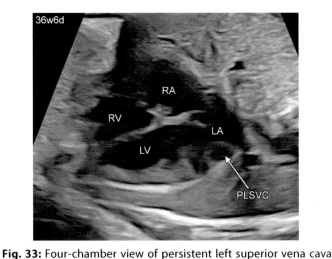

Fig. 33: Four-chamber view of persistent left superior vena cava (PLSVC) at 36 weeks and 6 days of gestation.
(LA: left atrium; LV: left ventricle; RA: right atrium; RV: right ventricle)

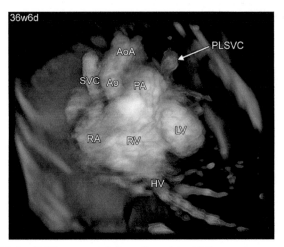

Fig. 34: Spatial three-vessel view of persistent left superior vena cava (PLSVC) depicted by HDlive Flow silhouette at 36 weeks and 6 days of gestation.
(Ao: aorta; AoA: aortic arch; HV: hepatic vein; LV: left ventricle; PA: pulmonary artery; RA: right atrium; RV: right ventricle; SVC: superior vena cava)
Source: Reprinted with permission from Jaypee Brothers Medical Publishers (P) Ltd.[20]

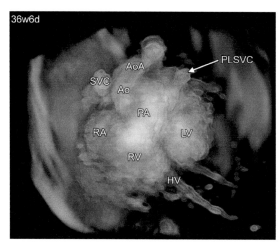

Fig. 35: Panoramic view of persistent left superior vena cava (PLSVC) depicted by HDlive Flow silhouette at 36 weeks and 6 days of gestation. (Ao: aorta; AoA: aortic arch; HV: hepatic vein; LV: left ventricle; PA: pulmonary artery; RA: right atrium; RV: right ventricle; SVC: superior vena cava)
Source: Reprinted with permission from Jaypee Brothers Medical Publishers (P) Ltd.[20]

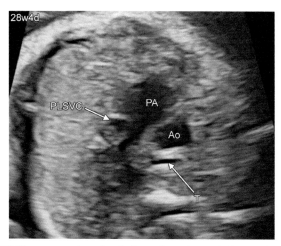

Fig. 36: Three-vessel tracheal view of persistent left superior vena cava (PLSVC) and absence of the superior vena cava at 28 weeks and 4 days of gestation.
(Ao: aorta; PA: pulmonary artery; T: trachea)

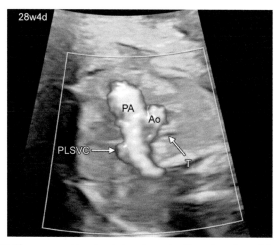

Fig. 37: Three-vessel tracheal view by color Doppler of persistent left superior vena cava (PLSVC) and absence of the superior vena cava at 28 weeks and 4 days of gestation.
(Ao: aorta; PA: pulmonary artery; T: trachea)

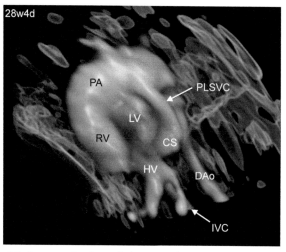

Fig. 38: Panoramic view of absent right superior vena cava and persistent left superior vena cava (PLSVC) at 28 weeks and 4 days of gestation.
(CS: coronary sinus; DAo: descending aorta; HV: hepatic vein; IVC: inferior vena cava; LV: left ventricle; PA: pulmonary artery; RV: right ventricle)
Source: Reprinted with permission from Jaypee Brothers Medical Publishers (P) Ltd.[26]

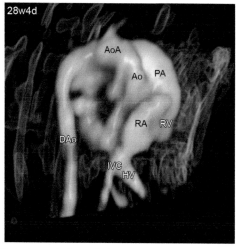

Fig. 39: Right lateral view of absent right superior vena cava and persistent left superior vena cava at 28 weeks and 4 days of gestation.
(Ao: aorta; AoA: aortic arch; DAo: descending aorta; HV: hepatic vein; IVC: inferior vena cava; PA: pulmonary artery; RA: right atrium; RV: right ventricle)
Source: Reprinted with permission from Jaypee Brothers Medical Publishers (P) Ltd.[26]

views by HDlive Flow clearly demonstrated absent right superior vena cava (ARSVC) and PLSVC connected to a dilated coronary sinus **(Figs. 38 and 39)**.[26]

■ CONCLUSION

HDlive Flow (silhouette) with STIC provides useful information for physicians and sonographers, and it can be used as an adjunct to conventional 2D fetal echocardiography when assessing normal cardiac structures and diagnosing CHD. However, it should be borne in mind that this technique has a marked learning curve because it may be unfamiliar to many beginners and some experts. More training may be necessary to use this technique easily in clinical settings. 3D/4D reconstruction of the normal fetal heart and CHD may become an important diagnostic tool for assessment of the normal fetal cardiac structures and antenatal diagnosis of CHD in clinical practice and future research.

Conflict of interest: The authors have no conflict of interest.

■ REFERENCES

1. Hata T, Kanenishi K, Tanaka H, Kimura K. Real-time 3-D echocardiographic evaluation of the fetal heart using instantaneous volume-rendered display. J Obstet Gynaecol. 2006;32:42-6.

2. Hata T, Yan F, Dai SY, Kanenishi K, Yanagihara T. Real-time 3-dimensional echocardiographic features of fetal cardiac tumor. J Clin Ultrasound. 2007;35:338-40.

3. Hata T, Dai SY, Inubashiri E, Kanenishi K, Tanaka H, Yanagihara T, Nukazawa T. Real-time three-dimensional color Doppler fetal echocardiographic features of congenital heart disease. J Obstet Gynaecol Res. 2008;34:670-3.

4. Hata T, Dai SY, Inubashiri E, Kanenishi K, Tanaka H, Yanagihara T, et al. Four-dimensional sonography with B-flow imaging and spatiotemporal image correlation for visualization of the fetal heart. J Clin Ultrasound. 2008;36:204-7.

5. Hata T, Mashima M, Ito M, Uketa E, Mori N, Ishimura M. Three-dimensional HDlive rendering images of the fetal heart. Ultrasound Med Biol. 2013;39:1513-7.

6. Lakshmy SR, Jain B, Rose N. Role of HDlive in imaging the fetal heart. J Ultrasound Med. 2017;36:1267-78.

7. Hata T, AboEllail MAM, Sajapala S, Ishimura M, Masaoka H. HDlive silhouette mode with spatiotemporal image correlation for assessment of the fetal heart. J Ultrasound Med. 2016;35:1489-95.

8. Dai SY, Inubashiri E, Hanaoka U, Kanenishi K, Yamashiro C, Tanaka H, et al. Three- and four-dimensional volume-rendered imaging of fetal double-outlet right ventricle using inversion mode. Ultrasound Obstet Gynecol. 2006;28:345-1.

9. Hata T, Tanaka H, Noguchi J, Dai SY, Yamaguchi M, Yanagihara T. Four-dimensional volume-rendered imaging of the fetal ventricular outflow tracts and great arteries using inversion mode for detection of congenital heart disease. J Obstet Gynaecol Res. 2010;36:513-8.

10. Turan S, Turan OM, Maisel P, Gaskin P, Harman CR, Baschat AA. Three-dimensional sonography in the prenatal diagnosis of aortic arch abnormalities. J Clin Ultrasound. 2009;37:253-7.

11. Hata T, Kanenishi K, Mori N, Yazon AO, Hanaoka U, Tanaka H. Four-dimensional color Doppler reconstruction of the fetal heart with glass-body rendering mode. Am J Cardiol. 2014;114:1603-6.

12. Hata T, AboEllail MAM, Sajapala S, Ito M. HDlive Flow in the assessment of fetal circulation. Donald School J Ultrasound Obstet Gynecol. 2015;9:462-70.

13. Ito M, AboEllail MAM, Yamamoto K, Kanenishi K, Tanaka H, Masaoka H, et al. HDlive Flow silhouette mode and spatiotemporal image correlation for diagnosing congenital heart disease. Ultrasound Obstet Gynecol. 2017;50:411-5.

14. AboEllail MAM, Kanenishi K, Tenkumo C, Mori N, Katayama T, Koyano K, et al. Four-dimensional power Doppler sonography with the HDlive silhouette mode in antenatal diagnosis of a right aortic arch with an aberrant left subclavian artery. J Ultrasound Med. 2016;35:661-3.

15. Yang PY, Sajapala S, Yamamoto K, Mori N, Kanenishi K, Koyano K, et al. Antenatal diagnosis of idiopathic dilatation of fetal pulmonary artery with 3D power Doppler imaging. J Clin Ultrasound. 2017;45:121-3.

16. Hata T, Ito M, Nitta E, Pooh R, Sasahara J, Inamura N. HDlive Flow silhouette mode for diagnosis of ectopia cordis with a left ventricular diverticulum at 15 weeks' gestation. J Ultrasound Med. 2018;37:2465-7.

17. Hata T, Hanaoka U, Kanenishi K. HDlive Flow Silhouette mode for fetal heart. Donald School J Ultrasound Obstet Gynecol. 2019;13:10-22.

18. AboEllail MAM, Kanenishi K, Tenkumo C, Kawanishi K, Kaji T, Hata T. Diagnosis of truncus arteriosus in first trimester of pregnancy using transvaginal four-dimensional color Doppler ultrasound. Ultrasound Obstet Gynecol. 2015;45:759-60.

19. Karmegaraj B, Rajeshkannan R, Kappanayil M, Vaidyanathan B. Fetal descending aortic tortuosity with ductal aneurysm. Ultrasound Obstet Gynecol. 2019;54:142-4.

20. Hata T, Hanaoka U, Kanenishi K. HDlive Flow silhouette mode for fetal heart. In: Merz E, Kurjak A (Eds). Donald School Textbook Current Status of Clinical Use of 3D/4D Ultrasound in Obstetrics and Gynecology. New Delhi: Jaypee Brothers Medical Publishers (P) Ltd.; 2018. pp. 137-51.

21. Hata T. HDlive Flow for fetal heart. In: Sen C, Stanojevic M (Eds). Fetal Heart: Screening, Diagnosis and Intervention. New Delhi: Jaypee Brothers Medical Publishers (P) Ltd.; 2019. pp. 201-17.

22. Hata T, Mori N, AboEllail MAM, Ito M, Nitta E, Miyake T, et al. Advances in color Doppler in obstetrics. J South Asian Feder Obst Gynae. 2019;11:1-12.

23. Tseng JJ, Peng HW, Jan SL. An in-depth perspective of aortic arch branching in fetal vascular rings using spatiotemporal image correlation combined with high-definition flow imaging. J Ultrasound Med. 2019;38:2217-24.

24. Ma B, Wu L, Zhang W. Rare vascular ring of right aortic arch and aberrant left subclavian artery in association with bilateral ductus arteriosus. Ultrasound Obstet Gynecol. 2020;55:132-9.

25. Hata T, Koyanagi A, Yamanishi T, Bouno S, Takayoshi R, Miyagi Y, et al. Success rate of five cardiac views using HDlive Flow with spatiotemporal image correlation at 18-21 and 28-31 weeks of gestation. J Perinat Med. 2020;48:384-8.

26. Hata T, Koyanagi A, Yamanishi T, Bouno S, Takayoshi R, Nakai Y, Miyake T. Three-dimensional fetal echocardiographic assessment of persistent left superior vena cava with absent right superior vena cava. Donald School J Ultrasound Obstet Gynecol. 2020;14:346-8.

27. Takayoshi R, Hata T, Bouno S, Koyanagi A, Yamanishi T, Nakai Y, et al. HDlive Flow for the diagnosis of double outlet right ventricle at 19 weeks of gestation. Donald School J Ultrasound Obstet Gynecol. 2020;14:351-4.

28. Hata T, Koyanagi A, Takayoshi R, Nakai Y, Miyake T. Transposition of great arteries diagnosed at 20 weeks of gestation: HDlive Flow features. Donald School J Ultrasound Obstet Gynecol. 2021;15:215-7.

29. Hata T, Koyanagi A, Takayoshi R, Miyake T. Recent topics in fetal echocardiography. Donald School J Ultrasound Obstet Gynecol. 2021;15(3):259-5.

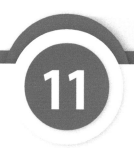

Microvasculature of Normal and Abnormal Placentas

Toshiyuki Hata, Aya Koyanagi, Riko Takayoshi, Takahito Miyake, Kenji Kanenishi

■ INTRODUCTION

Superb microvascular imaging (SMI) is a recent Doppler technology that uses a special algorithm to minimize motion artifacts by eliminating tissue motion (clutter), and can depict low-velocity blood flow in small vessels of the placenta by significantly reducing motion artifacts.[1] Superb microvascular imaging with Doppler luminance is advanced color Doppler technology, which shows three-dimensional (3D) SMI information on a two-dimensional (2D) gray-scale image by shading based on the amplitude of the color Doppler signal.[2] Smart 3D facilitates 3D reconstruction of the SMI placental microvasculature by fanning the routine 2D transducer.[1-4] There have been numerous SMI and 3D-SMI studies on normal and abnormal placental microvasculatures.[1-10] Recently, more detailed assessment of placental microvasculature has been reported using SMI and 3D-SMI with an 18-MHz probe.[11-14]

In this chapter, we present the latest state-of-the-art SMI and 3D-SMI of normal and abnormal placental microvasculatures using conventional SMI and SMI with an 18-MHz probe.

■ NORMAL PLACENTAL MICROVASCULATURE

As reported previously,[1] the ability of SMI to visualize low-velocity blood flow in small placental vessels was significantly improved due to reduce motion artifacts compared with conventional color/power Doppler ultrasound. As shown in **Figure 1**, SMI can clearly detect small placental vessels compared with color Doppler ultrasound.

In the first trimester of pregnancy, primary and secondary stem villous vessels could be identified **(Figs. 2 to 4)**.

The tertiary stem villous vessels could be seen early in the second trimester of pregnancy **(Figs. 5 to 7)**, and they showed increasing complexity during the second trimester **(Figs. 8 to 11)**. Spiral arteries could also be seen discharging blood into the intervillous space, and the terminal ends of these vessels suggested successful trophoblastic invasion.

The increased density of the placental microvasculature was evident in the third trimester of pregnancy using conventional SMI and SMI with an 18-MHz probe **(Figs. 12 to 19)**. Stem villous vessels in each cotyledon were thickly

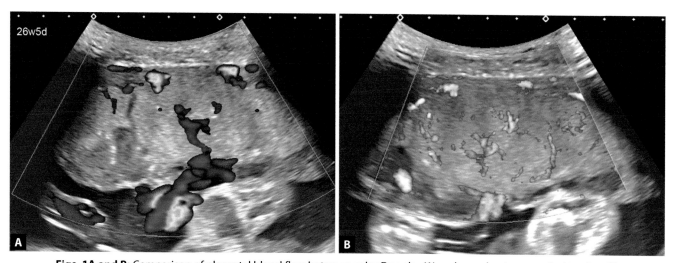

Figs. 1A and B: Comparison of placental blood flow between color Doppler (A) and superb microvascular imaging (B) at 26 weeks and 5 days of gestation.

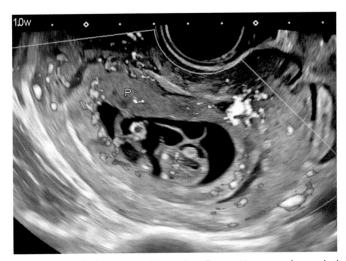

Fig. 2: Normal placenta at 10 weeks of gestation on color-coded superb microvascular imaging (SMI).
(P: placenta)
Source: Reprinted with permission from Jaypee Brothers Medical Publishers (P) Ltd.[11]

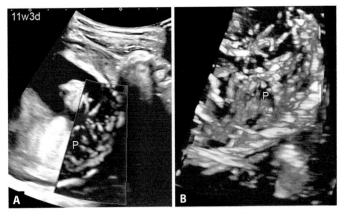

Figs. 3A and B: Normal placenta at 11 weeks and 3 days of gestation on superb microvascular imaging (SMI). (A) Monochrome SMI and (B) 3D-SMI.
(P: placenta)

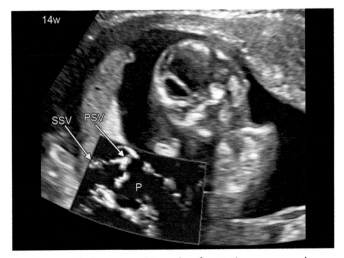

Fig. 4: Normal placenta at 14 weeks of gestation on monochrome superb microvascular imaging (SMI) with Doppler luminance.
(P: placenta; PSV: primary stem villous vessels; SSV: secondary stem villous vessels)

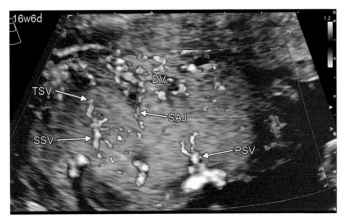

Fig. 5: Normal placenta at 16 weeks and 6 days of gestation on color-coded superb microvascular imaging (SMI) with an 18-MHz probe. (DV: decidual vessel; PSV: primary stem villous vessels; SAJ: spiral artery jet flow; SSV: secondary stem villous vessels; TSV: tertiary stem villous vessel)

branched. Superb microvascular imaging with an 18-MHz probe more clearly showed the placental microvasculature compared with conventional SMI **(Figs. 16 and 17)**.

■ DICHORIONIC DIAMNIOTIC TWIN PLACENTA

In a case of dichorionic diamniotic (DD) twin pregnancy, the border of two fused placentas was noted, and different microvasculatures between the two placentas were evident using monochrome **(Fig. 20)** and color-coded **(Fig. 21)** SMIs. SMI with an 18-MHz probe clearly showed the border of two fused placentas and their different microvasculatures **(Fig. 22)**.

■ FETAL GROWTH RESTRICTION PLACENTA

A thick heterogeneous (jellylike) placenta is specified as a thickened placenta with patchy echogenicity and sonolucent spaces by 2D sonography, wobbling like jelly under maternal abdominal pressure, and closely associated with intrauterine and neonatal death, hypertensive disorders of pregnancy, fetal growth restriction (FGR), and preterm labor.[15]

In a markedly thickened heterogeneous placenta **(Fig. 23A)** (placental thickness = 57.5 mm) with severe FGR [estimated fetal weight = 912 g, –3.8 standard deviation (SD)] at 31 weeks and 4 days of gestation, SMI depicted long primary stem villous vessels and reduced intermediate stem villous vessels **(Fig. 23B)**.[4] Moreover, 3D-SMI clearly demonstrated very sparse villous trees in the placenta, and each stem villous vessel became straight **(Fig. 23C)**.[4] Especially, primary stem villous vessels were thick and long. The umbilical artery pulsatility index (UAPI) was 1.48, and the middle cerebral artery pulsatility index (MCAPI) was 1.25. The amniotic fluid index (AFI) was 15.7 cm. There was no major fetal anomaly. On the same day, cardiotocographic monitoring showed decreased variability and prolonged deceleration, and emergency

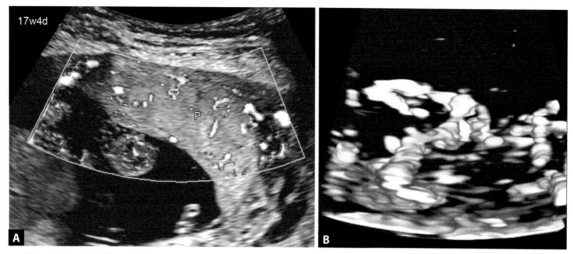

Figs. 6A and B: Normal placenta at 17 weeks and 4 days of gestation on superb microvascular imaging (SMI). (A) Color-coded SMI and (B) 3D-SMI. (P: placenta)

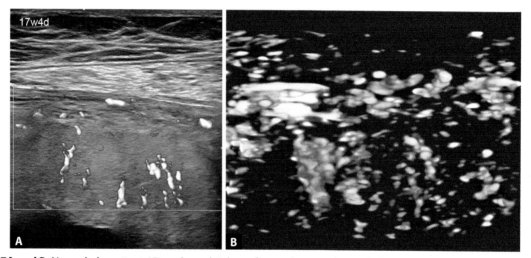

Figs. 7A and B: Normal placenta at 17 weeks and 4 days of gestation on color-coded superb microvascular imaging (SMI) with an 18-MHz probe. (A) Color-coded SMI; (B) 3D-SMI.

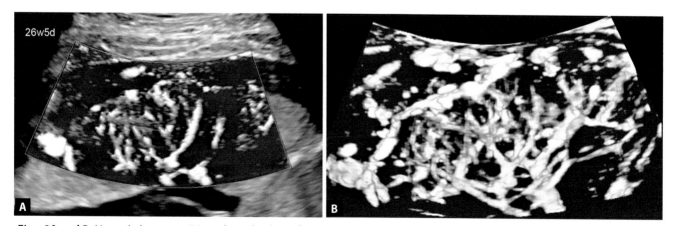

Figs. 8A and B: Normal placenta at 26 weeks and 5 days of gestation on superb microvascular imaging (SMI) with Doppler luminance. (A) Monochrome SMI; (B) 3D-SMI.

cesarean section was performed, resulting in a single female newborn weighing 832 g, with a length of 33 cm. The Apgar score was 3 at 1 minute and 8 at 5 minutes, with an umbilical artery pH of 7.267. The placental weight was 250 g **(Fig. 24)**, and the umbilical cord was 32 cm in length. The pathologic findings were placental infarcts, retroplacental hematoma, and chorioamnionitis (Blank classification, stage I-II).

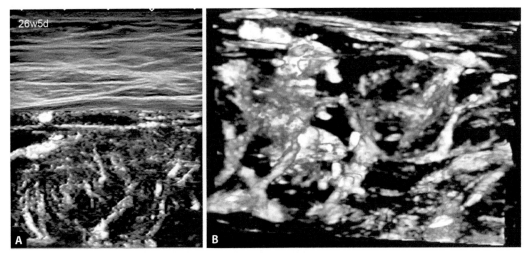

Figs. 9A and B: Normal placenta at 26 weeks and 5 days of gestation on monochrome superb microvascular imaging (SMI) with an 18-MHz probe. (A) Monochrome SMI with Doppler luminance; (B) 3D-SMI.

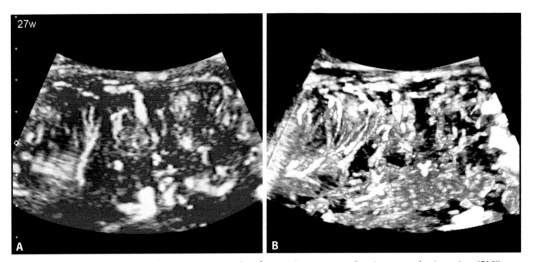

Figs. 10A and B: Normal placenta at 27 weeks of gestation on superb microvascular imaging (SMI). (A) Monochrome SMI; (B) 3D-SMI.

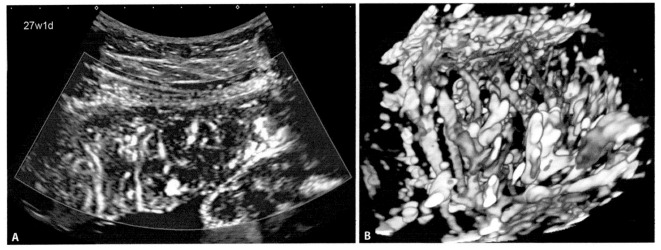

Figs. 11A and B: Normal placenta at 27 weeks and 1 day of gestation on superb microvascular imaging (SMI). (A) Monochrome SMI; (B) 3D-SMI.
Source: Reprinted with permission from Jaypee Brothers Medical Publishers (P) Ltd.[11]

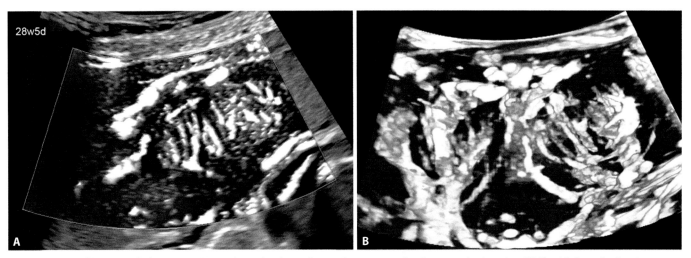

Figs. 12A and B: Normal placenta at 28 weeks and 5 days of gestation on superb microvascular imaging (SMI) with Doppler luminance. (A) Monochrome SMI; (B) 3D-SMI.

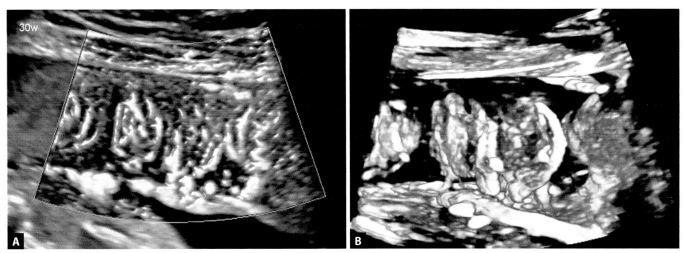

Figs. 13A and B: Normal placenta at 30 weeks of gestation on superb microvascular imaging (SMI). (A) Monochrome SMI with Doppler luminance; (B) 3D-SMI.

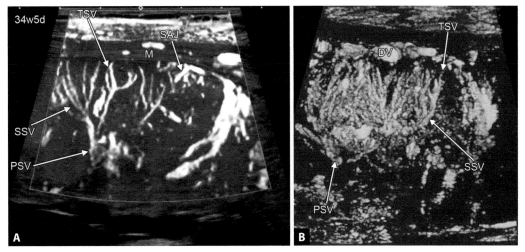

Figs. 14A and B: Normal placenta at 34 weeks and 5 days of gestation on superb microvascular imaging (SMI) with an 18-MHz probe. (A) Color-coded SMI; (B) 3D-SMI.

(DV: decidual vessel; M: myometrium; PSV: primary stem villous vessels; SAJ: spiral artery jet flow; SSV: secondary stem villous vessels; TSV: tertiary stem villous vessel)

Source: Reprinted with permission from Jaypee Brothers Medical Publishers (P) Ltd.[11]

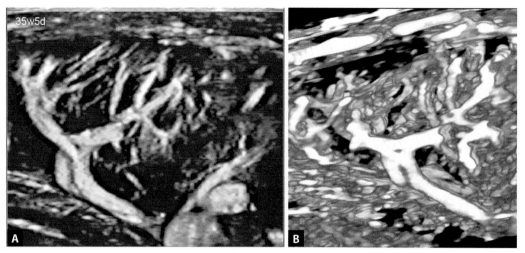

Figs. 15A and B: Normal placenta at 35 weeks and 5 days of gestation on superb microvascular imaging (SMI) with an 18-MHz probe. (A) Monochrome SMI; (B) 3D-SMI.

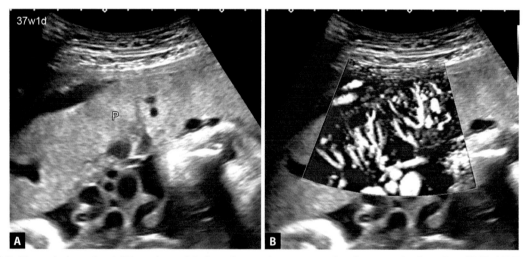

Figs. 16A and B: Normal placenta at 37 weeks and 1 day of gestation on superb microvascular imaging (SMI). (A) Two-dimensional sonography; (B) Monochrome SMI with Doppler luminance.
(P: placenta)
Source: Reprinted with permission from Jaypee Brothers Medical Publishers (P) Ltd.[14]

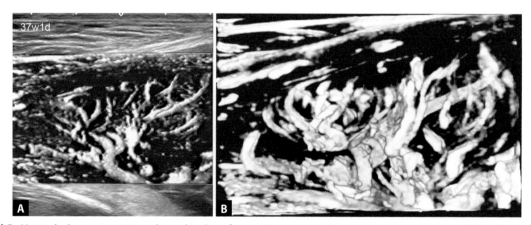

Figs. 17A and B: Normal placenta at 37 weeks and 1 day of gestation on superb microvascular imaging (SMI) with an 18-MHz probe. (A) Monochrome SMI with Doppler luminance; (B) 3D-SMI.
Source: Reprinted with permission from Jaypee Brothers Medical Publishers (P) Ltd.[14]

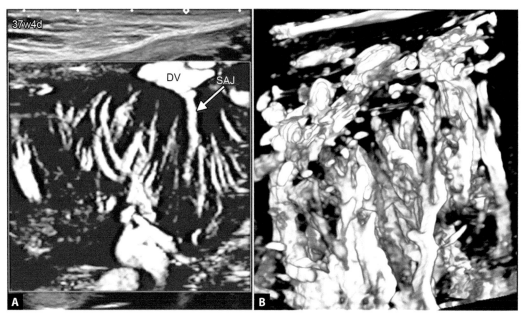

Figs. 18A and B: Normal placenta at 37 weeks and 4 days of gestation on superb microvascular imaging (SMI) with an 18-MHz probe. (A) Monochrome SMI with Doppler luminance; (B) 3D-SMI.
(DV: decidual vessel; SAJ: spiral artery jet flow)

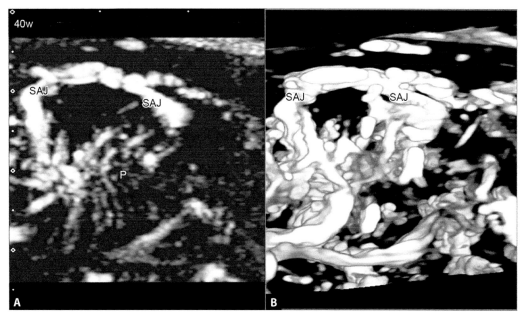

Figs. 19A and B: Normal placenta at 40 weeks of gestation on superb microvascular imaging (SMI) with an 18-MHz probe. (A) Monochrome SMI; (B) 3D-SMI.
(P: placenta; SAJ: spiral artery jet flow)

■ SUBCHORIONIC HEMATOMA

In a case of massive vaginal bleeding at 12 weeks and 5 days of gestation, an extremely large subchorionic hematoma was noted **(Fig. 25)**.[15] Conventional SMI and 3D-SMI showed an avascular area in the placenta adjacent to the hematoma **(Figs. 26 and 27)**.[15] Slightly increased echogenicity was noted in the placenta adjacent to the hematoma using high-resolution 2D sonography, and decreased vascularity was clearly recognized in the same area using SMI with an 18-MHz probe **(Fig. 28)**.[15] 3D-SMI using an 18-MHz probe also showed a few primary stem villous vessels in the avascular area of the placenta, whereas tertiary stem villous vessels were clearly identified in the normal-echogenicity placenta **(Fig. 29)**.[15]

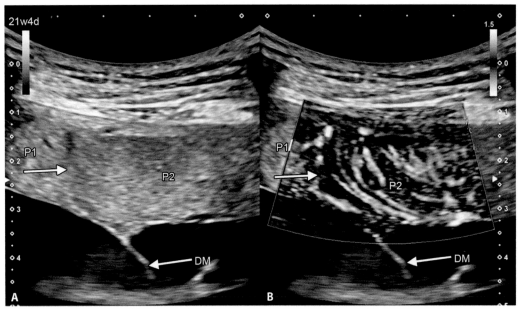

Figs. 20A and B: Dichorionic diamniotic (DD) twin placenta at 21 weeks and 4 days of gestation on superb microvascular imaging (SMI). Arrows indicate border of fused DD placenta. (A) Two-dimensional sonography; (B) Monochrome SMI.
(DM: dividing membrane; P1: one placenta of fused placentas; P2: another placenta of fused placentas)

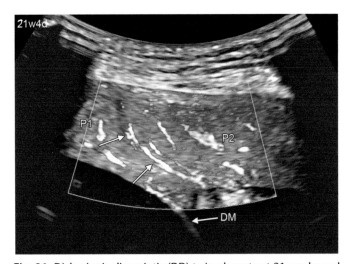

Fig. 21: Dichorionic diamniotic (DD) twin placenta at 21 weeks and 4 days of gestation on color-coded superb microvascular imaging (SMI). Arrows indicate border of fused DD placenta.
(DM: dividing membrane; P1: one placenta of fused placentas; P2: another placenta of fused placentas)

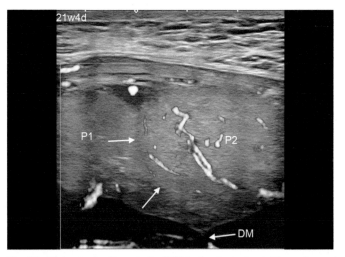

Fig. 22: Dichorionic diamniotic (DD) twin placenta at 21 weeks and 4 days of gestation on color-coded superb microvascular imaging (SMI) with an 18-MHz probe. Arrows indicate border of fused DD placenta. (DM: dividing membrane; P1: one placenta of fused placentas; P2: another placenta of fused placentas)

■ CIRCUMVALLATE PLACENTA

A thickened placenta with rolled up edges protruding into the uterine cavity was evident by 2D sonography at 28 weeks and 5 days of gestation, and normal stem villous vessels were noted using conventional SMI **(Fig. 30)**.[2] Conventional 3D-SMI spatially demonstrated intraplacental blood vessels, and the placental microvasculature using 3D-SMI with an 18-MHz SMI was more precisely depicted **(Fig. 31)**.[2] A gross specimen of the placenta after birth confirmed the diagnosis **(Fig. 32)**.[2]

■ PLACENTA ACCRETA SPECTRUM

In the case of placenta accreta spectrum (PAS) at 31 weeks and 4 days of gestation, significant dilatations of decidual vessels were evident using high-resolution 2D sonography, SMI, and 3D-SMI with an 18-MHz probe in the lower anterior segment of the uterus **(Figs. 33 and 34)**.[2]

Retained Placenta with Placenta Accreta Spectrum

In the retained placenta with placenta accreta, high-resolution 2D sonography clearly depicted irregular

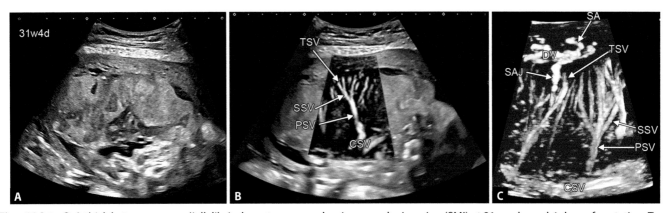

Figs. 23A to C: A thick heterogeneous (jellylike) placenta on superb microvascular imaging (SMI) at 31 weeks and 4 days of gestation. Two-dimensional (2D)-SMI presents long primary stem villous vessels (PSV) and reduced intermediate stem villous vessels. Three-dimensional (3D)-SMI clearly demonstrates very sparse villous trees in the placenta, and each stem villous vessel has become straight. Especially, PSV is thick and long on 2D/3D-SMI. (A) 2D sonography; (B) 2D-SMI; (C) 3D-SMI.

(CSV: chorionic surface vessels; DV: decidual vessels; SA: spiral artery; SAJ: spiral artery jet flow; SSV: secondary stem villous vessel; TSV: tertiary stem villous vessel)

Source: Reprinted with permission from John Wiley and Sons.[4]

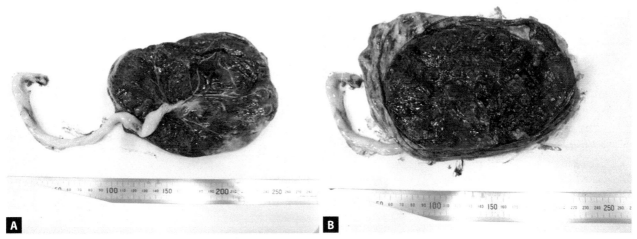

Figs. 24A and B: Gross specimen of a fetal growth restriction placenta. (A) Fetal surface; (B) Maternal surface.

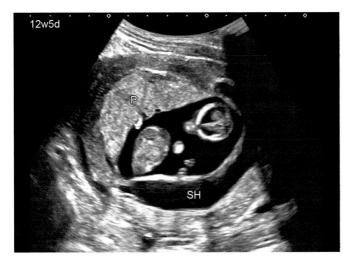

Fig. 25: Large subchorionic hematoma (SH) adjacent to the placenta (P) using two-dimensional sonography at 12 weeks and 5 days of gestation.
Source: Reprinted with permission from Jaypee Brothers Medical Publishers (P) Ltd.[14]

minimal invasion of the retained placenta into the anterior myometrium, and SMI with an 18-MHz probe also revealed disruption of decidual vessels at this pathological lesion with abnormal flow in the retained placenta **(Fig. 35)**.[12] Ultrasound-guided removal under general anesthesia was performed, and removal of the placenta was successful. Histopathological diagnosis of the removed placenta was placenta accrete (the villi attached directly to the myometrial tissue without intermediate decidua).

In the retained placenta with placenta percreta, conventional SMI revealed abundant blood flow in the placental bed adjacent to the uterine wall **(Figs. 36 and 37)**.[12] High-resolution 2D sonography demonstrated the loss of myometrium anterior to fundal lesions, and SMI with an 18-MHz probe clearly showed abnormally dilated, torturous, stem villous vessels invading until the uterine serosa (snow storm-like appearance) **(Fig. 38)**.[12]

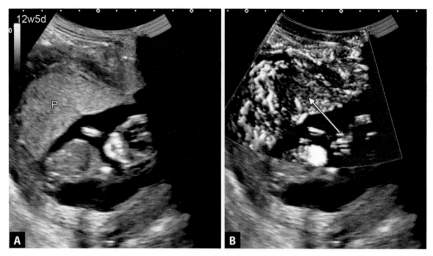

Figs. 26A and B: Large subchorionic hematoma adjacent to the placenta (P) at 12 weeks and 5 days of gestation. Superb microvascular imaging (SMI) with Doppler luminance reveals an avascular area (arrow) in the placenta adjacent to the hematoma. (A) Two-dimensional sonographic image; (B) SMI image with Doppler luminance.
Source: Reprinted with permission from Jaypee Brothers Medical Publishers (P) Ltd.[14]

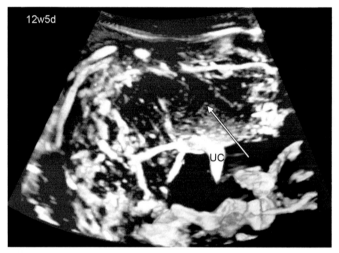

Fig. 27: Three-dimensional (3D) reconstruction of placental vasculature in the case of a large subchorionic hematoma using 3D superb microvascular imaging (SMI) at 12 weeks and 5 days of gestation. An avascular area (arrow) in the placenta adjacent to the hematoma can be clearly noted.
(UC: umbilical cord)
Source: Reprinted with permission from Jaypee Brothers Medical Publishers (P) Ltd.[14]

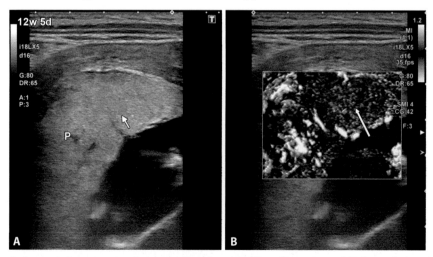

Figs. 28A and B: Large subchorionic hematoma adjacent to the placenta (P) at 12 weeks and 5 days of gestation. High-resolution two-dimensional (2D) sonography with an 18-MHz probe shows slightly increased echogenicity (small arrow) in an avascular area (large arrow) of the placenta adjacent to the hematoma. (A) High-resolution 2D sonography; (B) High-resolution SMI with Doppler luminance.
Source: Reprinted with permission from Jaypee Brothers Medical Publishers (P) Ltd.[14]

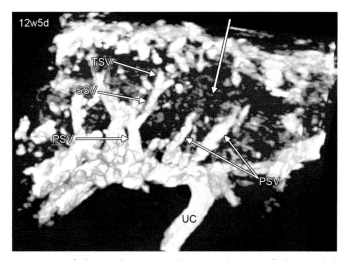

Fig. 29: Three-dimensional (3D) reconstruction of placental microvasculature in the case of a large subchorionic hematoma using 3D superb microvascular imaging (SMI) with an 18-MHz probe at 12 weeks and 5 days of gestation. 3D-SMI using an 18-MHz probe demonstrates a few primary stem villous vessels (PSV) in the avascular area of the placenta (large arrow), whereas tertiary stem villous vessels (TSV) were identified in the normal-echogenicity placenta.
(SSV: secondary stem villous vessel; UC: umbilical cord)
Source: Reprinted with permission from Jaypee Brothers Medical Publishers (P) Ltd.[14]

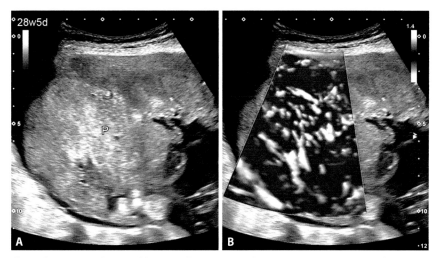

Figs. 30A and B: Circumvallate placenta (P) depicted by superb microvascular imaging (SMI) at 28 weeks and 5 days of gestation. (A) Two-dimensional sonography; (B) SMI image with Doppler luminance.
Source: Reprinted with permission from Jaypee Brothers Medical Publishers (P) Ltd.[2]

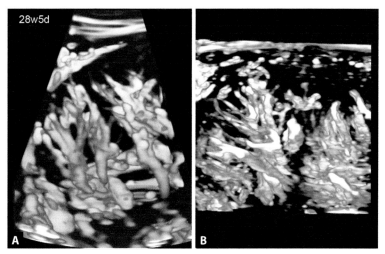

Figs. 31A and B: Three-dimensional (3D) reconstruction of placental vasculature in the case of a circumvallate placenta using 3D superb microvascular imaging (SMI) at 28 weeks and 5 days of gestation. (A) 3D-SMI; (B) 3D-SMI with an 18-MHz probe.
Source: Reprinted with permission from Jaypee Brothers Medical Publishers (P) Ltd.[2]

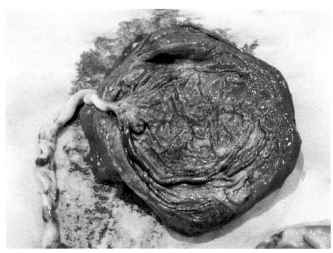

Fig. 32: Gross specimen of a circumvallate placenta.
Source: Reprinted with permission from Jaypee Brothers Medical Publishers (P) Ltd.[2]

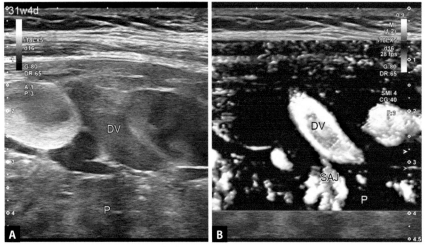

Figs. 33A and B: Placenta accreta spectrum depicted by superb microvascular imaging (SMI) with an 18-MHz probe at 31 weeks and 4 days of gestation. (A) High-resolution two-dimensional sonography; (B) High-resolution monochrome SMI with Doppler luminance.
(DV; decidual vessels; P; placenta; SAJ: spiral artery jet flow)
Source: Reprinted with permission from Jaypee Brothers Medical Publishers (P) Ltd.[2]

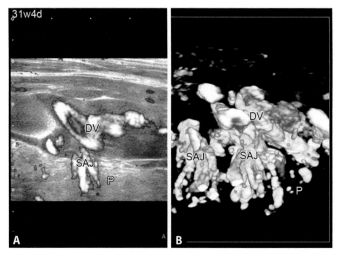

Figs. 34A and B: Placenta accreta spectrum depicted by superb microvascular imaging (SMI) with an 18-MHz probe at 31 weeks and 4 days of gestation. (A) High-resolution color-coded SMI; (B) High-resolution three-dimensional SMI.
(DV: decidual vessels; P: placenta; SAJ: spiral artery jet flow)
Source: Reprinted with permission from Jaypee Brothers Medical Publishers (P) Ltd.[2]

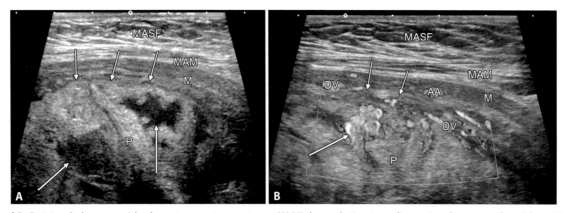

Figs. 35A and B: Retained placenta with placenta accreta spectrum. (A) High-resolution two-dimensional sonography with an 18-MHz linear probe clearly demonstrates irregular minimal invasion of the retained placenta into the anterior myometrium (small arrows), and a thin uterine wall is noted. Large echo-free spaces are evident (large arrows); (B) Color-coded superb microvascular imaging (SMI) with an 18-MHz probe reveals a minimally invasive placenta in the anterior myometrium (small arrows), and the disruption of decidual vessels (DV). Abnormal placental flow is also noted (large arrow).

(M: myometrium; MAM: maternal abdominal muscle; MASF: maternal abdominal subcutaneous fat; P: placenta)

Source: Reprinted with permission from Jaypee Brothers Medical Publishers (P) Ltd.[12]

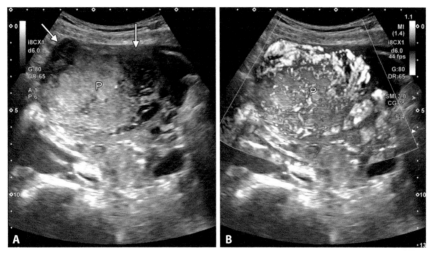

Figs. 36A and B: Retained placenta with placenta accreta spectrum. Two-dimensional sonography shows broad anechoic lesions in the uterus (arrows) (A), and color-coded superb microvascular imaging (SMI) reveals abundant blood flow in the placental bed adjacent to the uterine wall (B).
(P: placenta)

Source: Reprinted with permission from Jaypee Brothers Medical Publishers (P) Ltd.[12]

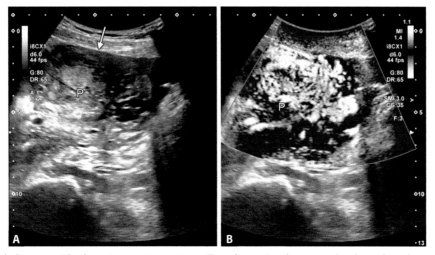

Figs. 37A and B: Retained placenta with placenta accreta spectrum. Two-dimensional sonography shows broad anechoic lesions in the uterus (arrow) (A), and monochrome superb microvascular imaging (SMI) reveals abundant blood flow in the placental bed adjacent to the uterine wall (B).
(P: placenta)

Source: Reprinted with permission from Jaypee Brothers Medical Publishers (P) Ltd.[14]

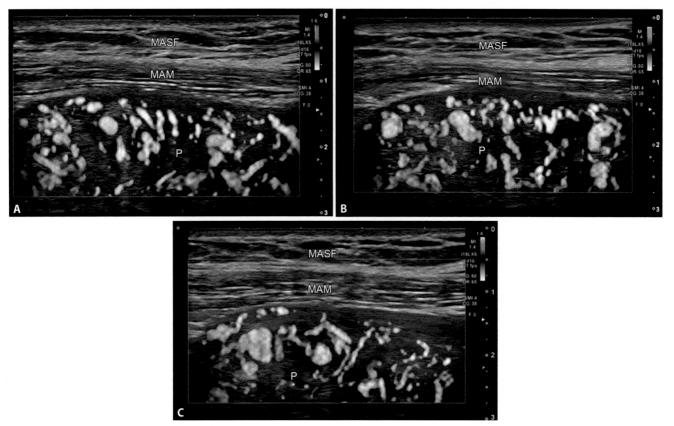

Figs. 38A to C: Retained placenta with placenta accreta spectrum. Superb microvascular imaging (SMI) with an 18-MHz probe clearly demonstrates the loss of myometrium anterior to fundal lesions. Abnormally torturous, abundant blood flow (snow storm-like appearance) invading until the uterine serosa is evident (A and B). Abnormally dilated vessels are also evident (C).
(MAM: maternal abdominal muscle; MASF: maternal abdominal subcutaneous fat; P: placenta)
Source: Reprinted with permission from Jaypee Brothers Medical Publishers (P) Ltd.[14]

■ CONCLUSION

With the advent of Doppler technology such as SMI, new scientific fields have developed, such as "placental microvasculature", heralding the dawn of a new era in placental science. Conventional SMI and SMI with an 18-MHz probe can clearly depict low-velocity blood flow and intraplacental microvasculature in normal and abnormal placentas. These techniques may provide new insights into understanding the pathophysiology of normal and abnormal placental microvasculatures in clinical practice and future research. Further studies with a larger sample size are needed to confirm the clinical relevance of SMI and SMI with an 18-MHz probe to assess placental physiology and pathology and diagnose abnormal placentas in clinical settings.

Conflict of interest: The authors have no conflict of interest.

■ REFERENCES

1. Hasegawa J, Suzuki N. SMI for imaging of placental infarction. Placenta. 2016;47:96-8.
2. Hata T, Mori N, AboEllail MAM, Nitta E, Miyake T, Kanenishi K. SMI with Doppler luminance in obstetrics. Donald School J Ultrasound Obstet Gynecol. 2019;13:69-77.
3. Hasegawa J, Yamada H, Kawasaki E, Matsumoto T, Takahashi S, Suzuki N. Application of superb micro-vascular imaging (SMI) in obstetrics. J Matern Fetal Neonatal Med. 2018;31:261-3.
4. Hata T, Kanenishi K, Yamamoto K, AboEllail MAM, Mashima M, Mori N. Microvascular imaging of thick placenta with fetal growth restriction. Ultrasound Obstet Gynecol. 2018;51:837-9.
5. Mack LM, Mastrobattista JM, Gandhi R, Castro EC, Burgess APH, Lee W. Characterization of placental microvasculature using superb microvascular imaging. J Ultrasound Med. 2019;38:2485-91.
6. Furuya N, Hasegawa J, Homma C, Kawahara T, Iwahata Y, Iwahata H, et al. Novel ultrasound assessment of placental pathological function using superb microvascular imaging. J Matern Fetal Neonatal Med. 2020;1-4.
7. Sainz JA, Carrera J, Borrero C, Garcia-Mejido JA, Fernandez-Placin A, Robles A, et al. Study of the development of placental microvascularity by Doppler SMI (superb microvascular imaging): a reality today. Ultrasound Med Biol. 2020;46:3257-67.
8. Inoue A, Horinouchi T, Yoshizato T, Kojiro-Sanada S, Kozuma Y, Ushijima K. Peculiar blood flow profiles among placental chorionic villous vessels of an abnormally thick placenta in a case of systemic lupus erythematosus characterized using microvascular imaging. J Obstet Gynaecol Res. 2020. doi: 10.1111/jog.14502.
9. Sun L, Li N, Jia L, Zhang C, Wang S, Jiao R, et al. Comparison of superb microvascular imaging and conventional Doppler

imaging techniques for evaluating placental microcirculation: A prospective study. Med Sci Monit. 2020;10:e926215.

10. Horinouchi T, Yoshizato T, Kojiro-Sanada S, Kozuma Y, Yokomine M, Ushijima K. Missing decidual Doppler signals as a new diagnostic criterion for placenta accreta spectrum: a case described using superb microvascular imaging. J Obstet Gynaecol Res. 2020;47(1):411-5.

11. Hata T, Mori N, AboEllail MAM, Ito M, Nitta E, Miyake T, et al. Advances in color Doppler in obstetrics. J South Asian Feder Obst Gynae. 2019;11:1-12.

12. Hata T, Hanaoka U, Mori A, Yamamoto K, Tenkumo C, Mori N, et al. Superb microvascular imaging of retained placenta with placenta accreta spectrum. Donald School J Ultrasound Obstet Gynecol. 2019;13:85-7.

13. Hasegawa J, Kurasaki A, Hata T, Miura A, Kondo H, Suzuki N. Sono-histological findings of the placenta accreta spectrum. Ultrasound Obstet Gynecol. 2019;54:705-7.

14. Hata T, Koyanagi A, Takayoshi R, Miyake T, Nitta E, Kanenishi K. Superb microvascular imaging assessment of placenta using 18-MHz probe. Donald School J Ultrasound Obstet Gynecol. 2021;15(3):312-22.

15. Raio L, Ghezzi F, Cromi A, Nelle M, Dürig P, Schneider H. The thick heterogeneous (jellylike) placenta: a strong predictor of adverse pregnancy outcome. Prenat Diagn. 2004;24:182-8.

Skeletal Dysplasias

Pamela Grant, Kenneth Ward

■ INTRODUCTION

A skeletal dysplasia is a generalized structural abnormality of the bone and cartilage groups. Skeletal dysplasias are a heterogeneous group of bone growth disorders resulting in abnormal shape and/or size of the skeleton. The current classification is based upon either descriptive findings or the presumed pathogenesis of the disease. The classification system most commonly used is the International Nomenclature and Classification of Constitutional Disorders of Bone (2001).[1] There are now over 33 osteochondrodysplasias groups and three genetically determined dysostoses.[1]

The prevalence of skeletal dysplasias identified at birth is approximately 2.4/10,000 births.[2] The overall frequency of skeletal dysplasias among perinatal deaths is approximately 9.1/1,000.[3] The frequencies of the different skeletal dysplasias are given in **Table 1**. The four most common skeletal dysplasias are: (1) thanatophoric dysplasia, (2) achondroplasia, (3) osteogenesis imperfecta, and (4) achondrogenesis. Thanatophoric dysplasia and achondrogenesis account for 62% of the lethal skeletal dysplasias.[4]

While >200 different skeletal dysplasias have been described, the number that can be recognized by ultrasound in the antenatal period is far fewer. The antenatal diagnosis of skeletal dysplasia can be difficult. The challenge involves not only accurately identifying the fetus affected with an abnormal skeleton but also accurately diagnosing the skeletal abnormality and predicting the fetal outcome. The first step in accurate diagnosis is establishing which aspect of bone development is abnormal.

Many dysplasias are named according to the part of the bone affected.

1. *Epiphysis:* This is an area of secondary ossification and is usually present at each end of the long bones. There is very limited ossification of the epiphyses by term, normally only the proximal tibial epiphysis and the distal femoral epiphysis is seen by birth. Disorders of epiphyseal development often cause pain and osteoarthritic complications in childhood and adult life.

2. *Metaphysis:* The metaphysis is immediately adjacent to the epiphysis and is the growing area of the long bone. Conditions that predominantly affect metaphyseal development, for example, achondroplasia, often lead to short stature.

3. *Diaphysis:* This forms the central shaft of the bone. Abnormalities involving the diaphysis may lead to abnormalities in the bone shape and fractures.

4. *Spondylo:* Involvement of the spinal column or vertebrae is present. Scoliosis, kyphosis or shortening of the spine may result.

Definitions of different skeletal abnormalities:

- *Micromelia:* Shortening of the entire limb
- *Rhizomelia:* Shortening of the proximal segment (arm and thigh)
- *Mesomelia:* Shortening of the intermediate segment (forearm and leg)
- *Acromelia:* Shortening of the distal segment (hands and feet)

TABLE 1: Incidence of skeletal dysplasias.	
Type of dysplasia	
Achondrogenesis	9%
Achondroplasia	15%
Campomelic dysplasia	2%
Chondrodermal dysplasia	2%
Chondrodysplasia punctata	4%
Osteogenesis imperfecta	14%
Thanatophoric dysplasia	29%
Other	19%

- *Polydactyly:* Presence of >5 digits, postaxial: extra digit on the ulnar or fibular side, preaxial: extra digit on the radial or tibial side
- *Syndactyly:* Soft tissue or bony fusion of the adjacent digits
- *Craniosynostoses:* Premature fusion of the sutures. Results in cloverleaf shape of the skull.

ULTRASOUND FINDINGS OF THE MOST COMMON DYSPLASIAS

Short Limbs

Thanatophoric dysplasia is a lethal skeletal dysplasia caused by a new dominant mutation in the *FGFR3* gene. Its incidence is 1 in 20,000. Ultrasound findings include: large head with prominent forehead, depressed nasal bridge, narrow chest and extremely short limbs (**Figs. 1 to 7**). There are two types: in type 1, the ends of the femurs are curved in a "telephone receiver appearance with mild mishappening of the skull; type 2 is associated with straight femurs but severe craniosynostosis producing a cloverleaf appearance to the skull. The risk of recurrence is very low.

Spondyloepiphyseal dysplasia congenita and Kniest dysplasia are autosomal dominant disorders resulting from mutations in the *COL2A1* gene. Mutation testing takes several months and is therefore unhelpful in the antenatal period.

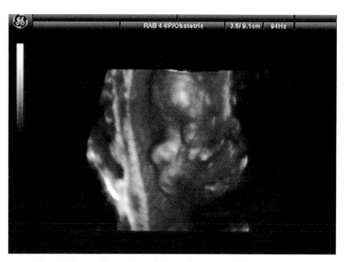
Fig. 3: Three-dimensional (3D) ultrasound demonstrating frontal bossing.

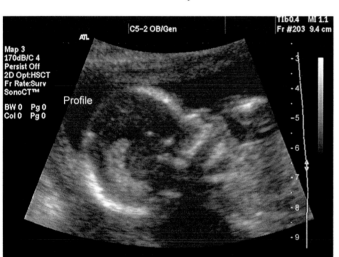
Fig. 1: Normal fetal profile.

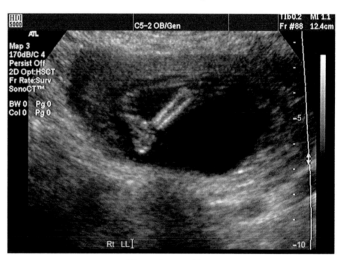
Fig. 4: Normal leg.

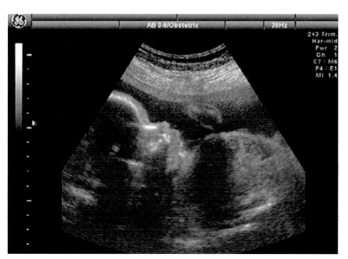
Fig. 2: Depressed nasal bridge.

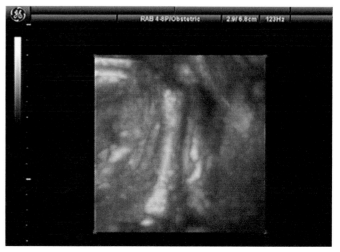
Fig. 5: Three-dimensional (3D) ultrasound of a femur with the "telephone receiver" appearance.

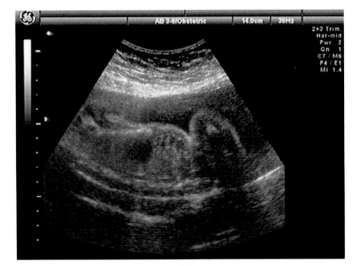

Fig. 6: Small chest.

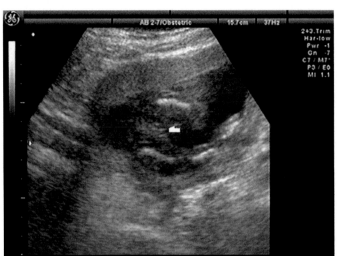

Fig. 8: Shortened and bowed femur.

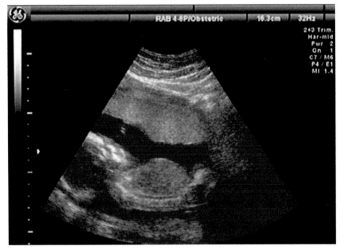

Fig. 7: Small thorax to abdomen.

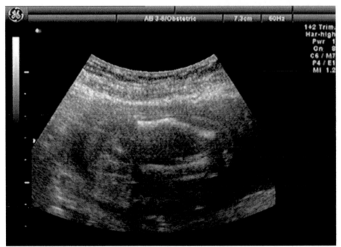

Fig. 9: Fractured femur.

Ultrasound findings may include: shortened long bones, cleft palate, talipes, kyphosis, and scoliosis.

Diastrophic dysplasia is a nonlethal dysplasia caused by an autosomal recessive mutation in the sulfate transporter gene *SLC26A2* or DTDST. Antepartum features include: angulation in the thumbs "hitch-hiker thumbs", severe bilateral talipes, scoliosis, cleft palate and shortened long bones.

Bowing of the Limbs

Campomelic dysplasia is caused by a mutation of the SRY-related gene *SOX9* or by rearrangements and deletions of the 17q24-5 region. The long bones, especially the tibia, are usually bowed **(Fig. 8)**. Sex reversal may be found in affected males.

Short, Bowed Limbs, and Reduced Bone Density

Osteogenesis imperfecta: There are four different forms. The prenatally identifiable form is the most severe—type 2 and

is considered lethal. Most cases are due to a new autosomal dominant mutation in the genes encoding type 1 collagen. Ultrasound findings include: severe shortening of the long bones, deformed limbs, often with bowing, angulation, and/or visible fractures **(Figs. 9 to 13)**. The bones may appear hypoechoic.

Infantile hypophosphatasia is an autosomal recessive condition characterized by severe deficiency of skeletal mineralization. It is caused by mutations in the tissue nonspecific alkaline phosphatase gene TNSALP on chromosome 1p34-36. Common ultrasound findings include: a hypoechoic, globular-shaped skull, deformity, and fractures in the long bones.

Short Ribs and/or Polydactyly

Short rib-polydactyly syndromes are a group of lethal skeletal dysplasias with autosomal recessive inheritance characterized by marked shortening of the long bones, short ribs, polydactyly and frequently the present of anomalies of other major organs. Four types have been recognized.

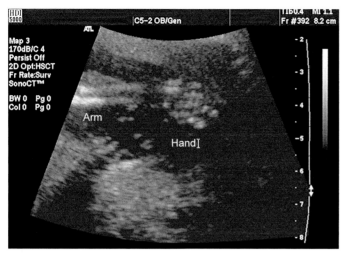

Fig. 10: Normal arm and hand.

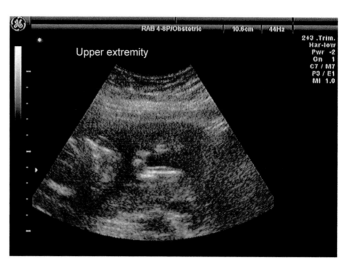

Fig. 12: Clubbed hand.

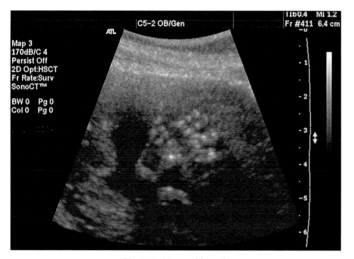

Fig. 11: Normal hand.

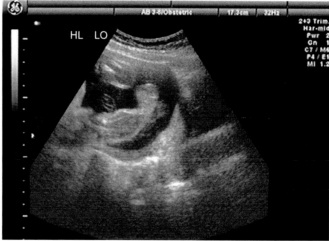

Fig. 13: Clubbed leg.

Ellis-van Creveld syndrome is characterized by postaxial polydactyly of the hands and occasionally the feet. Besides shortened limbs, a congenital heart defect is frequently present—most commonly and atrial septal defect. The ribs are short and the chest appears narrowed on ultrasound. The condition is caused by homozygous mutations in either EVC or EVC2 on chromosome 4p16.

Jeune syndrome is also known as asphyxiating thoracic dystrophy, characterized by rhizomelic limb shortening, a long narrow thorax with short ribs, 50% will have postaxial polydactyly. It is a genetically heterogeneous disorder.

Achondroplasia: It is the most frequently missed skeletal dysplasia in the antepartum period. It is the most common cause of short stature in children and adults. Prevalence at birth is approximately 1 in 27,000. During pregnancy the limb lengths are usually on or above the 5th percentile until 24 weeks with the head circumference at the 95th percentile. Other ultrasound findings may be a "trident" appearance to the fetal hands and frontal bossing. Achondroplasia is an autosomal dominant mutation in the *FGFR3* gene on chromosome 4p. 80% of affected individuals have a new mutation.

ULTRASOUND ACCURACY IN DIAGNOSING FETAL SKELETAL DYSPLASIAS

Several studies have assessed the accuracy of ultrasound (US) to antenatally diagnose the presence of a fetal skeletal dysplasia.[3,4] The majority of skeletal dysplasias are diagnosed after the first trimester. Approximately 50% will be diagnosed prior to 24 weeks. The accurate antenatal diagnosis of skeletal dysplasias is good at 60–65%, with approximately 19% being missed diagnosed, in 21% the diagnosis was imprecise but perhaps most importantly the prognosis was correctly predicted in 96% in the French study by Doray[4] and 100% in the series by Parilla et al.[3]

Distinguishing characteristics able to be identified by US that may help predict lethality include: a cloverleaf skull, severe micromelic bone shortening, multiple fractures, demineralization, a hypoplastic thorax, and an abnormal femur length/abdominal circumference (FL/AC) ratio of <0.16. Ramos et al.[5] first described the utility of the FL/AC ratio for prediction of fetal outcome in 27 pregnancies with skeletal dysplasias. Only one fetus survived the neonatal period with a FL/AC ratio of

<0.16. In that series and in Parilla's et al.[2] the only fetuses not correctly diagnosed by the FL/AC ratio were those with severe bowing of the FL that affected accurate measurements.

BIOMETRY IN THE DIAGNOSIS OF SKELETAL DYSPLASIAS

Significant shortening of the fetal long bones is the most common finding among all of the skeletal dysplasias. The nomograms available compare the long bones measured to the gestational age. Therefore, accurate assignment of the gestational age is critical. Therefore, patients known to be at risk for a skeletal dysplasia should seek care as soon in the pregnancy as possible for accurate dating. For patients presenting with unsure dates, comparison of the long bone measurements to the head circumference or the AC as noted by Ramus et al.[5]

CONCLUSION

Fetal skeletal dysplasias may be identified in the majority of cases by the second trimester of pregnancy. While the actual diagnosis of the specific skeletal dysplasia type by antenatal ultrasound may be limited; however, ultrasound is very accurate in predicting the likelihood of a lethal skeletal dysplasia. Thus ultrasound can be a highly valuable tool not only in identifying the potentially affected fetus but also in counseling the parents regarding the potential outcome and options for pregnancy management.

REFERENCES

1. Hall CM. International nosology and classification of constitutional disorders of bone (2001). Am J Med Genet. 2002;113:65-77.
2. Parilla BV, Leeth EA, Kambich MP, Chilis P, MacGregor SN. Antenatal detection of skeletal dysplasias. J Ultrasound Med. 2003;22:255-8; quiz 259-61.
3. Doray B, Favre R, Viville B, Langer B, Dreyfus M, Stoll C. Prenatal diagnosis of skeletal dysplasias: a report of 47 cases. Ann Genet. 2000;43:163-9.
4. Jeanty P, Valero G. (2006). The assessment of the fetus with skeletal dysplasia. [online] Available from: www.the fetus.net/files/skeletal_eng. [Last accessed April, 2022]
5. Ramus RM, Martin LB, Twickler DM. Ultrasonographic prediction of fetal outcome in suspected skeletal dyplasia with the use of femur length to abdominal circumference ratio. Am J Obstet Gynecol. 1998;179:1348-52.

Placenta

M Lisa Bartholomew, Ivica Zalud

■ INTRODUCTION

Placental morphology and function are the most important determinants of a healthy pregnancy outcome for an expectant mother as well as her developing fetus. The placenta is possibly the most unique organ in human physiology. The placenta is essentially disposable when compared to the lives of other human organs. During its short life the placenta is essential for maternal health and fetal life. If the placenta functions well, the newborn is most often normally grown and well equipped to meet the challenges of life outside the uterus. If the placenta functions poorly or the structure is abnormal, there is a higher risk of fetal death, hypoxic insult, or growth restriction. If the placenta is abnormally placed (i.e., placenta previa or accreta spectrum), there is a higher risk for maternal death by way of massive maternal hemorrhage. If the placenta is abnormally implanted, there is a higher risk for the development of preeclampsia, fetal growth restriction (FGR) or placental abruption.

Although visualization of the placenta is not foremost on the minds of expectant parents during an obstetrical ultrasound examination, it is best practice that ultrasound professionals fully evaluate the placental location, structure, and relationship to the umbilical cord. Practice guidelines from the American Institute of Ultrasound in Medicine (AIUM) for a basic obstetrical ultrasound (second and third trimester) indicate the following:

- The placental location, appearance, and relationship with the internal cervical os should be documented.
- The umbilical cord should be imaged and the number of vessels in the cord documented.
- The placental cord insertion site should be documented when technically possible.
- A transvaginal or transperineal ultrasound examination should be performed if the relationship between the cervix and the placenta cannot be assessed.
- A velamentous (also called membranous) placental cord insertion that crosses the internal os of the cervix

is suspicious for a vasa previa, a condition that has a high risk of fetal mortality if not diagnosed prior to labor. Color and pulsed Doppler ultrasound should be used to assess vasa previa or abnormal placental cord insertion.[1]

The use of three-dimensional (3D) and Doppler ultrasound technology is evolving rapidly and may become an important adjunct in the future evaluation of placental function throughout pregnancy. This chapter reviews ultrasound evaluation of the normal and abnormal placenta with clinical implications.

■ ULTRASOUND OF THE NORMAL PLACENTA

Size

The normally developing placenta increases in size and echogencity as pregnancy progresses. By convention, gestational age in this chapter will be referred to as menstrual weeks and not conceptual weeks. For example, six menstrual weeks is equivalent to four conceptual weeks since conception occurs approximately 2 weeks after the first day of the last menstrual period.

Before the embryo is visible with transvaginal sonography, early placental villi are visualized within the endometrium as an echogenic rim around a fluid-filled gestational sac at approximately four menstrual weeks of gestation. In early pregnancy, the diameter of the gestational sac normally grows 1 mm each day.[2] At approximately five menstrual weeks a yolk sac, umbilical cord, and a small mound of relatively echogenic chorionic villi consistent with the early placenta can be seen **(Figs. 1 and 2)**.[3] A normal yolk sac diameter measures between 3 and 5 mm **(Fig. 3)**. If the yolk sac diameter is >6 mm, there is an increased risk of embryonic demise.[4] The embryo with cardiac activity should be visualized when the crown rump length reaches 3–6 mm (approximately 5-6 menstrual weeks) **(Figs. 4 and 5)**. Cardiac activity is often visualized before the embryo is large enough to measure. If an embryo is not visualized

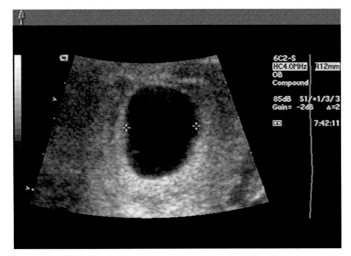

Fig. 1: Transvaginal ultrasound of an embryonic pregnancy.

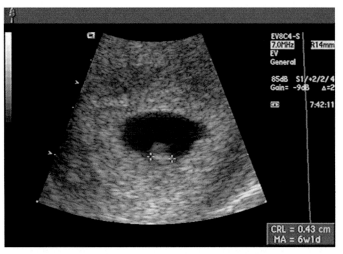

Fig. 4: Transvaginal ultrasound of normal gestational sac and fetal pole at approximately 6 menstrual weeks.

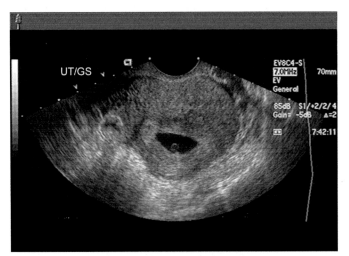

Fig. 2: Transvaginal ultrasound of normal gestational sac and yolk sac.

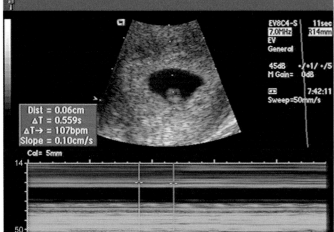

Fig. 5: Normal fetal cardiac activity at 6 menstrual weeks.

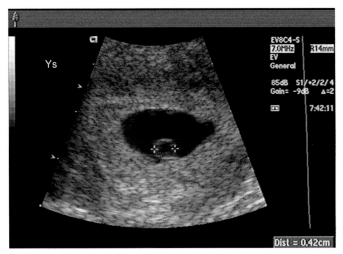

Fig. 3: Transvaginal ultrasound of gestational sac and normal size yolk sac.

with transvaginal sonography by the time the gestational sac reaches 16 mm, there is a significantly increased risk of an anembryonic pregnancy.[5]

After the first trimester, placental weight increases throughout normal gestation and correlates with birth weight. Overly small and overly large placentas have been associated with abnormal pregnancy outcomes. As a general rule, the placental thickness in millimeter should approximate the gestational age in weeks plus or minus 10 mm. Placentas >37 weeks gestational age should be not >40 mm thick.[6] Placentomegaly has been classically associated with hydrops fetalis and congenital viral infections **(Fig. 5)**. The ultrasound appearance of a thick heterogeneous placenta has been linked to other adverse pregnancy outcomes and fetal death.[7] Polyhydramnios may cause the placenta to appear thin because of compression **(Fig. 6)**.

When examining chromosomally normal fetuses with no additional anomalies, those found to have FGR also been noted to possess smaller placentas.[8,9] Several investigators have published data regarding two-dimensional placental volume measures in the first and second trimester in an effort to predict fetal outcomes. Wolf et al. concluded that small second trimester placental volumes estimated with

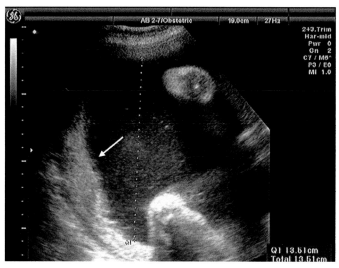

Fig. 6: A thin placenta caused from compression by polyhydramnios.

TABLE 1: Description of ultrasonographic placental grade.[26]	
Placental grade	**Description**
Grade 0	• No visible calcifications • Smooth chorionic plate
Grade 1	• Scattered tiny calcifications • Subtle indentations of chorionic plate
Grade 2	• Larger basal and comma like echodensities • Larger indentations of chorionic plate
Grade 3	• Extensive basal echogenicity and circular echodensities fully outlining cotyledons • Complete indentations of chorionic plate

two-dimensional ultrasound were more common in cases of adverse pregnancy outcome.[10] Thame et al. demonstrated that low birth weight was preceded by small placental volume in the second trimester and suggested that placental volume was a more reliable predictor of birth weight than fetal measurements.[11] Three-dimensional ultrasound volumes in the second trimester have been published in two series by Hafner et al. Three-dimensional placental volumes alone were not well correlated to the development of small for gestational age infants or preeclampsia.[12,13]

Grade

Calcium deposition occurs as part of the normal "aging" process of the placenta. The amount of calcium deposition is known as the placental grade. **Table 1** demonstrates the description of the placental grading system and **Figures 7 to 10** show ultrasound examples of grades 0–3. In the first 2/3 of pregnancy, the calcium deposition is microscopic. After 33 weeks more than half of placentas have macroscopic calcifications which then increases until term.[14] The appearance of a grade III placenta in the late third trimester has been associated with pulmonary maturity in nondiabetic pregnancies;[15] however the widespread use of first and second trimester ultrasound to accurately date pregnancies makes this potential marker redundant in most cases. Grade III placentas do not appear to predict intrauterine growth restriction when seen after 36 weeks.[16] Interobserver variation and debate over how much of the placenta must appear grade III are also confounders. There is conflicting information about the significance of grade III placentas seen prior to 34 weeks gestation. Several small studies have concluded that there is a relationship between early placental maturation and perinatal complications such as preeclampsia, intrauterine growth restriction and nonreasuring fetal testing.[17-21] Others have not found such

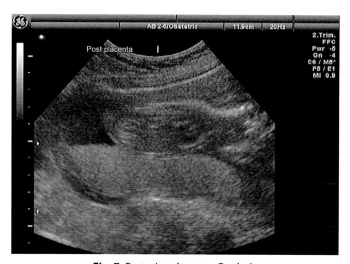

Fig. 7: Posterior placenta: Grade 0.

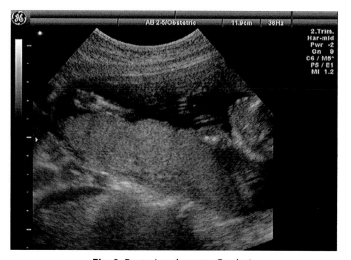

Fig. 8: Posterior placenta: Grade 1.

an association or disagree with the notion that advanced placental grade is associated with fetal maturation.[22,23] Maternal cigarette smoking has been associated with accelerated placental grade.[23-25] Reporting bias with regard to accurate smoking history during pregnancy may confound placental grading studies. There is no compelling evidence to suggest that premature placental maturation alone should

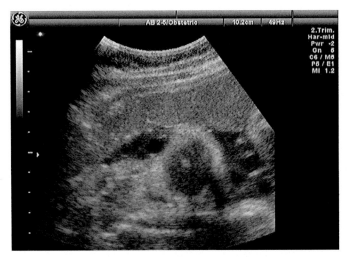

Fig. 9: Anterior placenta: Grade 2.

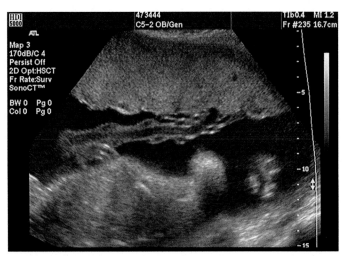

Fig. 11: Gray scale image of a normal placental cord insertion.

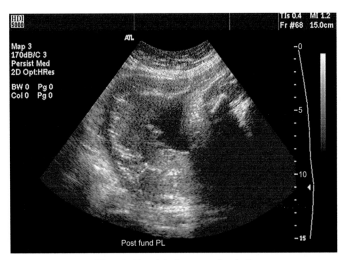

Fig. 10: Fundal placenta: Grade 3.

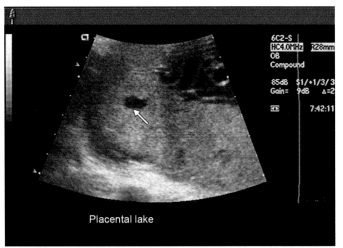

Placental lake

Fig. 12: Placental lake. Low velocity venous flow "swirling" is seen within the lake.

be used to guide obstetrical decisions. The entire clinical picture should be considered. Placental grading is shown in **Table 1.**[26]

Shape

The normal placental shape is a single round disk with a central cord insertion **(Fig. 11)**. The chorionic plate should be the same size as the basal plate so that the fetal membranes extend all the way to the edge.

Placental Lakes

Placental lakes are part of the normal appearance of the placenta in the second and third trimester. Placental lakes may be absent, few, or numerous. Lakes are anechoic and contain maternal blood which can be seen swirling and have low velocity venous blood flow within them. Placental lakes have little to no clinical significance. Some authors believe them to be precursors of perivillous fibrin deposition or intervillous thrombosis if venous flow decreases within the lake **(Fig. 12)**.[27]

ULTRASOUND OF THE ABNORMAL PLACENTA

Circumvallate Placenta

If the basal plate is smaller than the chorionic plate and the fetal membranes lie flat, this is known as a circummarginate placenta. A circummarginate placenta has no clinical significance. If the chorionic plate is smaller than the basal plate and the fetal membranes are folded into a circular ridge, this is called a circumvallate placenta. Circumvallate placentas are associated with pregnancy complications such as placental abruption, preterm labor, and stillbirth.[28,29] The accuracy of sonography for diagnosis of circumvallation appears to be limited with high false positive and false negative rates[30] (See **Figure 13** of a circumvallate placental edge).

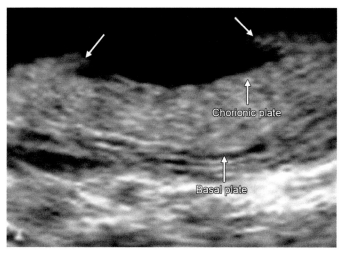

Fig. 13: Ultrasound appearance of circumvallate placenta. Note thickened edge where chorioamniotic membranes are folded and the difference in size between the chorionic and basal plate.

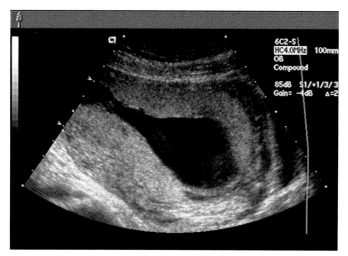

Fig. 15: Sagittal view of posterior placenta with anterior succenturiate lobe.

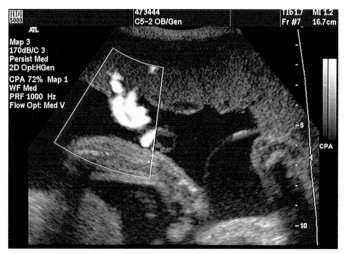

Fig. 14: Color Doppler image of an eccentric placental cord insertion.

If the cord inserts near the edge of the placenta, this is called an eccentric insertion **(Fig. 14)**. If it inserts on the edge and resembles a lollipop, it is called a battledore placenta. If the cord inserts into the membranes before entering the body of the placenta, this is known a membranous insertion. A battledore or membranous insertion may cause compromise to the integrity of the umbilical vessels because there is little support by the body of the placenta.

Succenturiate Lobes

Succenturiate lobes also known as accessory lobes are seen in almost 10% of placentas.[31,32] Another synonym is a bilobed placenta. The main lobe receives the umbilical cord insertion. The accessory lobe does not. Connecting vessels are usually present running through the membrane between the lobes. Documentation of the location of the connecting vessels is clinically relevant particularly if one of the lobes is in the lower

uterine segment. If connecting vessels traverse the cervical os, this is a form of vasa previa. If vasa previa is undiagnosed, rapid fetal hemorrhage and fetal death may occur at the time of ruptured membranes. Accessory lobes usually spontaneously deliver with the main lobe due to the membranes and vessels connecting them however; a retained placenta could occur if accessory lobes are not diagnosed antenatally. Care should be taken not to overdiagnose succenturiate lobes in placentas that are located laterally and wrap around from the anterior to posterior uterus. Succenturiate placentas are not continuous and demonstrate a significant gap in the placental body **(Fig. 15)**.

Placenta Membranacea

Placenta membranacea occurs when chorionic villi are spread all over the amniotic sac and are not located in one area. As a result, these very rare placentas are thin and may have abnormal implantation [placenta accreta spectrum (PAS)]. Reports of antenatal ultrasound diagnosis have been published.[33] Pregnancy outcomes are worse for the mother than the fetus. Over 30% of placenta membranaceas have associated abnormal implantation and 50% result in antepartum or postpartum hemorrhage. Fourteen of twenty six reported cases resulted in a live birth.[34]

Subchorionic Fibrin Deposition

Subchorionic fibrin deposition (SFD) occurs in 20% of placentas. SFD appears as complex cystic area located on the fetal side of the placenta where fibrin deposits under the chorion. The appearance may be large and dramatic. Color Doppler flow is not seen within the mass although low velocity swirling may be seen with direct visualization in the cystic areas. With gray scale ultrasound, they can be mistaken for chorioangiomas. Use of Doppler is critical to

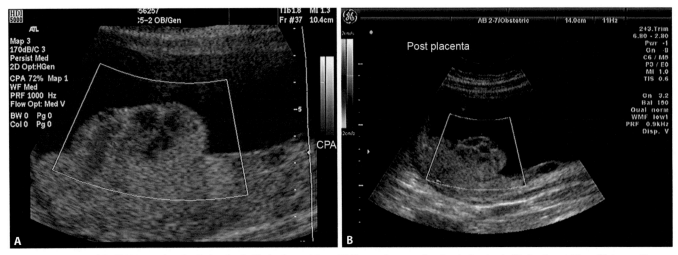

Figs. 16A and B: (A) Example of subchorionic fibrin deposition; (B) Second example of subchorionic fibrin deposition. Note cystic appearance and lack of color Doppler flow.

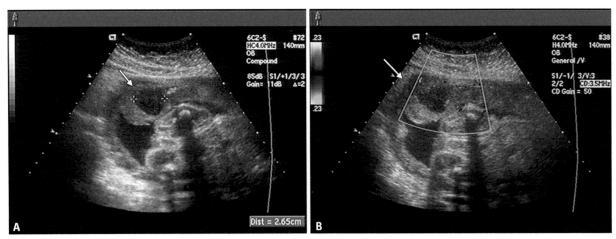

Figs. 17A and B: Placental infarct. Note absent color Doppler flow within infarct.

distinguish between the two. SFD has no clinical significance **(Figs. 16A and B)**.[35]

Infarcts

Placental infarcts occur when perfusion to an area of the placenta is reduced enough to cause necrosis of placental tissue. If necrosis causes liquefaction or bleeding, infarcts become visible with ultrasound therefore, many are not noted until pathological examination occurs. Infarcts are usually irregularly shaped and do not contain swirling blood upon direct visualization. Small infarcts are seen in 25% of normal pregnancies. If infarcts are large and/or extensive, placental function can be compromised as a refection of maternal vascular disease, preeclampsia, or poor placental implantation.[36] Such a placenta may be described as having a "moth eaten" appearance. Unexplained elevated maternal serum α-fetoprotein (AFP) has been associated with extensive placental infarction **(Figs. 17A and B)**.[37]

Molar Pregnancy

Molar pregnancy occurs when normal placental villi are replaced by profuse hydropic villi. The incidence of molar pregnancy in the United States is 1/1,000 pregnancies.[38] If a fetus is also present, this is known as a partial molar pregnancy. If a fetus is not present, this is known as a complete molar pregnancy. A complete mole occurs when an empty ovum is fertilized by a single spermatozoon or two spermatozoa resulting in a 46 XX or 46 XY karyotype. A partial mole is characterized by fertilization of a normal ovum by two spermatozoa resulting in a 69 XXX or 69 XXY karyotype. The fetus in a partial mole is almost always triploid or aneuploid and usually has multiple congenital anomalies and or growth restriction.

Ultrasound of a complete molar pregnancy classically demonstrates echogenic material filling the endometrium giving the typical snowstorm appearance **(Figs. 18A and B)**. Cystic anechoic areas may also be seen. If a fetus is visualized in addition to the amorphous material, this

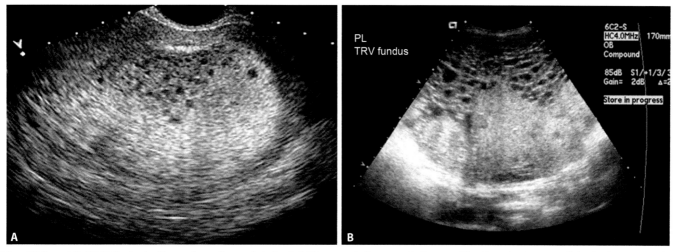

Figs. 18A and B: (A) Pathologically confirmed complete hydatidiform mole in second trimester. The fetus is absent and the hydropic vesicles have typical grape-like appearance; (B) Pathologically confirmed placental mesenchymal dysplasia in the second trimester. A fetus is present. There is a thickened placenta with apparent hydropic vesicles that can resemble a molar pregnancy. The differential diagnosis includes placental mesenchymal dysplasia, a complete molar pregnancy with a twin, a partial molar pregnancy, or a chorioangioma.

represents a partial mole. High β-human chorionic gonadotropin (β-hCG) levels (>100,000) and the presence of theca lutein cysts (enlarged ovaries with multiple small cysts throughout) can support the diagnosis of molar pregnancy. If a fetus is present, it is important to entertain alternative diagnoses such as placental mesenchymal dysplasia, complete molar pregnancy with a co-twin, or chorioangioma which have better prognoses than does a partial molar pregnancy **(Table 2)**.[39]

Most of the classic descriptions of the ultrasound appearance of molar pregnancies have come later in pregnancy when the patient develops bleeding or a rapidly enlarging uterus. First trimester diagnosis of molar pregnancy does not appear to be exactly the same as second trimester diagnosis and may become a more common challenge for the sonographer as first trimester ultrasound becomes more common. Only 56% of pathologically confirmed molar pregnancies had the diagnosis suspected during a first trimester ultrasound (mean gestational age at sonography was 10.5 weeks). In 38%, the diagnosis was not considered. 100% of the cases examined after 13 weeks were correctly identified. No theca lutein cysts were identified.[40] A second ultrasound series of pathologically confirmed molar pregnancies noted the classically described echogenic cystic intrauterine mass in 71% of cases between 5 and 12 menstrual weeks.[41]

Chorioangioma

Chorioangiomas are benign vascular (capillary filled) lesions that form within the placental body or protrude from the fetal side. The incidence of chorioangioma is 1% (all sizes). Larger chorioangiomas >5 cm are considerably rarer.[42] If chorioangiomas are large there is a significant risk

for maternal or fetal complications such as fetal anemia, fetal heart failure, hydrops, polyhydramnios, preeclampsia, fetal death, etc.[43] The ultrasound appearance of a chorioangioma is round, well circumscribed, mostly hypoechoic, and solid appearing with generous color Doppler flow. There may be hyperechoic components as well. If calcifications, cystic areas, and minimal color flow are noted, this is more characteristic of a teratoma which has little to no clinical significance. Frequent fetal surveillance with ultrasound is recommended if a near 5 cm chorioangioma is suspected to detect the development of fetal anemia and or hydrops.[44] Middle cerebral artery peak systolic velocity could be used for surveillance of fetal anemia.[45] Fetal anemia can be treated with intrauterine transfusions in the face of chorioangioma.[46]

Placental Abruption

Placental abruption occurs in up to 1% of pregnancies and is defined as the premature separation of the placenta from the myometrium usually in the late second and third trimester. Risk factors include tobacco smoking, hypertension, cocaine use, abdominal trauma, etc. If large enough, a placental abruption may present with symptoms of abdominal pain, vaginal bleeding, shock, coagulopathy, uterine contractions, nonreassuring fetal heart rate pattern, or intrauterine fetal demise. Concealed abruptions may also occur without the traditional description of painful vaginal bleeding.

Abruptions may be partial, complete, acute, or chronic. The most common location for placental separation is at the margin (edge) and may extend into a subchorionic collection although they may occur in any area of the placental bed. It is important to distinguish between subchorionic collections and retroplacental collections because subchorionic collections are not commonly referred

TABLE 2: Cystic appearing placenta: ultrasound and pathologic differentiation.

Variable	Placental mesenchymal dysplasia	Complete molar pregnancy with co-twin	Partial molar pregnancy	Normal pregnancy with chorioangioma
Ultrasound scan of the placenta	Placenta with hypoechoic/multicystic areas: may see normal area of placenta; may be thickened	Placenta in 1 sac with hypoechoic/multicystic areas: may or may not see separating membrane; may be thickened; placenta in second sac with fetus appears normal	Placenta with hypoechoic/multicystic areas: thickened	Located on the fetal placental surface with different echogenicity than the rest of the placenta; contains copious Doppler flow in mass
Ultrasound scan of the fetus	May appear normal	May appear normal with a second normal-appearing placenta	Usually abnormal-appearing fetus	May appear normal
Gross pathologic condition of the placenta	Large for gestational age with cystically dilated vesicles	Large for gestational age with cystically dilated vesicles and normal-appearing placenta	Large for gestational age with cystically dilated vesicles	Usually normal placenta with smooth round mass on fetal surface of the placenta
Microscopic characteristics of placenta	Dilated stem vessels and lack of trophoblastic proliferation	Dilated stem vessels with trophoblastic proliferation	Less prominent dilated stem vessels than a complete molar pregnancy with trophoblastic proliferation	Dilated small vessels and capillaries lined with a single layer of endothelial cells with normal placenta

Source: Adapted from Woo GW, Rocha FG, Gaspar-Oishi M, Bartholomew ML, Thompson KS. Placental mesenchymal dysplasia. Am J Obstet Gynecol. 2011;205(6):e3-5.

to as placental abruptions and do not have the same clinical risk or connotation to obstetricians. Subchorionic bleeds are more commonly described in the first and second trimesters and are usually managed expectantly. Small subchorionic bleeds (<15–60 mL) seen in the first half of pregnancy do not appear to in part adverse pregnancy outcome unlike larger bleeds.[47,48] Placental abruptions are more commonly a concern in later pregnancy when survival of the neonate becomes possible (after 24 weeks) and intervention could protect the fetus from hypoxia or death. If >50% of the placenta appears detached, the risk of adverse pregnancy outcome is significantly increased.[49]

Ultrasound has a poor (50%) sensitivity to detect placental abruption[50] and should not be used to "rule out" a placental abruption. The passage of time and clinical findings are the methods used to correctly diagnose placental abruption. If a retroplacental collection is noted on ultrasound, attempts should be made to quantify the amount of retroplacental hemorrhage seen on ultrasound. Retroplacental collections should be distinguished from the normal retroplacental complex that contains decidua, vessels, and myometrium and is usually not >1–2 cm thick in sagittal plane.[43]

The sonographic appearance of placental hemorrhage is variable. Fresh acute blood will appear hyperechoic. It becomes isoechoic in 3–7 days. In 1–2 weeks it becomes hypoechoic and after 2 weeks it becomes anechoic.[51]

See **Figure 18A and Table 2** for an example of a clinically significant retroplacental collection (abruption).

Placenta Previa

Placenta previa generally refers to the presence of placenta lying over or near the internal cervical os. Placenta previa is clinically significant only if there is significant bleeding or when the pregnancy reaches the point at which fetal survival outside the uterus is possible (approximately 24 weeks). The incidence of placenta previa after 20 weeks is 4 per 1,000 pregnancies.[52] Strictly speaking, there are three types of placenta previa [(1) complete, (2) partial, and (3) marginal].[53] The low-lying placenta is not technically a previa because the placental tissue does not cover the os and is usually described as the placental edge within 2 cm of the internal cervical os.[54] Low-lying placentas do impart a mildly increased risk of bleeding but not as dramatically as do the true previas. Bleeding during delivery is rare. Vaginal delivery is not contraindicated if the placental edge is at least 10 mm superior to the internal cervical os. Ninety percent of placenta previas diagnosed between 10 and 20 weeks will "migrate" and resolve by the third trimester. The amount of cervical overlap implies likelihood of resolution. Forty percent of previas will persist is there is ≥25 mm overlap of the internal os.[55]

A complete placenta previa is diagnosed when the placenta completely covers the internal cervical os.

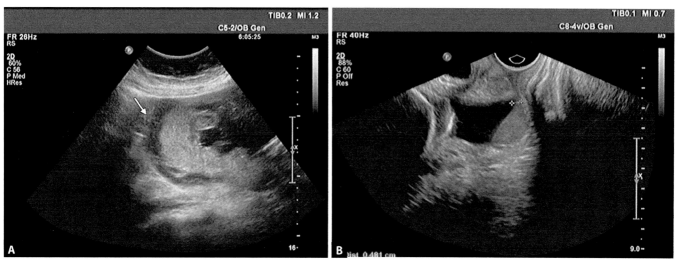

Figs. 19A and B: (A) Ttransabdominal image of a retroplacental collection consistent with a placental abruption; (B) Transvaginal ultrasound of the cervix in the same patient. Retroplacental bleeding caused preterm labor and cervical change with cervical dilation and funneling of membranes. This patient spontaneously delivered a preterm infant within 24 hours of this examination.

A subgroup of complete previa includes central previas in which the cervix appears in the center of the placenta. Partial placenta previa is described when the placenta partially covers the internal os, but not completely. Marginal placenta previa is described as the placenta that only reaches the edge of the internal os.

Although transabdominal ultrasound is 95% accurate if the placenta appears well away from the lower uterine segment, there is an overall 7% false positive rate.[56] Transvaginal sonography is considered safe and the method of choice for evaluating a suspected placenta previa with an accuracy of 99%.[57] Transvaginal sonography is performed with an empty bladder by convention which removes the confounder of the full bladder giving the false appearance of an anterior previa seen during an abdominal examination. Transvaginal sonography reduces the shadowing resulting from an engaged fetal presenting part during the third trimester and is better at evaluating the cervical involvement of a lateral or wrap around placenta. Gentle transvaginal sonography does not appear to incite placental bleeding in the setting of placenta previa and is not comparable to a digital examination.[57] Translabial imaging is also an alternative. See **Figures 19A and B** for an example of a transvaginal image of a complete placenta previa that migrated to a low-lying placenta.

Placenta Accreta Spectrum

Placenta accreta spectrum in general is defined as placental tissue that is abnormally and firmly attached to the myometrium. The normal decidua basalis and fibrinoid layer (Nitabuch's layer) are defective and as a result the placental villi adhere to the myometrial layer and may penetrate through it to reach other structures in the pelvis, most commonly the maternal bladder. There are three levels of invasive placentas called PAS. The first is accreta where the placenta adheres to the fetal surface of the myometrium. The second is increta where the placenta invades into the myometrium. The third is placenta percreta where the placenta invades all the way through the myometrium and often into the bladder wall and/or into the bladder cavity itself. All forms of PAS are associated with significant antenatal and/or intrapartum hemorrhage at the time of placental separation/removal. Most cases require cesarean hysterectomy for control or prevention of massive obstetrical hemorrhage. Nearly half of placenta percreta patients require massive transfusion. The maternal mortality rate is 13%. Other complications include uterine rupture, fetal death, need for a neobladder, fistula formation, and infection.[58]

Risk factors for PAS include prior uterine surgery, placenta previa, maternal smoking, and advanced maternal age.[59] A high index of suspicion by the sonographer could be lifesaving for women with risk factors. Women with a documented placenta previa after 24 weeks should be asked about prior uterine surgery particularly the number of cesarean deliveries. If there is prior uterine surgery and an anterior placenta previa, transabdominal and transvaginal ultrasound with a full bladder should be performed to assess ultrasonographic signs of accreta/percreta.[58]

Placenta accreta spectrum was rare 50 years ago occurring in 1 in 30,000 deliveries. The incidence has risen approximately 1 in 500 deliveries (50-fold increase) largely due to the marked increase in the rate of cesarean delivery. Women without scared uteruses have a 1–5% risk of placental invasion.[59] As the number of cesarean deliveries increase so does the risk of placenta previa (another risk factor). One prior cesarean delivery increases the risk of

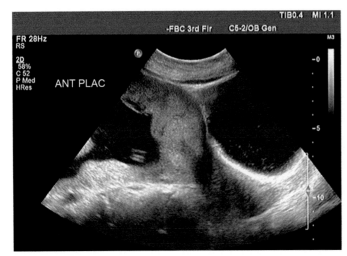

Fig. 20: Transvaginal sonography of a complete placenta previa.

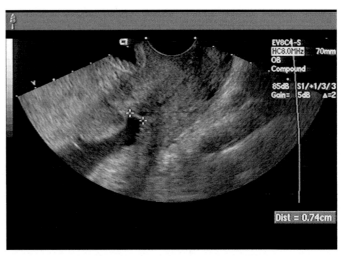

Fig. 21: Transvaginal ultrasound of a low-lying placenta and normal cervical length. Note edge of placenta lies <20 mm from the internal cervical os.

placenta previa by a factor of two-three.[60] More concerning is the combination of previous cesarean and placenta previa. The incidence of PAS among women with one, two, and four or more cesareans and a concomitant placenta previa is 25, 47, and 67%, respectively.[61]

Ultrasound is 85% sensitive for the detection of PAS in high risk women. The normal hypoechoic placental-myometrial interface is obscured and the placenta appears continuous with the myometrium. See **Figure 20** for a normal placental-myometrial interface. Cystic lacunae may be observed near the area of invasion.[62] Color Doppler is also sensitive (82%) and specific (97%) for the diagnosis of placenta previa/accreta when four criteria are used. The criteria are diffuse and focal intraparenchymal placental lacunar flow, hypervascularity of the bladder and uterine serosa, prominent subplacental venous complex, and loss of subplacental Doppler vascular signals.[63] Hematuria may also support the diagnosis of placenta percreta. See **Figures 21 to 24** for gray scale and color Doppler of placenta percreta. MRI of the uterus is shown to be helpful for diagnosis of the presence and extent of placenta increta/percreta and operative planning with a 97% accuracy in one series.[64] Planned cesarean hysterectomy is the delivery method of choice for most women with placenta increta or percreta while focal accreta may be managed without hysterectomy. For the best maternal outcome, multidisciplinary care in a tertiary placenta accreta center of excellence is recommended.

Placental Three-dimensional Power Doppler

During pregnancy, the spiral arteries are transformed into distended low-resistance channels capable of increasing the blood supply to the fetal-placental unit 10 times that of the nonpregnant uterus. This uteroplacental vascular adaptation is dependent on invasion of the spiral arteries by trophoblast which becomes incorporated into the vessel

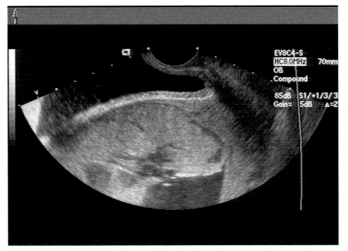

Fig. 22: Transvaginal image of a normal placental-myometrial interface. Note the thin homogeneous hypoechoic line indicating a normal Nitabuch's layer.

wall. This invasion occurs in a stepwise fashion starting with plugging of the distal ends of the arteries followed by migration into the decidual segments and, after several weeks' delay, into the myometrial segments. The first phase of this process starts from at least 8 weeks of gestation and continues to the 10th week, and the second phase is at 14–24 weeks. Establishment of the uteroplacental circulation in the second trimester is not a random phenomenon, but rather a consequence of events in the first trimester.[65]

One of the major weaknesses of more traditional Two-dimensional Doppler studies is the reproducibility of results. Three-dimensional power Doppler has the ability to evaluate placental volume, vascularity, and blood flow with greater detail than conventional ultrasound, which has led to its investigation in preeclampsia, FGR, and other placental vascular abnormalities. **Figures 25 to 31** show different forms of placental and spiral arteries 3D power Doppler evaluations. The virtual organ computer-aided

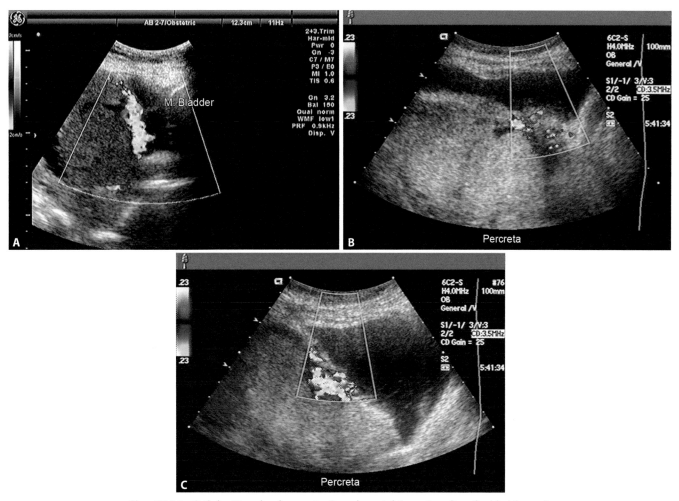

Figs. 23A to C: Color Doppler demonstrating placental tissue invading the bladder wall.

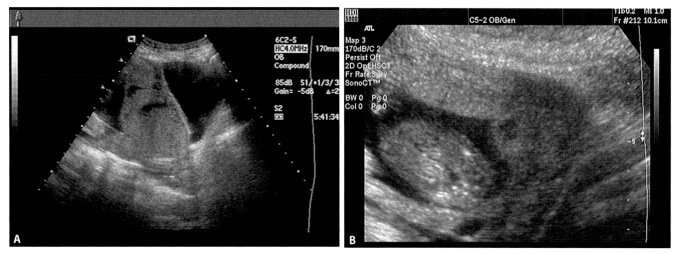

Figs. 24A and B: Gray scale images of placenta accreta/percreta. Note cystic lacunae and absence of echogenic layer between placenta and myometrium. Placenta previa is also seen. This patient had a history of four prior cesarean deliveries.

analysis (VOCAL) imaging program can be used to calculate vascularization index (VI), flow index (FI) and vascularization flow index (VFI). The VI gives information in percentages about the amount of color values in the placenta and spiral arteries. Flow index is a dimensionless index (0-100) with information about the intensity of blood flow. It is calculated as a ratio of weighted color values (amplitudes) to the number of color values. Vascularization flow index is the combined information of vascularization and mean blood flow intensity. It is also a dimensionless index (1-100) calculated by dividing weighted color values (amplitudes) by the total voxels minus background voxels.

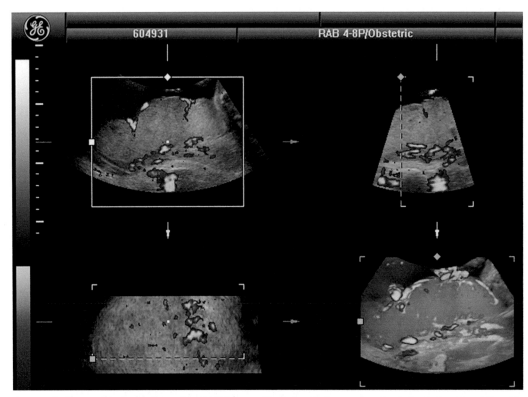

Fig. 25: Three orthogonal planes with three-dimensional (3D) power Doppler of placental and spiral arteries blood flow. Three-dimensional reconstruction of the placenta was shown in the lower right corner.

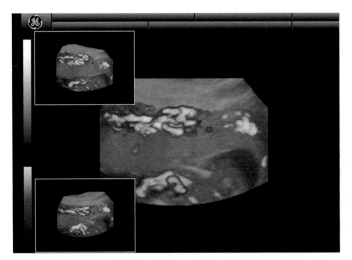

Fig. 26: Another three-dimensional (3D) power Doppler reconstruction of the placental (mid), spiral arteries (upper), and umbilical cord (lower) blood flow.

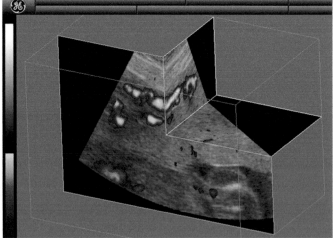

Fig. 27: Placental blood flow shown in Niche mode.

Three-dimensional Doppler is aimed to minimize operator influence on obtained results and allows assessment of the blood flow in real volume and remotely. While more data are needed on the optimal imaging protocol and its predictive ability for clinical outcomes, 3D power Doppler is emerging as a promising new technology that will improve the evaluation of placental function.[66-68]

Another potential application of 3D Doppler is investigations in PAS. In elegant recently published paper, Calì G et al. described 3D ultrasound and 3D power Doppler in the evaluation of PAS.[69] Due to the increased rate of cesarean sections in the last decades, the anomalies of placental implantation and invasion have become an emerging pathology. Undetected prenatally, severe forms of invasive placentation can lead to dramatic consequences such as a uterine rupture in labor, peripartum hemorrhage, necessity of hysterectomy, and massive blood transfusions. That is the reason why the prenatal diagnosis of impaired placentation plays a key role to detect patients at risk, who should be referred to tertiary perinatal centers. If the diagnosis of

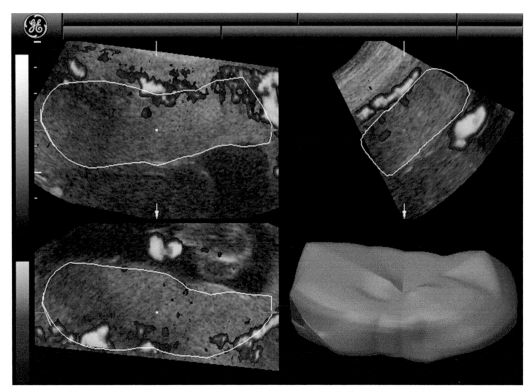

Fig. 28: Three-dimensional (3D) placental volume calculations (lower right corner).

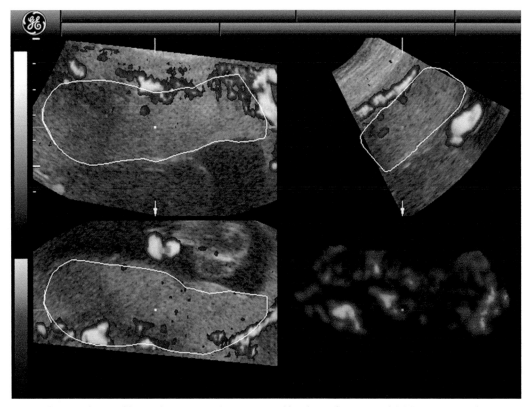

Fig. 29: Placental "virtual angiogram" as presented by three-dimensional (3D) power Doppler.

abnormal placentation is confirmed, the next step should be to define the degree of placental invasion. Two-dimensional ultrasonography is the technique mainly used to diagnose the PAS, but its accuracy could be possibly increased by the complementary use of the 3D ultrasound and 3D power Doppler. Only a few prospective studies are available on the role of 3D US in the detection of PAS without establishing objective, universally acceptable ultrasonographic diagnostic

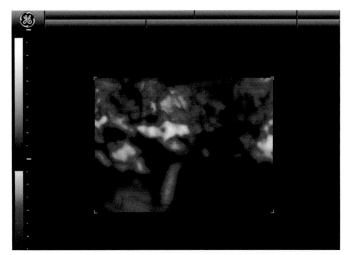

Fig. 30: Another example of placental and spiral arteries "virtual angiogram" obtained by three-dimensional (3D) power Doppler.

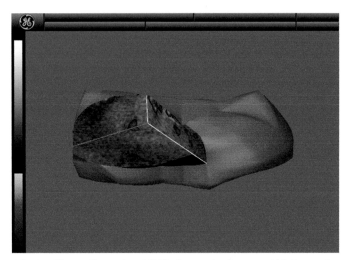

Fig. 31: Three-dimensional (3D) placental volume and Niche mode of placental vascular network.

criteria. Moreover, diagnosis is subjective with accuracy depending on the experience of the operator. Three-dimensional power Doppler technique seems to have a good intraoperator but low interoperator reproducibility, because it needs a rigorous standardization of predetermined machine settings. Multicentric studies are needed to identify common and objective 3D US and 3D power Doppler diagnostic criteria for PAS, to reduce interoperator variability.[69]

PLACENTAL IMAGING SUMMARY: PAST MEETS THE FUTURE

The placenta is many times referred as forgotten organ but yet holds so many keys to understanding what went wrong during pregnancy resulting in poor maternal, fetal, or outcome in both. Ultrasound evaluation of the placenta went long way from the landmark study by Kurjak and Barsic published in 1977 on the concept of placental migration to today's virtual angiogram of placenta presented by recent advances in placental imaging.[70,71]

Kurjak and Barsic reviewed 7,137 localizations of placenta.[70] In 67 patients on the first examination, it was found that the lower margin of placenta reached the internal os of the uterus. All these patients were followed up by examinations every 2 or 4 weeks. In 63 of the 67 patients, placental migration was found involving a change in the level of the lower placental edge from the cervix toward the fundus. All four cases where the placenta extended from anterior to posterior wall ended as placenta previa. The authors concluded that, ultrasonic proof of placental migration shows the necessity for ultrasonic examination shortly before the birth, as only then is the final diagnosis of placenta previa possible.

The most recent study by Hata et al. described that superb microvascular imaging (SMI) can detect low-velocity blood flow in the placenta by significantly reducing motion artifacts.[71] Moreover, SMI using an 18-MHz probe generates a high-resolution image of the placental microvasculature in normal and abnormal placentas. In the normal placenta, the increased density of the placental microvasculature with advancing gestation was evident using SMI with an 18-MHz probe. The placental baseline between the placenta and myometrium was also clearly identified. In the first-trimester placenta with an extremely large subchorionic hematoma, decreased vascularity in the placenta adjacent to the hematoma was clearly recognized. In the circumvallate placenta, the placental microvasculature using 18-MHz SMI was more precisely noted compared with conventional SMI. In a case of pregnancy after a previous uterine fundal incision, a high-resolution SMI with an 18-MHz probe could clearly identify the very thin uterine wall. In cases of PAS during pregnancy and in the retained placenta after birth, various types of placentas were noted, and unique microvasculature was also demonstrated using SMI with an 18-MHz probe. Superb SMI with an 18-MHz probe may become a future modality to provide novel information on the antenatal evaluation of normal and abnormal placentas, and the physiologic progress of normal placental microvascular development, and precise pathologic findings of placental abnormality in clinical practice and future research.

■ REFERENCES

1. AIUM–ACR–ACOG–SMFM–SRU Practice Parameter for the Performance of Standard Diagnostic Obstetric Ultrasound Examinations. J Ultrasound Med. 2018;37:E13-E24.
2. Nyberg DA, Laing FC, Filly RA. Threatened abortion: Sonographic distinction of normal and abnormal gestational sacs. Radiology. 1987;158:397-400.
3. deCrespigny L, Cooper D, McKenna M. Early detection of intrauterine pregnancy with ultrasound. J Ultrasound Med. 1988;7:129-35.
4. Kurtz AB, Needleman L, Pennell RG, Baltarowich O, Vilaro M, Goldberg BB. Can detection of yolk sac in the first trimester

be used to predict the outcome of pregnancy? A prospective sonographic study. Am J Roentgenol. 1992;158:843-7.

5. Levi CS, Lyons EA, Lindsay DJ. Early diagnosis of nonviable pregnancy with transvaginal US. Radiology. 1988;167:383-5.

6. Hoddick WK, Mahony BS, Callen PW, Filly RA. Placental thickness. J Ultrasound Med. 1985;4:479-82.

7. Raio L, Ghezzi F, Cromi A, Nelle M, Dürig P, Schneider H. The thick heterogeneous (jellylike) placenta: a strong predictor of adverse pregnancy outcome. Prenat Diagn. 2004;24(3):182-8.

8. Aherne W. A weight relationship between the human fetus and placenta. Biol Neonate. 1966;10:113-8.

9. Molteni RA, Stys SJ, Battaglia FC. Relationship of fetal and placental weight in human beings: fetal/placental weight ratios at various gestational ages and birth weight distributions. J Reprod Med. 1978;21:327-34.

10. Wolf H, Oosting H, Treffers PE. Second-trimester placental volume measured by ultrasound: prediction of fetal outcome. Am J Obstet Gyncol. 1989;160:121-6.

11. Thame M, Osmond C, Wilks R, Bennett FI, Forrester TE. Thame M, et al. Second-trimester placental volume and infant size at birth. Obstet Gynecol. 2001;98:279-83.

12. Hafner E, Phillip T, Schucter K, Dillinger-Paller B, Philipp K, Bauer P. Second-trimester measurements of placental volume by three-dimensional ultrasound to predict small-for-gestational age infants. Ultrasound Obstet Gynecol. 1998;12:97-102.

13. Hafner E, Metzenbauer M, Höfinger D, Munkel M, Gassner R, Schuchter K, et al. Placental growth from the first to the second trimester of pregnancy in SGA-foetuses and pre-eclamptic pregnancies compared to normal foetuses. Placenta. 2003;24:336-42.

14. Sprit BA, Cohen WN, Weinstein HM. The incidence of placental calcification in normal pregnancies. Radiology. 1982;142:707-11.

15. Kazzi GM, Gross TL, Rosen MG. The relationship of placental grade, fetal maturity, and neonatal outcome in normal and complicated pregnancies. Am J Obstet Gynecol. 1984;148(1):54-8.

16. Vosmar MB, Jongsma HW, van Dongen PW. The value of ultrasonic placental grading: no correlation with intrauterine growth restriction or with maternal smoking. J Pernat Med. 1989;17(2):137-43.

17. Quinlan RW, Cruz AC, Buhi WC, Martin M. Changes in placental ultrasonic appearance. Pathologic significance of Grade III placental changes. Am J Obstet Gynecol 1982;144(4):471-3.

18. Kazzi GM, Gross TL, Sokol RJ, Kazzi NJ. Detection of intrauterine growth retardation: a new use for sonographic placental grading. Am J Obstet Gynecol 1983;145(6):733-7.

19. Hopper KD, Komppa GH, Bice P, Williams MD, Cotterill RW, Ghaed N. A reevaluation of placental grading and its clinical significance. J Ultrasound Med. 1984;3(6):261-6.

20. Chitlange SM, Hazari KT, Joshi JV, Shah RK, Mehta AC. Ultrasonographically observed preterm grade III placenta and perinatal outcome. Int J Gynaecol Obstet. 1990;31(4):325-8.

21. McKenna D, Tharmaratnam S, Mahsud S, Dornan J. Ultrasonic evidence of placental calcification at 36 weeks' gestation: maternal and fetal outcomes. Acta Obstet Gynecol Scand. 2005;84:7-10.

22. Spirt BA, Gordon LP. The placenta as an indicator of fetal maturity—fact and fancy. Semin Ultrasound. 1984;5:290-2.

23. Montan S, Jörgensen C, Svalenius E, Ingemarsson I. Placental grading with ultrasound in hypertensive and normotensive pregnancies. A prospective, consecutive study. Acta Obstet Gynecol Scand. 1986;65(5):477-80.

24. Brown HL, Miller JM, Khawli O, Gabert HA. Premature placental calcification in maternal cigarette smokers. Obstet Gynecol. 1988;71:914-7.

25. Pinette M, Loftus-Brault K, Nard D. Maternal smoking and accelerated placental maturation. Obstet Gynecol. 1989; 73:379-82.

26. Grannum PA, Berkowitz RL, Hobbins JC. The ultrasonic changes in the maturing placenta and their relation to fetal pulmonic maturity. Am J Obstet Gynecol. 1979;133:915-22.

27. Spirt BA, Gordon LP. Sonography of the placenta. In: Fleischer AC, Manning FA, Jeanty P, Romero R (Eds). Sonography in Obstetrics and Gynecology, 6th edition. New York: McGraw Hill; 2001. pp. 195-245.

28. Wilson D, Paalman RJ. Clinical significance of circumvallate placenta. Obstet Gynecol. 1967;29(6):774-8.

29. Naftolin F, Khudur G, Benirschke K, Hutchinson DL. The syndrome of chronic abruption placentae, hydrorrhea, and circumvallate placenta. Am J Obstet Gynecol. 1973; 116(3):347-50.

30. Harris RD, Wells WA, Black WC, Chertoff JD, Poplack SP, Sargent SK, et al. Accuracy of prenatal sonography for detecting circumvallate placenta. Am J Roentgenol. 1997;168(6): 1603-8.

31. Spirt BA, Kagan EH, Gordon LP, Massad LS. Antepartum diagnosis of a succenturiate lobe: sonographic and pathologic correlation. J Clin Ultrasound. 1981;9(3):139-40.

32. Chihara H, Obsubo Y, Ohta Y, Araki T. Prenatal Diagnosis of succenturiate lobe by ultrasonography and color Doppler imaging. Arch Gynecol Obstet. 2000;263(3):137-8.

33. Molloy CE, McDowell W, Armour R, Crawford W, Bernstine R. Ultrasonic diagnosis of placenta membranacea in utero. J Ultrasound Med. 1983;2:377-9.

34. Greenburg JA, Sorem KA, Shifren JF, Riley LE. Placenta membranacea with placenta increta: a case report and literature review. Obstet Gynecol. 1991;78(3 part 2): 512-4.

35. Spirt BA, Kagan EH, Rozanski RM. Sonolucent areas in the placenta: sonographic and pathologic correlation. Am J Roentgenol. 1978;131:961-5.

36. Fox H. Pathology of the placenta. Clin Obstet Gynecol. 1986;13:501-19.

37. Fleischer A, Kurtz A, Wapner R, Ruch D, Sacks GA, Jeanty P, et al. Elevated alpha-fetoprotein and a normal fetal sonogram: association with placental abnormalties. Am J Roentgenol. 1988;150:881-3.

38. Smith HO. Gestational trophoblastic disease epidemiology and trends. Clin Obstet Gynecol. 2003;46(3):541-56.

39. Woo GW, Rocha FG, Gaspar-Oishi M, Bartholomew ML, Thompson KS. Placental mesenchymal dysplasia. Am J Obstet Gynecol. 2011;205:6 e3-5.

40. Lazarus E, Hulka C, Siewert B, Levine D. Sonographic appearance of early complete molar pregnancies. J Ultrasound Med. 1999;18(9):589-94.

41. Benson CB, Genest DR, Bernstein MR, Soto-Wright V, Goldstein DP, Berkowitz RS. Sonographic appearance of first trimester complete hydatidiform moles. Ultrasound Obstet Gynecol. 2000;16(2):188-91.

42. Hadi HA, Finley J, Strickland D. Placental chorioangioma: prenatal diagnosis and clinical significance. Am J Perinatol. 1993;10 (2):146-9.

43. Battaglia MC, Woolever CA. Fetal and neonatal complications associated with recurrent chorioangiomas. Pediatrics. 1967; 41:62-6.

44. Harris RD, Alexander RD. Ultrasound of the placenta and umbilical cord. In: Callen PW (Ed). Ultrasonography in Obstetrics and Gynecology, 4th edition. Philadelphia: WB Saunders; 2000. pp. 597-625.

45. Detti L, Mari G, Akiyama M, Cosmi E, Moise KJ Jr, Stefor T, et al. Longitudinal assessment of the middle cerebral artery peak systolic velocity in healthy fetuses and in fetuses at risk for anemia. Am J Obstet Gynecol. 2002;187(4):937-9.

46. Haak MC, Oosterhof H, Mouw RJ, Oepkes D, Vandenbussche FP. Pathophysiology and treatment of fetal anemia due to placental chorioangioma. Ultrasound Obstet Gynecol. 1999;14:68-70.

47. Stabile I, Campbell S, Grudzinskas J. Threatened miscarriage and intrauterine hematomas. J Ultrasound Med. 1989;8:289-92.

48. Sauerbrei EE, Pham DH. Placental abruption and subchorionic hemorrhage in the first half of pregnancy: US appearance and clinical outcome. Radiology. 1986;160(1):109-12.

49. Nyberg D, Cyr D, Mack L, Wilson DA, Shuman WP. Sonographic spectrum of placental abruption. Am J Roentgenol. 1987;148:161-4.

50. Sholl J. Abruptio placentae: clinical management in nonacute cases. Am J Obstet Gynecol. 1987;156:40-51.

51. Nyberg D, Mack LA, Benedetti TJ, Cyr DR, Schuman WP. Placental abruption and placental hemorrhage: correlation of sonographic findings with fetal outcome. Radiology. 1987;164:357-61.

52. Faiz AS, Anath CV. Etiology and risk factors for placenta previa: an overview and meta-analysis of observational studies. J Matern Fetal Neonatal Med. 2003;13:175-90.

53. Lavery JP, Placenta previa. Clin Obstet Gynecol. 1990;33:414-21.

54. Oppenheimer LW, Farine D, Ritchie JW, Lewinsky RM, Telford J, Fairbanks LA. What is a low-lying placenta. Am J Obstet Gynecol. 1991;165:1036-8.

55. Becker RH, Vonk R, Mende BC, Ragosch V, Entezami M. The relevance of placental location at 20-23 gestational weeks for prediction of placenta previa at delivery: evaluation of 8650 cases. Ultrasound Obstet Gynecol. 2001;17:496-501.

56. Cotton DB, Read JA, Paul RH, Quilligan EJ. The conservative aggressive management of placenta previa. Am J Obstet Gynecol. 1980;137:687-95.

57. Leerentveld RA, Giberts EC, Arnold MJ, Wladimir JW. Accuracy and safety of transvaginal sonographic placental localization. Obstet Gynecol. 1990;76:759-62.

58. Timor-Tritsch IE, Yunis RA. Confirming the safety of transvaginal sonography in patients suspected of placenta previa. Obstet Gynecol. 1993;81;742-4.

59. O'Brian JM, Barton JR, Donaldson ES. The management of placenta percreta: conservative and operative strategies. Am J Obstet Gynecol. 1996;175:1632-8.

60. Wu S, Kocherginsky M, Hibbard JU. Abnormal placentation: twenty year analysis. Am J Obstet Gynecol. 2005;192: 1458-61.

61. Miller DA, Diaz FG, Paul RH. Incidence of placenta previa with previous cesarean. Am J Obstet Gynecol. 1996;174:345.

62. Clark SL, Koonings PP, Phelan JP. Placenta previa/accreta and prior cesarean section. Obstet Gynecol. 1985;66:89-92.

63. Finberg HJ, Williams, JW. Placenta accreta: prospective sonographic diagnosis in patients with placenta previa and prior cesarean section. J Ultrasound Med 1992;11:333-43.

64. Chou MM, Ho ES, Lee YH. Prenatal Diagnosis of placenta accreta by transabominal color Doppler ultrasound. Ultrasound Obstet Gynecol. 2000;15(1):28-35.

65. Jaraquemada JM, Bruno CH. Magnetic resonance imaging in 300 cases of placenta accreta: surgical correlation of new findings. Acta Obstet Gynecol Scand. 2005;84:716-24.

66. Zalud IZ, Shaha S. Evaluation of the utero-placental circulation by three-dimensional Doppler ultrasound in the second trimester of normal pregnancy. J Matern Fetal Neonatal Med. 2007;20(4):299-305.

67. Hata T, Tanaka H, Noguchi J, Hata K. Three-dimensional ultrasound evaluation of the placenta. Placenta. 2011; 32(2):105-15.

68. Yamasato K, Zalud I. Three-dimensional power Doppler of the placenta and its clinical applications. J Perinat Med. 2017;45(6):693-700.

69. Calì G, Forlani F, Minneci G. Three-dimensional ultrasonography and three-dimensional power Doppler in the evaluation of placenta accreta spectrum. Donald School J Ultrasound Obstet Gynecol. 2019;13(1):4-9.

70. Kurjak A, Barsic B. Changes of placental site diagnosed by repeated ultrasonic examination. Acta Obstet Gynecol Scand. 1977;56:161-5.

71. Hata T, Koyanagi A, Takayoshi R, Miyake T, Nitta E, Kanenishi K. Superb microvascular imaging of retained placenta with placenta accreta spectrum. Donald School J Ultrasound Obstet Gynecol. 2019;13(3):85-7.

Congenital Cardiac Tumors

Aleksandar Ljubić, Ida Jovanović, Dušan Damnjanović, Milica Đurđić,
Andjela Perović, Milena Srbinović, Dušica Petrović, Tatjana Božanović

◼ INTRODUCTION

Congenital cardiac tumors are rare in infants and children. Among the pediatric population, more than 90% of cardiac neoplasms are histologically benign, malignant, and metastatic tumors are also described, although they are very rare.[1,2] However, they have the potential for serious consequences, like cardiac arrhythmias, inflow or outflow tract obstruction, heart failure, hydrops, and even sudden death. Early prenatal diagnosis is important for careful fetal monitoring and therapy during pregnancy and adequate management of the pregnancy and labor.

◼ INCIDENCE AND ETIOLOGY

Estimated incidence of cardiac tumors is 1–2:10.000 patients.[3] The occurrence rate in infants and children varies from 0.0017 to 0.25% of pediatric autopsies.[4,5] Tumors are seen more frequently in fetal series than in unselected neonates due to recent changes in clinical practice and advance in sonographic imaging. In one of the large multicentric study, cardiac tumors were recognized in 0.14% pregnancies referred for fetal echocardiography.[6]

Etiology of congenital cardiac tumors is unknown.

◼ PATHOLOGY

Tumor can be located in ventricular or atrial walls or in the pericardium. It can be singular or multiple, solid (homogeneous) or cystic. Majority of tumors are unencapsulated, but some are encapsulated.

Primary cardiac tumors can be divided into two subcategories—benign tumors (rhabdomyomas, teratomas, fibromas, hemangiomas, hamartomas, and myxomas) and malignant tumors (rhabdomyosarcomas and fibrosarcomas).[1] Some authors added oncocytic (histiocytoid) cardiomyopathy into the category.[2] Malignant fetal cardiac tumors are extremely rare.

TABLE 1: Cardiac tumors and tumor-like conditions of the fetus and neonate.[9-13]

Primary	Metastatic tumors	Miscellaneous tumor-like conditions
• Rhabdomyoma • Teratoma • Fibroma • Myxoma • Oncocytic (histiocytoid) cardiomyopathy • Hemangioma • Lymphangioma • Hemangiopericytoma • Intravascular fasciitis • Rhabdomyosarcoma • Fibrosarcoma	• Neuroblastoma • Leukemia	• Epithelial cysts • Blood cyst of heart valves

Rhabdomyoma is the most common tumor, occurring in 62–89% of cases, *teratoma* in 7–21%, but *fibroma, hemangioma, hamartoma,* and *myxoma* are very rare **(Table 1)**.[2,5-9]

▮ PRENATAL DIAGNOSIS OF CARDIAC TUMORS

Fetal echocardiography is a well-established tool for the prenatal diagnosis of cardiac tumors.

Diagnosis of fetal heart tumor is almost always recognized during routine obstetric ultrasound examination. Clinical manifestation of tumor depends on size, location, and number of cardiac tumors. Usual types of presentation are:
- Abnormal cardiac mass seen during regular obstetric ultrasound
- Irregular fetal heart rhythm
- Fetal hydrops
- Pericardial effusion.

There are a lot of differences in morphology, clinical presentation, and particularly prognosis between different

TABLE 2: Main pathologic characteristic of fetal cardiac tumors.

Tumor location	Number of tumors	Morphology	Histology
• Atrial • Ventricular • Pericardial	• Single • Multiple	• Solid • Cystic • Unencapsulated • Encapsulated	• Rhabdomyoma • Teratoma • Fibroma • Hamartoma • Hemangioma • Myxoma

types of tumors **(Table 2)**. This is important for differential diagnosis and pregnancy management.

In a recent study, the magnetic resonance imaging (MRI) was found to be very promising technique for diagnosing solitary tumors, because it assists in tissue characterization if different sequences are applied and helps define the relationship with normal structures.[14,15]

◼ FETAL CARDIAC TUMORS

Rhabdomyoma

Rhabdomyoma is the most common congenital cardiac tumor. The reported incidence for cardiac rhabdomyoma varies from 0.002 to 0.25% in autopsy, 0.02 to 0.08% in live-born infants, and 0.12% in prenatal fetal studies.[2,16]

It is an anomalous benign proliferation of embryonal myoblasts displaying typical "spider cells" on histopathology, with positive immunoreactivities to periodic acid–Schiff, myoglobin, desmin, actin, and myogenin.[17]

The tumors tend to appear as early as at 17th week, but typically between 20 and 30 weeks of gestation.[1,7] Rhabdomyomas grow slowly in utero under the influence of maternal hormones. The tumor mass is solid, circumscribed, unencapsulated, and of variable size **(Figs. 1 to 5)**. It may arise anywhere in the myocardium, most commonly the ventricle, but not from a valve, and may project into the

cardiac chamber, or extracardiacally.[18,19] Dependent on size and location, tumor may cause variety of arrhythmias, usually supraventricular tachycardia (SVT) **(Fig. 1B)** or may grow within the cardiac chambers obstructing inflow to or outflow from either ventricle **(Fig. 6A)**. In utero, however, cardiac problems such as pericardial effusion or arrhythmia occurred regardless of tumor size.[16]

The tumors can be single, but are more commonly multiple (up to 90%) **(Fig. 6B)**.[8,16] It can be the reason for nonimmune hydrops.[20-22] Small pericardial effusion is common. In some cases, cardiac rhabdomyoma is associated with congenital heart abnormalities, complicating treatment, and outcomes. Tetralogy of Fallot with a missing tricuspid valve, Ebstein's malformation with an atrial septal defect, and hypoplastic left heart syndrome are examples.[6]

There is a very strong connection between cardiac rhabdomyomas and tuberous sclerosis, occurring in 50% fetuses with a single tumor and 100% of patients with multiple cardiac rhabdomyomas.[5,6,23,24] In utero, rhabdomyoma is the first clinical sign of tuberous sclerosis.[2,25] Tuberous sclerosis is a familial disease inherited as an autosomal dominant trait, with a high degree of penetrance and variable expressivity. However, it is thought that between 50 and 80% of cases are caused by novel mutations.[26] The genes, *TSC1* on chromosome 9q34, encoding hamartin, and *TSC2* on chromosome 16p13.3, encoding the tuberin are responsible for tuberous sclerosis.[27] Quest for finding the cause of mutations is very difficult due to their random distribution over the genes.

Skin lesions are one of the clinical symptoms of tuberous sclerosis (hypomelanotic macules—usually present at birth, adenoma sebaceum, shagreen patches), along with cerebral malformations (periventricular calcifications or nodules, seizures, cerebral atrophy) and retinal phakomata. Renal angiomyolipomas and hamartomas are common in tuberous sclerosis patients, however, they typically appear

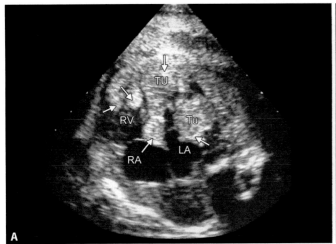
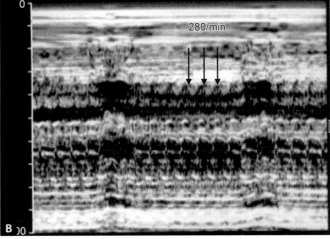

Figs.1A and B: (A) Four-chamber view of the fetal heart with a typical appearance of multiple rhabdomyoma (arrows); (B) M-mode recording of supraventricular tachycardia at 280 beats/min in the same fetus.
(LA: left atrium; RA: right atrium; RV: right ventricle; Tu: tumor)

later in life and advance slowly. Up to 80% of infants with tuberous sclerosis will have seizures and mental retardation, which are the most serious long-term complications of the disease. There is evidence of an unexpected link between prenatally diagnosed cardiac rhabdomyoma and Down's syndrome in fetuses with tuberous sclerosis.[28]

With the exception of tuberous sclerosis, there is no link between cardiac rhabdomyoma and any hereditary or familial illnesses. More than half of rhabdomyomas detected antenatally are asymptomatic and identified through regular obstetric screening sonography.[6] On sonograms, rhabdomyomas are rounded, homogeneous, hyperechogenic regions.[2]

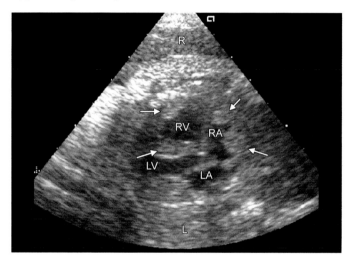

Fig. 2: Multiple rhabdomyomas in fetus referred due to extrasystolic arrhythmia; two tumors were located at the roof of the right atria and two additional small tumors were in the right ventricle, of similar echo texture as surrounding myocardium.
(LA: left atrium; LV: left ventricle; R: right; RA: right atrium; RV: right ventricle)

In utero prognosis depends on the number, size, and location of tumors as well as the presence of hemodynamic abnormalities, cardiac arrhythmias, and hydrops. After birth most rhabdomyomas show some degree or complete regression.[29,30] The clinical spectrum ranges from completely asymptomatic to severely ill neonates. In utero 75% of rhabdomyomas stayed stable in size and 25% of rhabdomyomas showed progression.[16]

However, although spontaneous tumor regression has been observed, sudden death is not uncommon.[31-34] The 29% mortality rate has been reported[35] for infants operated on within the first year of life. Up to 80% of infants with tuberous sclerosis will have seizures and mental retardation, which are the most severe long-term complications of the disease. For neonates with cardiac symptoms on birth, surgical intervention is required. Everolimus (mammalian target of rapamycin inhibitor) can be used for inoperable multifocal cardiac rhabdomyomas.[36-38]

Teratoma

Teratomas are the second most common tumors reported prenatally, detected by imaging studies more often antenatally than postnatally.[2,35,39-41] They are diagnosed on average in mid-gestation, significantly earlier compared to rhabdomyomas and fibromas.[42]

Teratomas are rare primary tumors of the heart that emerge from the pericardium, although they can be found in the auricle or ventricle. They usually emerge from the heart's base and receive sustenance from the aorta or pulmonary artery. The tumor consists of multiple cysts within solid areas that can be projected through the chambers of the heart.[43]

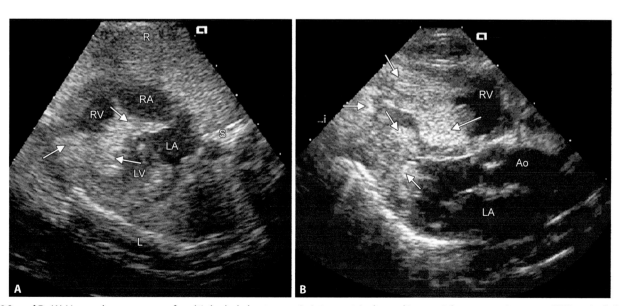

Figs. 3A and B: (A) Unusual appearance of multiple rhabdomyomas in interventricular and interatrial septa arteriovenous (AV) node, followed by complete AV block; (B) Postnatal long-axis view with apparent tumors growth.
(Ao: aorta; L: left; LA: left atrium; LV: left ventricle; R: right; RA: right atrium; RV: right ventricle; S: spine)

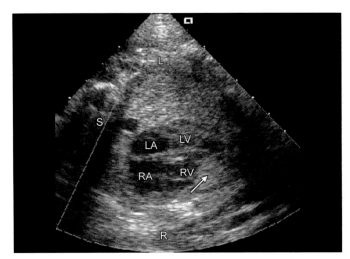

Fig. 4: Solitary tumor into the right ventricular apex. The father and the sister of the fetus have cutaneous changes suspicious for tuberous sclerosis. After the birth, diagnosis of tuberous sclerosis in the child was confirmed.
(L: left; LA: left atrium; LV: left ventricle; R: right; RA: right atrium; RV: right ventricle; S: spine)

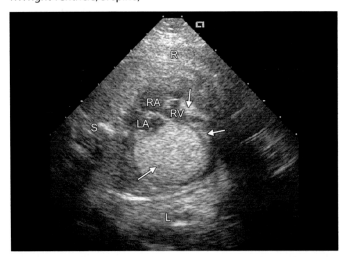

Fig. 5: A huge cardiac rhabdomyoma occupying almost the entire cavity of the left ventricle (surprisingly with no inflow- or outflow-tract obstruction) and few small additional tumors.
(L: left; LA: left atrium; R: right; RA: right atrium; RV: right ventricle; S: spine)

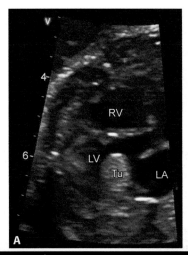

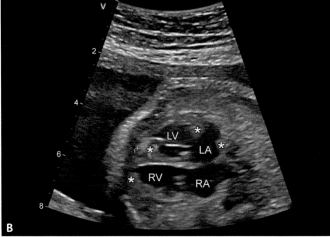

Figs. 6A and B: (A) Fetal echocardiography (three-chamber view) showing large rhabdomyoma (Tu) located in the left ventricular (LV) inlet portion; (B) Fetal echocardiography (four-chamber view) at 24 weeks, showing a multiple rhabdomyomas (asterix).
(LA: left atrium; RA: right atrium; RV: right ventricle; Tu: tumor)

Teratomas are usually single, encapsulated tumors attached to the base of the heart. On imaging study, the main presenting findings in the fetus are the tumor and pericardial effusion **(Figs. 7A and B)**.[44-48] Fetal hydrops and stillbirth are less common.[46]

Pericardial teratomas in fetuses cause more or less severe pericardial effusions, which can be worsened by cardiac compression and/or hydrops fetalis. Pericardial teratomas are a type of teratoma that can be treated. However, due to mediastinal disease (compression and hydrops fetalis), they may become life-threatening. Occasionally, the sole indicators of fetal pericardial teratomas are significant pericardial effusions.[1,49]

In addition, computerized tomography and MRI are helpful in determining the diagnosis. Solid and multicystic areas, sometimes with foci of calcification are diagnostic on imaging studies.[35]

Prognosis depends on the size, hemodynamic status, and the amount of pericardial effusion. The development of fetal hydrops requires treatment with in utero pericardiocentesis or early delivery.[46-48,50] Pericardial teratomas have been successfully removed in neonates, with the highest survival rate after surgical excision; hemangioma is the exception.[2,48] In situations of polyhydramnios, aspiration of intrapericardial or pleural fluid and amniodrainage are less intrusive approaches to relieve cardiac compression and tamponade and to reduce the risk of preterm labor due to overdistension.[49] Cardiac teratoma may cause stillbirth or sudden unexpected death in the perinatal period.[46,51] Cardiac teratomas are more common among twins.[52]

Fibroma

Cardiac fibroma is a rare, benign tumor that occurs predominately in infants and children.[5,53]

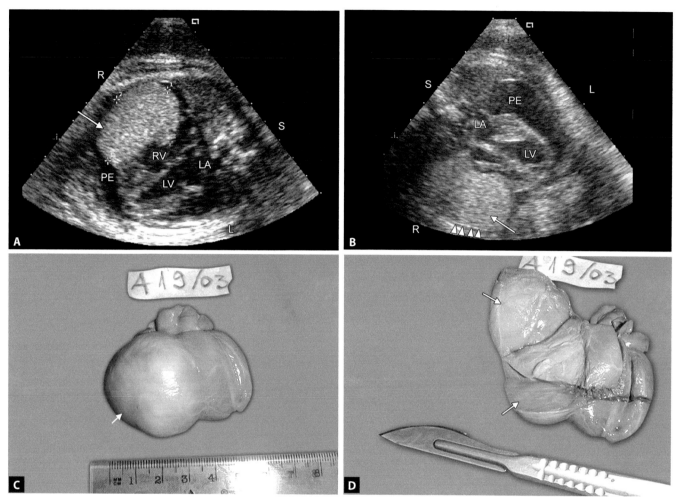

Figs. 7A to D: (A) Very large intrapericardial tumor (arrow) from the base of the heart of homogeneous appearance; (B) In this view, additional information characteristic for teratoma was obtained: large pericardial effusion (PE), presence of tumor capsule (arrowheads), and hypodense zone in the tumor; (C and D) Autopsy findings confirmed diagnosis of teratoma.
(L: left; LA: left atrium; LV: left ventricle; R: right; RA: right atrium; RV: right ventricle; S: spine)

Cardiac fibromas are connective tissue tumors arising from fibroblasts and myofibroblasts having similar gross and microscopic features and biologic behavior as their soft tissue counterpart.[35] Synonyms for cardiac fibroma are fibromatosis, myofibromatosis, fibrous hamartoma, congenital mesoblastic tumor.[10] The tumor may be either circumscribed or unencapsulated, blending imperceptively with the adjacent myocardium, thus making it difficult to remove from the adjacent myocardium.[2]

They are single intracardiac tumors, usually in the interventricular septum or left or right from the ventricular free wall. A typical sonographic finding is a homogeneous echogenic mass. However, the tumors can show the nonhomogeneous echogenicity in a case of cystic degeneration, which may help to distinguish this tumor from a single rhabdomyoma. MRI provides additional information on the characterization of the tissue components.[54]

Fibromas can cause left ventricular outflow obstruction and ventricular dysfunction, leading to congestive heart failure, or they can cause cardiac arrhythmias due to conduction abnormalities.[50] Extracardiac abnormalities or syndromes may be present in some cases. For example, cardiac fibroma has been linked to cleft lip and palate,[55,56] Beckwith–Wiedemann syndrome,[57,58] and, most commonly, Gorlin syndrome (nevoid basal cell carcinoma syndrome).[58]

Fibroma does not regress postnatally and may need surgical resection, or the affected patient can even be the candidate for cardiac transplantation.[7]

Hamartoma

Cardiac hamartomas are very rare. Some authors consider the hamartoma as a synonym for rhabdomyoma, but there are differences between them.

Hamartomas consist of a mixture of spindle cells and cardiac myocytes arranged in haphazard way. They do not have spider cells like rhabdomyomas. The hamartoma has been recognized in a fetus at 32 weeks of gestation like a tumor predominantly involving the left ventricle and associated with pericardial effusion.[7] The precise diagnosis has been made at autopsy, after birth.

Hemangioma

Cardiac hemangiomas are benign vascular tumors and have yet to be identified in utero.

Hemangiomas can involve any chamber of the heart, although the right atrium is most frequent location.[2] This tumor has been recognized in a fetus at 28 weeks' gestation. With the use of fetal echocardiography, a mixed echogenic mass protruding outward from the right atrial wall was observed. Moderate amounts of pericardial effusion were also found. Although no apparent blood flow signal was detected in the mass, fetal echocardiography showed signs suggestive of a hemangioma.[59,60]

Magnetic resonance imaging can be of more diagnostic value in determining the possible tumor type.[61]

Intrauterine pericardiocentesis may be needed. Vascular tumors have tendency to regress without therapy, but for patients with rapid growth and heart failure treatment option is surgical resection. Steroid therapy is used in case of an inoperable tumors.[6,59]

Myxoma

Myxoma, a benign neoplasm derived from cardiac multipotential mesenchymal cells, is the most common primary tumor of the heart in adults but is very rare in the fetus and neonate.[10,12] Only a few cases have been reported.[9,10]

Prenatal echocardiography is a safe and effective diagnostic tool that can detect cardiac myxomas as early as 18 weeks of pregnancy.[62]

Myxomas arise from the endocardium, occurring most frequently in the left atrium. They are characteristically polypoid, soft, gelatinous, friable grayish-white mucoid in appearance, with a broad base of attachment. When a soft, echogenic, pedunculated mass is found within the fetal heart, this diagnosis should be considered.[9]

When a tumor appears on the left side of the heart, it produces mitral valve disease, specifically mitral stenosis, as well as other symptoms. It causes tricuspid or pulmonary valvular disease, as well as conduction abnormalities, when it comes from the right side.[2]

Complete surgical excision, if possible, is the treatment option. Valve replacement may be required.[10]

■ DIFFERENTIAL DIAGNOSIS AND PITFALLS

It is impossible to make a histologic diagnosis in utero, but several ultrasonographic criteria may help narrow the differential diagnosis. These criteria are:
- Number of tumors
- Size
- Location
- Nature of the mass.

The presence of *multiple tumors* is suggestive of rhabdomyoma, with 100% association with tuberous sclerosis.

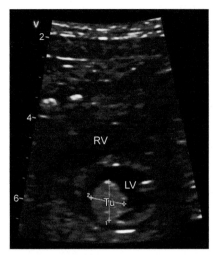

Fig. 8: Fetal echocardiography (short-axis view) at 26 weeks, showing large tumor (Tu) in the left ventricle.
(LV: left ventricle; RV: right ventricle)

Size is variable in all types of tumors. But, a large, singular tumor, heterogenous, lobulated, and encapsulated, is characteristic for teratoma. The most distinguishing feature of intrapericardial teratoma can be its huge size, followed by pericardial effusion. Rhabdomyoma can also be very large, but one should carefully search for additional small tumors.

Location is variable. A pericardial tumor, particularly attached to the base of the heart is characteristic for teratoma. If the tumor is arising from the endocardium, especially from the left atrium and is a soft, pedunculated mass, it is strongly indicated of myxoma. Hemangioma and teratoma are both cystic tumors, but hemangioma more often occurs in the atrium, while teratoma is more frequently located within the pericardial space.[42]

If the *nature* of tumor is cystic, it could be teratoma, fibroma with degeneration, hemangioma, and hamartoma. If the tumor is homogeneous, it could be rhabdomyoma or fibroma.

Echotexture is almost always hyperechoic **(Fig. 8)**. Some fibromas can be isoechoic.

The *pitfalls* associated to prenatal echocardiographic diagnosis of cardiac tumors include:
- They may be too small to be visualized.
- Intracardiac echogenic foci may imitate tumors.
- Echogenicity resulting from extracardiac structures or neoplasms near the heart may falsely appear as tumors.

■ MANAGEMENT AND COUNSELING

Early prenatal diagnosis is important for adequate management of pregnancy.

Death of neonate is connected to the fetal hydrops, larger tumor (≥40 mm), premature delivery (≤31 weeks of gestation), and treatment resistant SVT.[42]

Management of pregnancy depends on gestation at diagnosis, patient's wishes, and the likely histologic type of tumor.[7] If a rhabdomyoma is recognized, it is of the utmost importance to inform the future parents of the virtually constant perspective of tuberous sclerosis complex. If diagnosis is made within the legal time limit, termination of pregnancy may be suggested.

Ultrasonic evaluations should be performed regularly to identify signs of hemodynamic compromise, congestive heart failure or arrhythmias. Standard obstetrical management is appropriate for uncomplicated cases.

In utero fetal therapy or preterm delivery should be considered if cardiac function is severely impaired.

There is no therapeutic guideline for cases of fetal cardiac tumors exhibiting hydrops fetalis so far. However, several investigators have indicated some therapeutic methods. In cases of hydrops fetalis caused by SVT, elevated preload condition and successful transplacental therapy have been reported.[22,63]

Pericardiocentesis is indicated for cardiac decompression in fetuses with pericardial effusion in cases with teratoma.[45] Furthermore, in utero open surgery has been suggested for an intrapericardial teratoma.[64]

The delivery should take place in a tertiary care facility with access to a pediatric cardiologist. In the asymptomatic patient, conservative neonatal management is recommended, with surgery reserved for those with hemodynamic impairment.

■ REFERENCES

1. Yuan SM. Fetal primary cardiac tumors during perinatal period. Pediatr Neonatol. 2017;58(3):205-10.
2. Isaacs H Jr. Fetal and neonatal cardiac tumors. Pediatr Cardiol. 2004;25(3):252-73.
3. McAllister HA Jr. Primary tumors of the heart and pericardium. Pathol Annu. 1979;14 Pt 2:325-55.
4. Nadas AS, Ellison RC. Cardiac tumors in infancy. Am J Cardiol. 1968;21(3):363-6.
5. Groves AM, Fagg NL, Cook AC, Allan LD. Cardiac tumours in intrauterine life. Arch Dis Child. 1992;67(10 Spec No):1189-92.
6. Holley DG, Martin GR, Brenner JI, Fyfe DA, Huhta JC, Kleinman CS, et al. Diagnosis and management of fetal cardiac tumors: a multicenter experience and review of published reports. J Am Coll Cardiol. 1995;26(2):516-20.
7. Allan L. Fetal cardiac tumors. In: Sharland G, Allan L, Hornberger L, Hornberger LK (Eds). Textbook of Fetal Cardiology. London: Greenwich Medical Media; 2000. pp. 358-65.
8. Manco-Johnson ML, Drose JA. Congenital cardiac tumors. In: Drose JA (Ed). Fetal Echocardiography. Philadelphia: WB Saunders; 1998. pp. 241-51.
9. Paladini D, Tartaglione A, Vassallo M, Martinelli P. Prenatal ultrasonographic findings of a cardiac myxoma. Obstet Gynecol. 2003;102(5 Pt 2):1174-6.
10. Burke A, Virmani R (Eds). Tumors of the Heart and Great Vessels, Fascicle 16, third series. Washington, D.C.: Armed Forces Institute of Pathology; 1996.
11. Isaacs Jr H. Tumors. In: Gilbert-Barness E (Ed). Potter's Pathology of the Fetus and Infant, Vol. 2. Mosby: St. Louis; 1997. pp. 1319-23.
12. Isaacs Jr H (Ed). Tumors of the Fetus and Newborn, Vol. 35. Philadelphia: Saunders; 1997. pp. 330-43.
13. Isaacs Jr H (Ed). Tumors of the Fetus and Infant: An Atlas. New York: Springer-Verlag; 2002. pp. 377-86.
14. Kivelitz DE, Mühler M, Rake A, Scheer I, Chaoui R. MRI of cardiac rhabdomyoma in the fetus. Eur Radiol. 2004; 14(8):1513-6.
15. Araoz PA, Mulvagh SL, Tazelaar HD, Julsrud PR, Breen JF. CT and MR imaging of benign primary cardiac neoplasms with echocardiographic correlation. Radiographics. 2000; 20(5):1303-19.
16. Altmann J, Kiver V, Henrich W, Weichert A. Clinical outcome of prenatally suspected cardiac rhabdomyomas of the fetus. J Perinat Med. 2019;48(1):74-81.
17. Philip S, Thampy L. A solitary fetal cardiac rhabdomyoma: a hemodynamically unstable left ventricular tumor with autopsy and histopathology findings. J Fetal Med. 2021;8:163-8.
18. Meyer WJ, Gauthier DW, Font G. (1993). Cardiac rhabdomyoma. [online] Available from: https://thefetus.net/content/cardiac-rhabdomyoma/. [Last accessed April, 2022].
19. Lethor JP, de Moor M. Multiple cardiac tumors in the fetus. Circulation. 2001;103(10):E55.
20. Calhoun BC, Watson PT, Hegge F. Ultrasound diagnosis of an obstructive cardiac rhabdomyoma with severe hydrops and hypoplastic lungs. A case report. J Reprod Med. 1991; 36(4):317-9.
21. Guereta LG, Burgueros M, Elorza MD, Alix AG, Benito F, Gamallo C. Cardiac rhabdomyoma presenting as fetal hydrops. Pediatr Cardiol. 1986;7(3):171-4.
22. Nakata M, Fujiwara M, Ishikawa Y, Sumie M, Hasegawa K, Miwa I, et al. Prenatal diagnosis and management for a large fetal cardiac tumor complicated with hydrops fetalis. J Obstet Gynaecol Res. 2005;31(5):476-9.
23. Harding CO, Pagon RA. Incidence of tuberous sclerosis in patients with cardiac rhabdomyoma. Am J Med Genet. 1990;37(4):443-6.
24. Webb DW, Osborne JP. Incidence of tuberous sclerosis in patients with cardiac rhabdomyoma. Am J Med Genet. 1992;42(5):754-5.
25. Bussani R, Rustico MA, Silvestri F. Fetal cardiac rhabdomyomatosis as a prenatal marker for the detection of latent tuberous sclerosis. An autopsy case report. Pathol Res Pract. 2001;197(8):559-61.
26. Chitayat D, McGillivray BC, Diamant S, Wittmann BK, Sandor GG. Role of prenatal detection of cardiac tumours in the diagnosis of tuberous sclerosis—report of two cases. Prenat Diagn. 1988;8(8):577-84.
27. Rosner M, Freilinger A, Lubec G, Hengstschläger M. The tuberous sclerosis genes, TSC1 and TSC2, trigger different gene expression responses. Int J Oncol. 2005;27(5):1411-24.
28. Krapp M, Baschat AA, Gembruch U, Gloeckner K, Schwinger E, Reusche E. Tuberous sclerosis with intracardiac rhabdomyoma in a fetus with trisomy 21: case report and review of literature. Prenat Diagn. 1999;19(7):610-3.
29. Smith HC, Watson GH, Patel RG, Super M. Cardiac rhabdomyomata in tuberous sclerosis: their course and diagnostic value. Arch Dis Child. 1989;64(2):196-200.
30. Alkalay AL, Ferry DA, Lin B, Fink BW, Pomerance JJ. Spontaneous regression of cardiac rhabdomyoma in tuberous sclerosis. Clin Pediatr (Phila). 1987;26(10):532-5.

31. Valdés-Dapena M, Gilbert-Barness E. Cardiovascular causes for sudden infant death. Pediatr Pathol Mol Med. 2002;21(2):195-211.

32. Grellner W, Henssge C. Multiple cardiac rhabdomyoma with exclusively histological manifestation. Forensic Sci Int. 1996;78(1):1-5.

33. Rigle DA, Dexter RD, McGee MB. Cardiac rhabdomyoma presenting as sudden infant death syndrome. J Forensic Sci. 1989;34(3):694-8.

34. Pipitone S, Mongiovì M, Grillo R, Gagliano S, Sperandeo V. Cardiac rhabdomyoma in intrauterine life: clinical features and natural history. A case series and review of published reports. Ital Heart J. 2002;3(1):48-52.

35. Corno A, de Simone G, Catena G, Marcelletti C. Cardiac rhabdomyoma: surgical treatment in the neonate. J Thorac Cardiovasc Surg. 1984;87(5):725-31.

36. Hoshal SG, Samuel BP, Schneider JR, Mammen L, Vettukattil JJ. Regression of massive cardiac rhabdomyoma on everolimus therapy. Pediatr Int. 2016;58(5):397-9.

37. Demir HA, Ekici F, Erdem AY, Emir S, Tunç B. Everolimus: a challenging drug in the treatment of multifocal inoperable cardiac rhabdomyoma. Pediatrics. 2012;130(1):e243-7.

38. Yamamura M, Kojima T, Koyama M, Sazawa A, Yamada T, Minakami H. Everolimus in pregnancy: case report and literature review. J Obstet Gynaecol Res. 2017;43(8):1350-2.

39. Guerrero D, Olavarría S. (2000). Pericardial teratoma. [online] Available from: https://thefetus.net/content/pericardial-teratoma [Last accessed April, 2022].

40. Aldousany AW, Joyner JC, Price RA, Boulden T, Watson D, DiSessa TG. Diagnosis and treatment of intrapericardial teratoma. Pediatr Cardiol. 1987;8(1):51-3.

41. Alegre M, Torrents M, Carreras E, Mortera C, Cusí V, Carrera JM. Prenatal diagnosis of intrapericardial teratoma. Prenat Diagn. 1990;10(3):199-202.

42. Yinon Y, Chitayat D, Blaser S, Seed M, Amsalem H, Yoo SJ, et al. Fetal cardiac tumors: a single-center experience of 40 cases. Prenat Diagn. 2010;30(10):941-9.

43. Brabham KR, Roberts WC. Cardiac-compressing intra-pericardial teratoma at birth. Am J Cardiol. 1989;63(5):386-7.

44. de Bustamante TD, Azpeitia J, Miralles M, Jiménez M, Santos-Briz A, Rodríguez-Peralto JL. Prenatal sonographic detection of pericardial teratoma. J Clin Ultrasound. 2000;28(4):194-8.

45. Daniels CJ, Cohen DM, Phillips JR, Rowland DG. Prenatal detection of a pericardial teratoma. Circulation. 1999;99(2):1-2.

46. Catanzarite V, Mehalek K, Maida C, Mendoza A. Early sonographic diagnosis of intrapericardial teratoma. Ultrasound Obstet Gynecol. 1994;4(6):505-7.

47. Benatar A, Vaughan J, Nicolini U, Trotter S, Corrin B, Lincoln C. Prenatal pericardiocentesis: its role in the management of intrapericardial teratoma. Obstet Gynecol. 1992;79(5 (Pt 2)):856-9.

48. Sepulveda W, Gómez E, Gutiérrez J. Intrapericardial teratoma. Ultrasound Obstet Gynecol. 2000;15(6):547-8.

49. Nassr AA, Shazly SA, Morris SA, Ayres N, Espinoza J, Erfani H, et al. Prenatal management of fetal intrapericardial teratoma: a systematic review. Prenat Diagn. 2017;37(9):849-63.

50. Beghetti M, Gow RM, Haney I, Mawson J, Williams WG, Freedom RM. Pediatric primary benign cardiac tumors: a 15-year review. Am Heart J. 1997;134(6):1107-14.

51. Bruch SW, Adzick NS, Reiss R, Harrison MR. Prenatal therapy for pericardial teratomas. J Pediatr Surg. 1997;32(7):1113-5.

52. Sklansky M, Greenberg M, Lucas V, Gruslin-Giroux A. Intrapericardial teratoma in a twin fetus: diagnosis and management. Obstet Gynecol. 1997;89(5 Pt 2):807-9.

53. Muñoz H, Sherer DM, Romero R, Sanchez J, Hernandez I, Diaz C. Prenatal sonographic findings of a large fetal cardiac fibroma. J Ultrasound Med. 1995;14(6):479-81.

54. Kim TH, Kim YM, Han MY, Kim WH, Oh MH, Han KS. Perinatal sonographic diagnosis of cardiac fibroma with MR imaging correlation. AJR Am J Roentgenol. 2002;178(3):727-9.

55. Back LM, Brown AS, Barot LR. Congenital cardiac tumors in association with orofacial clefts. Ann Plast Surg. 1988;20(6):558-61.

56. de León GA, Zaeri N, Donner RM, Karmazin N. Cerebral rhinocele, hydrocephalus, and cleft lip and palate in infants with cardiac fibroma. J Neurol Sci. 1990;99(1):27-36.

57. Reddy JK, Schimke RN, Chang CH, Svoboda DJ, Slaven J, Therou L. Beckwith-Wiedemann syndrome. Wilms' tumor, cardiac hamartoma, persistent visceromegaly, and glomerulo-neogenesis in a 2-year-old boy. Arch Pathol. 1972;94(6):523-32.

58. Coffin CM. Congenital cardiac fibroma associated with Gorlin syndrome. Pediatr Pathol. 1992;12(2):255-62.

59. Tseng JJ, Chou MM, Lee YH, Ho ES. In utero diagnosis of cardiac hemangioma. Ultrasound Obstet Gynecol. 1999;13(5):363-5.

60. Sebastian V, Einzig S, D'Cruz C, Costello C, Kula M, Campbell A. Cardiac hemangioma of the right atrium in a neonate: fetal management and expedited surgical resection. Images Paediatr Cardiol. 2005;7(4):5-9.

61. Kiaffas MG, Powell AJ, Geva T. Magnetic resonance imaging evaluation of cardiac tumor characteristics in infants and children. Am J Cardiol. 2002;89(10):1229-33.

62. Yuan SM. Fetal cardiac myxomas. Z Geburtshilfe Neonatol. 2017;221(4):175-9.

63. Strasburger JF, Cuneo BF, Michon MM, Gotteiner NL, Deal BJ, McGregor SN, et al. Amiodarone therapy for drug-refractory fetal tachycardia. Circulation. 2004;109(3):375-9.

64. Sydorak RM, Kelly T, Feldstein VA, Sandberg PL, Silverman NH, Harrison MR, et al. Prenatal resection of a fetal pericardial teratoma. Fetal Diagn Ther. 2002;17(5):281-5.

15

Congenital Lung Anomalies

Aleksandar Ljubić, Ida Jovanović, Dušan Damnjanović, Milica Đurđić,
Andjela Perović, Milena Srbinović, Dušica Petrović, Tatjana Božanović

■ INTRODUCTION

Congenital lung abnormalities (CLA) are a group of abnormalities of the lungs and bronchial tree, which can consist of isolated bronchopulmonary anomalies, vascular anomalies, or a mixture of these.[1]

Estimated incidence of all CLAs is 1:35,000 pregnancies[2] and 1:2,400 live births.[3]

Most frequent CLAs include congenital pulmonary airway malformation (CPAM), pulmonary sequestration, bronchial atresia, bronchogenic cyst, and congenital lobar overinflation [(CLO); previously called lobar emphysema].[4] These entities represent more than 95% of all lung anomalies.[5]

Congenital lung abnormalities' prenatal diagnosis has increased significantly in recent years as a result of more extensive and effective prenatal ultrasound (US) screening. Although a well-performed US may offer a proper diagnosis in most circumstances, supplementary magnetic resonance imaging (MRI) or computed tomography (CT) is increasingly being used in certain cases to provide additional information. Ultrasonic and CT findings appears to have a high degree of consistency.[6]

Due to overlapping symptoms between distinct lesions and the existence of complex, hybrid lesions with integrated vascular and bronchopulmonary abnormalities, prenatal diagnosis of CLA is challenging. Prenatal diversity in clinical evolution and outcome is high, ranging from complete involution in utero to progressive growth and secondary complications. Postnatal clinical spectrum varies from the asymptomatic infant to the child with increasing severe respiratory distress requiring prompt intervention.[5,7]

▌ CONGENITAL PULMONARY AIRWAY MALFORMATION

Congenital pulmonary airway malformation is a heterogeneous set of lesions caused by overgrowth of mesenchymal components and disruption of normal alveolar development. It was previously known as congenital

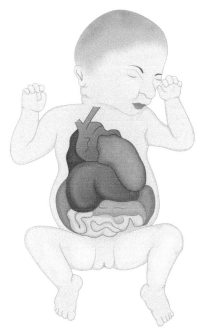

Fig. 1: Schematic illustration of the pathophysiology of large congenital pulmonary airway malformations.
Source: https://childrenswi.org/medical-care/fetal-concerns-center/ conditions/infant-complications/congenital-pulmonary-airway-malformation

cystic adenomatoid malformation (CCAM). Because neither cysts nor adenomatoid elements are present, the term CCAM is no longer deemed suitable.[5] The majority of CPAMs are in the pulmonary vascular circuit and communication with the bronchial tree is normal. The respiratory ciliated epithelium lines the CPAM cysts.[5] The condition can be bilateral, affecting all lung tissues, but it is usually limited to a single lung or lobe.[8] The prevalence of cystic adenomatoid malformation of the lungs is not high **(Fig. 1)**.

Congenital pulmonary airway malformation is slightly more common in males and may affect any lobe of the lung. In 80–95% of cases, the lesion is unilobar, and is bilateral in less than 2% of cases. Unlike bronchopulmonary sequestration (BPS), CPAMs have a communication with the

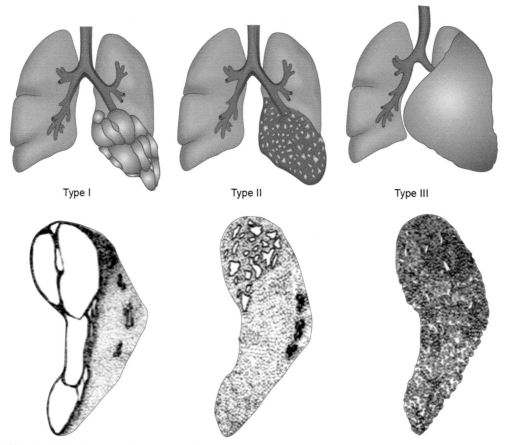

Type I   Type II   Type III

Fig. 2: Depiction of Stocker's classification of type I, II, and III congenital pulmonary airway malformation.
Source: Stocker JT, Madewell JE, Drake RM. Congenital cystic adenomatoid malformation of the lung. Classification and morphologic spectrum. Hum Pathol. 1977;8(2):155-71.

tracheobronchial tree, albeit via a minute tortuous passage. In contrast to BPS, normal pulmonary circulation provides arterial blood supply and venous drainage for CPAMs, but abnormal arterial and venous drainage of CPAM has been also reported.

Stocker et al. proposed a classification of CPAM into three subtypes according to the size of the cysts—type I has large cysts, type II has multiple small cysts of <1.2 cm in diameter, and type III consists of a noncystic lesion producing mediastinal shift.[9] The worst prognosis is seen in type III lesions. Associated anomalies are frequently present in type II **(Fig. 2)**.

Adzick[10] has proposed a revision of Stocker's classification of CPAMs, based on anatomy and sonographic appearance to aid in predicting outcome in cases detected in utero. In this classification, macrocystic CPAMs have single or multiple cysts >5 mm in diameter. Microcystic CPAMs are more solid and bulky, with cysts that are <5 mm in diameter. In the fetus, this differentiation can be easily made sonographically. Macrocystic lesions appear sonographically as fluid-filled cysts, while microcystic lesions appear solid due to fine interfaces with the US beam creating an almost homogeneous appearance.

One theory holds that CPAM occurs around the fifth or sixth week of pregnancy, during the pseudoglandular stage of lung development, when bronciolar structures fail to mature. Others have considered CPAM to represent a focal pulmonary dysplasia, since skeletal muscle has been identified within the cyst walls.

Although the actual cause is unknown, Langston[11] recently suggested in utero airway obstruction as a possible cause, leading to the creation of a more comprehensive classification that includes a large-cyst type comparable to Stocker type I and a small-cyst type equivalent to Stocker type II. Stocker type III is a type of pulmonary hyperplasia that should not be included in the CPAM group, according to this classification.

The rapid growth of the chest mass is compressing the lungs, depressing the diaphragm, shifts the mediastinum, compromising venous return to the heart. Ascites, placentomegaly, and anasarca of nonimmune hydrops develop. Polyhydramnios can be found in up to 70% of CPAMs diagnosed antenatally. The pathogenesis of polyhydramnios is not completely understood, however, it is assumed to be related to esophageal obstruction caused by mediastinal shift and difficulty with fetal amniotic fluid swallowing. The absence of fluid in the stomachs of many of these fetuses supports this theory. Although some prenatal indicators (mediastinal shift, hydrops, etc.) can point to CPAM, the diagnosis of CPAM relies on the demonstration of a solid or cystic, nonpulsatile intrathoracic tumor.[7]

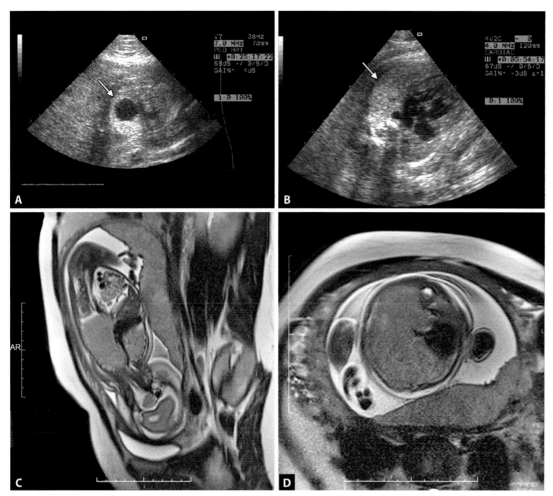

Figs. 3A to D: Prenatal sonographic cross-sectional sonographic image of a fetal chest, demonstrating a large type I congenital pulmonary airway malformation (A—arrow) and type III congenital pulmonary airway malformation (B—arrow) filling the right chest, displacing the mediastinum to the left, as well as magnetic resonance imaging image (C and D).

Congenital pulmonary airway malformations are diagnosed prenatally by the demonstration of a lung tumor that may be solid or cystic in the absence of vascular flow detected by Doppler studies. Types I and II CPAM appear as cystic or echolucent pulmonary masses. It is important to note that on US examination, diaphragmatic hernias, cystic hygromas, and other cystic lesions, such as bronchogenic or enteric cysts, and pericardial cysts, can be mistaken for type I or type II congenital pulmonary airway malformation. When compared to normal pulmonary parenchyma, the implicated lung in some fetuses with Stocker type II or III lesions is homogeneously hyperechoic and hyperintense. Other CLAs, such as BPS and CLO, cannot be distinguished from these lesions.[11] A type III CPAM typically appears as a large hyperechogenic mass, often associated with mediastinal shift and hydrops.

Unilateral lesions are frequently associated with contralateral mediastinum deviation. The heart may be substantially compressed in bilateral disease, which is generally coupled with ascites due to venocaval blockage or cardiac failure.[8]

In about 85% of cases CPAM is unilateral and approximately half are microcystic and the other half macrocystic. Polyhydramnios may develop during the third trimester, which is a result of decreased fetal swallowing, the consequence of esophageal compression by the mass or there may be increased fetal lung fluid production by the abnormal tissue **(Figs. 3 and 4)**.[8]

The condition is usually isolated but in around 10% of cases, additional malformations, such as renal, abdominal wall, or central nervous system abnormalities, are present. There is no significant evidence of association with chromosomal defects **(Fig. 5)**.[8]

Prognosis

The outcome of CPAM is unpredictable; however, there has been evidence of a characteristic evolution in utero. Lesions, which are most typically identified during the second trimester, rise in volume between 20 and 25 weeks of pregnancy before stabilizing toward the conclusion of the trimester.[12] During the mid-third trimester, usually at 29–34 weeks' gestation, 20–50% of women experience further

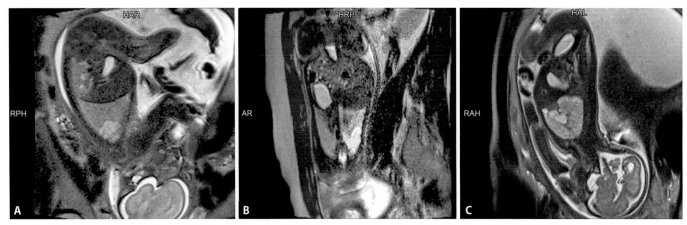

Figs. 4A to C: (A) 28 gestational weeks, T2W sequence, sagittal plane of the upper lung field on the right is lobulated, elevated intensity signal relative to the normal lung wing; (B) 29 gestational weeks T2W sequence, the coronal plane of the upper lung field on the right is lobulated, elevated intensity signal relative to the normal lung wing; (C) 29 gestational weeks, T2W sequence, parasagittal plane left lung is lobulated, pseudocystically altered, enlarged, elevated intensity signal relative to normal lung.

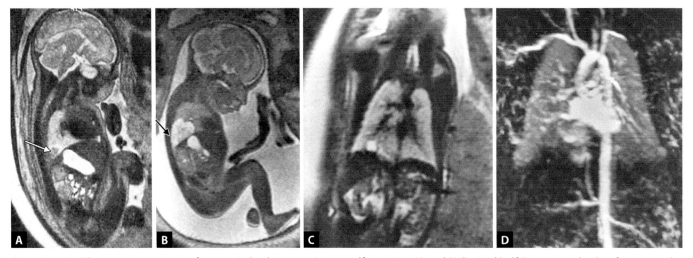

Figs. 5A to D: Changing appearance of congenital pulmonary airway malformation. (A and B) Sagittal half-Fourier single-shot fast spin-echo MR images (96-msec effective echo time, 40 × 40-cm field of view, 512 × 256 matrix, 3-mm section thickness) of a fetus at (A) 23 and (B) 34 weeks gestation. The lesion (arrow) is of high signal intensity at 23 weeks gestation but has shrunk to a small residual mass at 34 weeks gestation, at which time it is no longer visible at ultrasound; (C and D) Type II cystic adenomatoid malformation in a 29-week-old fetus. (C) Coronal single-shot fast spin-echo MR image shows multiple small cysts in the lower lobe of the right lung. (D) Coronal gadolinium-enhanced MR angiogram obtained 4 days after birth clearly shows an aberrant artery from the abdominal aorta
Source: Shinmoto H, Kashima K, Yuasa Y, Tanimoto A, Morikawa Y, Ishimoto H, et al. MR imaging of non-CNS fetal abnormalities: a pictorial essay. Radiographics. 2000;20(5):1227-43.

regression.[12,13] Microcystic lesions succumbed to regression more likely than macrocystic.[14]

Microcystic lesions are almost invariably fatal. Microcystic lesions have a significant mortality rate due to their large size and subsequent complications such as mediastinal shift, pulmonary hypoplasia, polyhydramnios, and nonimmune hydrops. Regardless of the type of lesion, the overall prognosis is mostly determined by the size of the lesion.

Bilateral CPAM is a lethal condition. Unilateral CPAM is associated with a good prognosis—it either stays the same size or shows signs of spontaneous prenatal resolution in the majority of cases, and it enlarges in the minority of cases. Recent investigations have indicated that pregnancies that are allowed to continue have a good

prognosis, with around half of the cases concluding in spontaneous regression.[13,15,16]

In the majority of cases with antenatal resolution, postnatal study with chest X-ray, CT, and MRI will reveal residual lung illness.

The diagnosis of CPAM may also have implications for the health of the mother. There have been reports of mothers with a fetus with CPAM that developed the "mirror syndrome", a hyperdynamic preeclamptic state that may be life-threatening. Molar pregnancies, sacrococcygeal teratoma, and prenatal abnormalities that result in inadequate placental perfusion, which leads to endothelial cell injury, have all been linked to the "mirror syndrome". The sole treatment for this syndrome is immediate delivery of the baby.

Therapy

The management of CPAM and hydrops depends on the gestational age of the fetus at detection. In the fetus with CPAM presenting with or developing hydrops at 32–34 weeks of gestation, consideration should be given to treating the mother with corticosteroids and early delivery for immediate postnatal resection.

Fetuses in which hydrops develops prior to 32 weeks can be considered for treatment in utero. Nicolaides reported the first case of CCAM treated in utero. In 1987, percutaneous placement of a thoracoamniotic catheter shunt was used to decompress a very large cystic lung lesion in a 20-week-old fetus. The surgery resolved both the mediastinal shift and the hydrops, resulting in a successful delivery at 37 weeks of pregnancy. Survivors have had marked respiratory insufficiency and some have required extracorporeal membrane oxygen (ECMO) or high-frequency ventilation.[17,18]

Postnatally, thoracotomy and lobectomy may be performed for symptomatic neonates, but the decision and timing of an excision in an asymptomatic patient remains controversial among pediatric surgeons. At present, there is uncertainty whether there is need for elective surgery in asymptomatic infants or it may be better in such cases to adopt expectant management if serial radiographs demonstrate regression of the tumor.[19] Argument for the routine resection is the probability that the lesion is not benign CPAM but rather a type I pleuropulmonary blastoma.[20] *However, whether resected or not, a considerable number of asymptomatic cases have failed to show evidence of malignancy.*[21,22]

In summary, in absence of nonimmune fetal hydrops, in cases of prenatally diagnosed CPAM, counseling should emphasize the prevalence of a positive outcome, even circumstances where surgical intervention may be needed.[23] If this diagnosis is made before viability, the option of pregnancy termination should be offered. After viability, management and prognosis depend on the presence of associated hydrops. In patients without hydrops, delivery can wait until fetal and pulmonic maturity is reached. Serial scans are recommended to monitor the growth of the lesion and to look for early signs of hydrops. To date, fetuses with hydrops have had a 100% mortality rate. Nonaggressive management may be offered to the parents in these cases. Repeated thoracentesis do not seem to guarantee long-lasting decompression of the chest. In utero surgery for fetuses with hydrops and large lesions in early pregnancy has been suggested but has not been carried out at the time of this writing. In situations of isolated congenital unilateral cystic adenomatoid malformation of the lung, conservative therapy appears to be an adequate medical practice.[24] Antenatal diagnosis of CPAM mandates delivery in a tertiary care center, where immediate thoracic surgery can be performed.

◼ LUNG SEQUESTRATION

Pulmonary sequestration is a malformation in which a segment of nonfunctioning bronchopulmonary tissue is isolated from the normal lung tissue. They account for up to 6% of congenital lung anomalies.[25]

It can be extra- or intralobar, with extralobar lesions presenting a separate pleural investment. It usually does not communicate with an airway and receives its blood supply from the systemic circulation, rather than the pulmonary artery.[5,6,26]

These are systemic arteriovenous malformations that, if hemodynamically substantial, might cause cardiovascular symptoms.[27]

The arterial supply coming from the aorta is a pathognomonic feature of the sequestration. In both intra- and extralobar sequestrations, the artery comes from various sites of the aorta. In intralobar sequestration, the venous drainage takes place in the pulmonary vein, whereas in the extralobar sequestration it occurs in the azygos system.

Extralobar sequestration accounts for 25%[28] of CLAs and has been linked to other congenital systemic defects like diaphragmatic hernia and cardiac malformations. This form has the potential to involute in utero. The lesion is most commonly found at the left costophrenic angle, inferior to the lung, or even within or beneath the diaphragm. Neuroblastoma, adrenal hemorrhage, and other main abdominal anomalies are among the differential diagnoses of BPS in the left subphrenic region during pregnancy.

Intralobar sequestration (which accounts for about 75% of all intralobar sequestration) is frequently found in a normal lobe.[10] It is a bronchial atresia with systemic vascular supply, according to Langston.[29]

In fetal extralobar sequestration, hyperechogenicity of the sequestre characteristically contrasts with the rest of the lung; in intralobar sequestration, normal echogenicity of the sequestre accounts for diagnosis underestimation.[30]

On prenatal US the abnormal lung appears as an echogenic intrathoracic or intra-abdominal mass. In about 50% of cases, there is an associated pleural effusion. Polyhydramnios is a frequent complication. The extralobar sequestration may be supradiaphragmatic (90%) or subdiaphragmatic (10%). Visualization of a systemic feeding artery arising from the thoracic or abdominal aorta is a useful finding that distinguishes a sequestration from other masses such as CPAM, bronchial atresia, and CLO.[31,32] Color and spectral Doppler sonography can be helpful in visualizing the feeding artery, but visualization may still be difficult **(Fig. 6)**.[26]

In some cases, severe fetal complications such as oligohydramnios with nonimmune hydrops fetalis leading to fetal death can be observed. Overcirculation across the sequestration can induce heart failure and edema.[30]

About 6–10% of fetuses with extralobar sequestration have an ipsilateral pleural effusion, which may be related to the

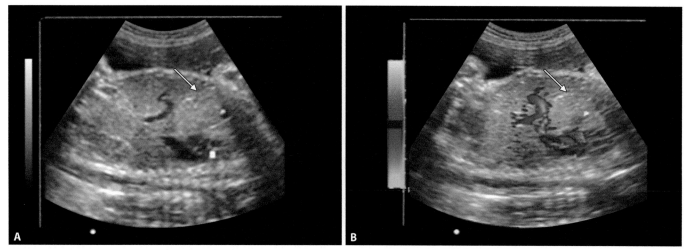

Figs. 6A and B: B mode and color Doppler mapping of sequestration. Hyperechogenic mass in the posteroinferior part of the thorax (A—arrow), with systemic arterial blood supply (B—arrow).

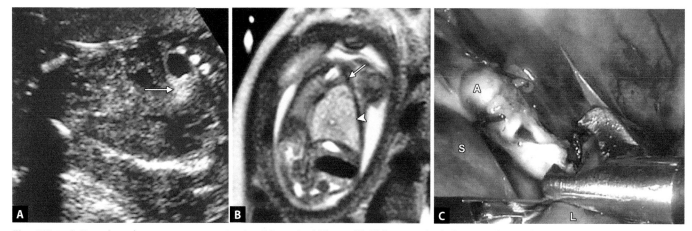

Figs. 7A to C: Bronchopulmonary sequestration in a 23-week-old fetus. (A) Oblique sagittal ultrasound scan shows cystic structures (arrow) in a hyperechoic left lung (the cranial direction of the fetus is on the right). This appearance was diagnosed as cystic adenomatoid malformation; (B) Oblique coronal single-shot fast spin-echo MR images show the left side of the thorax mostly occupied by an abnormal mass with small cysts (arrowhead), which compresses the hypoplastic left lung superiorly (arrow); (C) Thoracoscopic view—intralobar pulmonary sequestration: stepwise cutting of an atypical artery originating from the aorta. S indicates intralobar pulmonary sequestration; A, atypical artery; L, normal lung. *Source:* (A and B) Dhingsa R, Coakley FV, Albanese CT, Filly RA, Goldstein R. Prenatal sonography and MR imaging of pulmonary sequestration. AJR Am J Roentgenol. 2003;180(2):433-7. (C) Jesch NK, Leonhardt J, Sumpelmann R, Gluer S, Nustede R, Ure BM. Thoracoscopic resection of intra- and extralobar pulmonary sequestration in the first 3 months of life. J Pediatr Surg. 2005;40(9):1404-6.

typical pathologic finding of dilated subpleural lymphatics or to torsion around the connecting vasculature and fibrous pedicle. An extralobar sequestration is suggested by the presence of a unilateral pleural effusion in combination with a prenatal thoracic mass and in case of pleural effusion fetal therapy is required because it improves postnatal prognosis.[30,33]

Therapy

After birth, embolization, sequestration resection, lobe resection, or thoracoscopic ligature of the vasculature are possible, depending on tumor size, heart failure, respiratory distress, repeated infections, hemoptysis, or aneurysm **(Fig. 7)**.[30,34,35]

Detailed sonographic evaluation of the entire fetus should be done, since extrapulmonary anomalies are found in about 60% of cases with extralobar sequestration and 10% of those with intralobar sequestration. The most common abnormalities are diaphragmatic hernia, CCAMs, and cardiac, renal, cerebral, or vertebral defects.[34,36,37]

Because it can be difficult to tell the difference between a sequestration and other congenital pulmonary anomalies, MRI is increasingly used as an addition to obstetric sonography in prenatal imaging of fetuses with complex anomalies, including thoracic lesions such as a sequestration.[31] Because they are filled with amniotic fluid, normal fetal lungs appear homogeneous on MRI and have a relatively high T2 signal intensity.[31,38] A sequestration usually manifests as a well-defined mass in the chest with a T2 signal intensity that is higher than the normal lung but lower than the free amniotic fluid.[31,38]

The true value of MRI over sonography is still being researched, and it may be helpful in complex cases in which an associated anomaly, such as congenital diaphragmatic hernia, or in differentiating subdiaphragmatic sequestration from a neuroblastoma or an adrenal hemorrhage.[26]

BRONCHOGENIC CYSTS

Bronchogenic cysts are foregut malformations and are derived from an anomalous division of the embryonic foregut. They account for 11–18% of mediastinal masses and 40–50% of congenital intrathoracic cysts.[39] They are caused by aberrant tracheobronchial tree branching and are most commonly found at the carina of trachea (70%), but they can also be found paratracheal, in the hila, or even within the lung.[4] The cysts are filled with mucinous material and lined with ciliated respiratory columnar epithelium. Bronchogenic cysts are much more often single than multiple and may be of different sizes.

Antenatal diagnosis of bronchogenic cysts is rare and they may be suspected when an anechoic uni- or bilocular intrathoracic cyst is seen.[40] On fetal MRI T2-weighted images, they exhibit uniform high signal intensity, while T1-weighted pictures have low signal intensity.[5] They can occasionally cause secondary bronchial compression, which results in morphological alterations in the lung distal to the obstruction, such as an increase in volume and the retention of fetal lung fluid. On T2-weighted MRI, the retained fluid is homogeneously hyperechoic and hyperintense.[31]

The prenatal differential diagnosis of cysts of the fetal chest is complex and includes cystic adenomatoid malformation, diaphragmatic hernia, lung sequestration, bronchogenic cyst, laryngeal atresia, neuroenteric cyst, duplication of the oesophagus, congenital lobar emphysema, Swyer–James syndrome, and other mediastinal tumors. If the bronchial obstruction is involved, differential diagnosis may include bronchial atresia **(Fig. 8)**.[5]

Prognosis

The fetal prognosis depends mainly upon the origin of the cyst, which is often impossible to establish antenatally, and also on the presence of combined anomalies.[41] Associated anomalies may be found—tracheoesophageal fistula, esophageal diverticulum, esophageal cyst, and lung sequestration. Vertebral abnormalities (hemivertebrae) are often associated with bronchogenic cyst of mediastinal origin.

Prognosis is generally good and the cysts are often asymptomatic. Infection, rupture, bleeding, and compression are all frequent long-term cyst complications.

There is also the possibility of malignant degeneration. A prenatal diagnosis of a thoracic or abdominal cyst does not need any changes in the management of pregnancy or delivery.

CONGENITAL LOBAR OVERINFLATION OR EMPHYSEMA

Congenital lobar overinflation is a rare lung malformation (1/20,000–300,000 live births),[42] and is characterized by postnatal lobar enlargement that causes normal lung compression. A localized cartilaginous bronchial wall irregularity is the most common cause[4]—bronchomalacia—most likely due to cartilaginous deficit.[20] The restricted airway may have a one-way valve effect after birth, trapping air in the distal lung.[32]

Antenatally CLO is visible as hyperechoic lung segments, without aberrant blood flow. Prenatal ultrasonography may reveal a single cystic lesion.[20] Mediastinal shift or polyhydramnios can be associated with CLO.[43] Fluid-overloaded, enlarged lung tissue with homogeneous hyperechogenicity, and MRI hyperintensity may be difficult to identify from other lung anomalies, such as lung sequestration, bronchial atresia, and small cystic type CPAM, on prenatal US and MRI. The lung structure is usually retained, and stretched blood vessels can be seen.[44]

Therapy

In mild and moderate cases of CLO, conservative treatment should be favored, while lobectomy should be considered in severe cases. However, as a result of higher antenatal diagnosis and intrauterine regression, conservative treatment of the disease appears to be increasing.[44]

BRONCHIAL ATRESIA

Bronchial atresia is a rare malformation, characterized by focal obliteration of a lobar, segmental or subsegmental bronchus, with peripheral mucus impaction (bronchocele or mucocele), and hyperinflation distal of the obstruction.[45] Recent studies shown a close link between bronchial atresia and other CLAs, such as intralobar BPS and CPAM, implying that they share a same embryological genesis.[10,29,32]

Antenatally, on T2-weighted MRI, the lung (segment or subsegment) affected is enlarged, has increased echogenicity, and has a strong signal. In the case of proximal bronchial obstruction, US and MRI may reveal a centrally dilated bronchus or bronchocele.[5]

Therapy

Treatment for bronchial atresia should be conservative, and regular follow-up chest X-ray should be performed. Surgical treatment should be reserved for following indications: recurrent and severe infections, ineffective

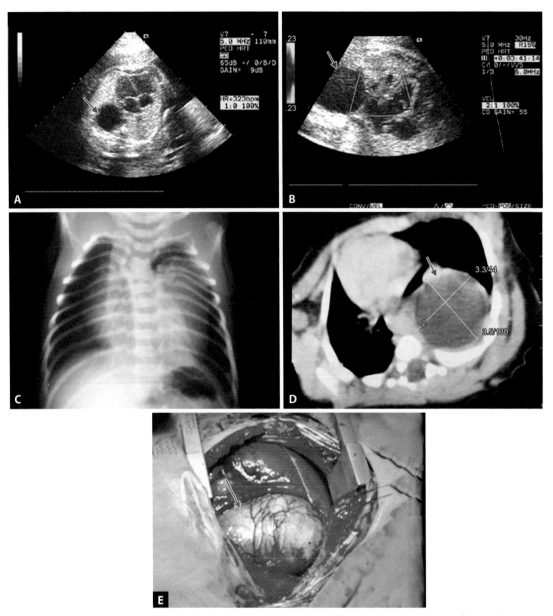

Figs. 8A to E: Sonographic, Roentgen, magnetic resonance imaging, and operative appearance of bronchogenic cyst.

medical treatment, malignant alteration of the affected lung. For those patients, if possible, minimally invasive surgery is recommended (thoracoscopic surgery).[35,45]

■ PULMONARY AGENESIS

Pulmonary agenesis is a rare developmental disorder in which one or both lungs are completely absent or have significant hypoplasia. In some cases, bilateral pulmonary agenesis was an isolated finding. In other cases, pulmonary agenesis was found in association with other anomalies in the gastrointestinal, genitourinary, and ocular systems.

In experimental animals fed a vitamin A-deficient diet, lung aplasia has been found. Some researchers have proposed a vascular etiology for pulmonary agenesis, similar to the one proposed for intestinal atresia.[46] Other researchers have proposed that pulmonary agenesis is caused by a genetic mutation.

Schneider (1909) created a classification system for determining the degree of lung underdevelopment, which has since been adopted by a number of authors. Agenesis of the lung or entire absence of the bronchus and lung characterize Class I. Class II is aplasia in which there is a rudimentary bronchus but there is no lung tissue. Bronchial hypoplasia and a variable amount of lung tissue are found in Class III hypoplasia. Bilateral agenesis of the lung is incompatible with life and, luckily, quite uncommon. Bilateral lung agenesis is an uncommon condition characterized by a cessation in the outgrowth of the respiratory primordium during the embryonic developmental stage of the lung.[47] Unilateral agenesis occurs about 25 times more commonly, and it may be compatible with a normal life. Agenesis and hypoplasia are the most acceptable terms for this classification scheme, with Class I and II representing agenesis and Class III representing hypoplasia.

The incidence of agenesis, either unilateral or bilateral, in newborns is uncertain, but certainly very rare, with prevalence of 0.0034–0.0097%. There is no estimate of the prenatal incidence of pulmonary aplasia; however, it has been estimated an incidence of 1 in 15,000 based on autopsies.[48] Both lungs are affected, right side is more common,[47] and patients with left lung aplasia have a much better prognosis.

Often, the diagnosis of pulmonary agenesis is made only after the body has been autopsied. However, examples of unilateral pulmonary agenesis have been identified prenatally in recent years.[49,50]

Sonographically, the mediastinum is shifted toward the afflicted side and the diaphragm on the ipsilateral side is lifted. It is important to identify compression-induced pulmonary hypoplasia from a diaphragmatic hernia or CPAM from unilateral agenesis. Medial mediastinal shift to the side of agenesis and enlarged echogenic lung herniating into the contralateral chest anterior and/or posterior to the mediastinum are sonographic signs of unilateral pulmonary agenesis. Scoliosis with a curvature toward the side of agenesis, with or without hemivertebrae, may be present **(Fig. 9)**.

A thorough sonographic examination, including scanning of the vertebrae, heart, and limbs, as well as the genitourinary and central nervous systems, should be conducted due to the high frequency of concomitant anomalies in pulmonary agenesis impacting other organ systems. Hemifacial microsomia and ipsilateral radial ray abnormalities have been linked. Bilateral pulmonary agenesis may be accompanied by bilateral facial or radial ray abnormalities. Renal abnormalities including dysplasia and horseshoe kidney have been reported with unilateral pulmonary agenesis, as has encephalocele. In pulmonary agenesis, both polyhydramnios and oligohydramnios have been described.

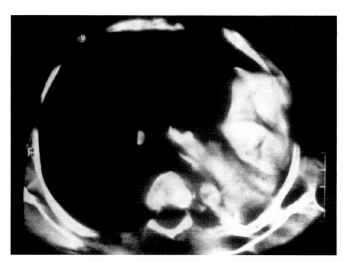

Fig. 9: Axial computed tomography section of chest shows absence of left lung parenchyma and herniation of right lung across the midline to left side anteriorly.

Bilateral pulmonary agenesis is not generally mistaken for other conditions. Unilateral agenesis, however, must be distinguished from other conditions that cause mediastinal shift, including diaphragmatic hernia, CPAM, and BPS.

■ MANAGEMENT OF PREGNANCY

Any fetus in which bilateral pulmonary agenesis is suspected should have a detailed sonographic assessment to confirm the diagnosis. If bilateral pulmonary agenesis is confirmed, the parents should be advised of the uniformly fatal outcome. Termination is an option. If the diagnosis is made later in the pregnancy, the delivery should be planned without monitoring for fetal distress. In addition, the neonatologist should be aware of the diagnosis.

■ PLEURAL EFFUSIONS

Pleural effusions represent accumulation of fluid in the pleural space.

Prenatal pleural effusion may be part of a generalized immune or nonimmune fetal hydrops, accompanying a structural anomaly or, more rarely, an isolated finding—primary or secondary. Most primary congenital effusions are chylous and occur on the right.[51]

Pleural effusions may be unilateral, bilateral, isolated, or occur in association with other manifestations of hydrops, most usually subcutaneous skin edema, pericardial effusion, or ascites. Fetal hydrops is a nonspecific finding in a wide variety of fetal and maternal disorders—hematological, chromosomal, cardiovascular, pulmonary, gastrointestinal, hepatic and metabolic abnormalities, congenital infection, neoplasms, and malformations of the placenta or umbilical cord.[52] While comprehensive US scanning can often reveal the underlying reason, the aberration often goes unexplained even after fetal blood collection or expert postmortem investigation.

Pleural effusion is seen as fluid that surrounds the lung on one (unilateral) or both (bilateral) sides. Associated anomalies depend on underlying cause, which may be of fetal or maternal origin **(Fig. 10)**.[53]

Prognosis

Irrespective of the underlying cause, infants affected by pleural effusions usually present in the neonatal period with severe, and often fatal, respiratory insufficiency. This is either a direct result of pulmonary compression caused by the effusions, or due to pulmonary hypoplasia secondary to chronic intrathoracic compression. The overall mortality of neonates with pleural effusions increases from low in infants with isolated pleural effusions to very high in those with gross hydrops. Chromosomal abnormalities, mainly trisomy 21, are found in about 5% of fetuses with apparently isolated pleural effusions **(Fig. 11)**.[53]

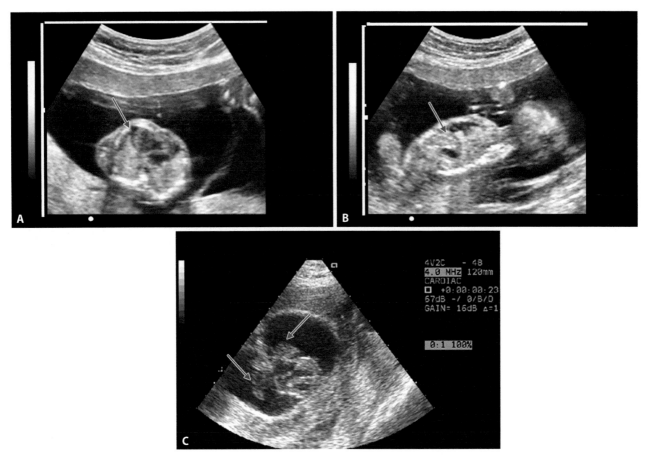

Figs. 10A to C: Transverse and oblique scan of unilateral pleural effusion (A and B) and bilateral pleural effusion (C, arrows indicate collapsed lungs).

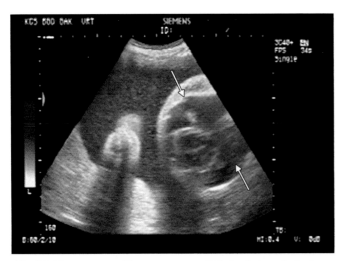

Fig. 11: Ultrasonographic appearance of bilateral pleural effusions increases with gross hydrops.

In the human, isolated fetal pleural effusions may resolve spontaneously antenatally, or they may persist. In some cases, postnatal thoracocentesis may be sufficient but in others the chronic compression of the fetal lungs can result in pulmonary hypoplasia and neonatal death. Additionally, mediastinal compression may lead to the development of fetal hydrops and polyhydramnios which are associated with a high risk of premature delivery and subsequent perinatal death.[52] Parameters associated with a better prognostic include later gestational age at diagnosis, spontaneous resolution of the effusion prior to delivery, lack of hydrops, isolated effusion, and unilateral effusion.[54]

Therapy

One option in the management of such fetuses is thoracocentesis and drainage of the effusions. However, in the majority of cases the fluid reaccumulates within 24 hours needing repeated procedures and it is therefore preferable to achieve chronic drainage by the administration of pleural-amniotic shunts.

Pleural effusion is among the most common indications for in utero shunting since it has been introduced.[17] Pleural-amniotic shunting is used for both, diagnosis and therapy[55,56] and is an effective and safe method of chronic drainage of fetal pleural effusions to reverse fetal hydrops, resolve polyhydramnios, and potentially prevent the development of pulmonary hypoplasia.[52,57,58]

A cardiac anomaly or some other abnormality in the chest may be seen only after the lungs have been decompressed and the whole chest returns to a normal state. It also helps to differentiate hydrops due to primary accumulation of pleural effusions, when the ascites and skin edema will resolve after shunting, and other causes of hydrops such as infection, in

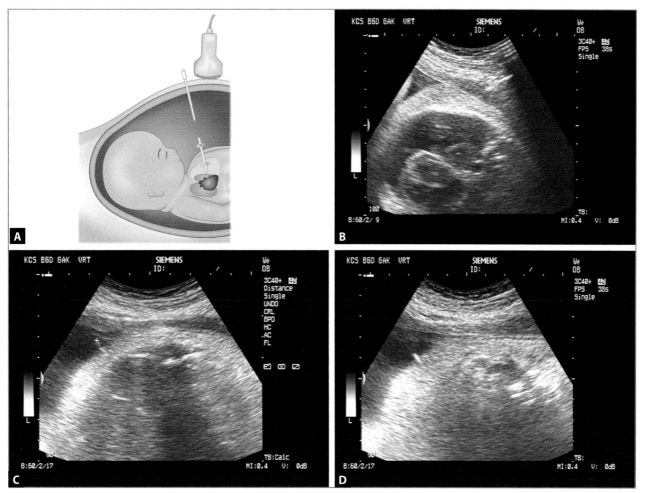

Figs. 12A to D: (A) Schematic representation of thoracoamniotic shunting and (B to D) application of thoracoamniotic shunt in sequences.

which drainage of the effusions does not prevent worsening of the hydrops **(Fig. 12)**.

Although complications of fetal shunting that include shunt migration, hypoproteinemia,[59] scars,[60] and limb constriction,[61] the outcome of fetuses with isolated effusions after shunting is excellent with survival rates of >95%. In hydropic fetuses, the survival rate is only 50%, because pleural-amniotic shunting obviously does not cure the underlying disease.[44] The efficacy of thoracoamniotic shunting was supported by several studies.[18,62-65]

■ CONCLUSION

A new classification system of fetal lung anomalies has recently been suggested, using two-dimensional US and color and power Doppler technology, with the claim that new approach enabled prenatal evaluation of each lung component and facilitated cogent management of the fetus with congenital lung dysplasia—it remains to be seen if it will be broadly adopted.[66,67]

As sole US fails to correctly predict histology in around 25% of prenatally discovered congenital lung anomalies, and it has a low sensitivity for systemic feeding arteries that are

pathognomonic for BPS, there is need for additional cross-sectional imaging, especially a postnatal CT scan.[68]

In recent years, evidence has accumulated that most CLAs have a common developmental basis. With bronchial atresia seen in many cases of BPS and CPAM, early airway obstruction in utero is now regarded the most likely underlying embryological etiology for a wide range of pathologies.[5]

Associated anomalies were found in 14%[69] of all patients with a CLA, especially those with lung agenesis and bronchogenic cysts. Suggestion would be that, during the newborn examination, special attention should be given to the cardiovascular and gastrointestinal tracts. An anteroposterior and lateral chest and abdominal radiograph may be useful to assess signs of major associated anomalies, regardless of the CLA type or clinical course, as the definitive CLA diagnosis is determined after cross-sectional imaging.

In summary, congenital lung malformations are more and more diagnosed antenatally, and sometimes necessitate prompt surgical resection. The natural history is variable. All infants with a prenatal diagnosis require postnatal evaluation. Patients should be evaluated for associated disorders. The presence of mass effects is an indication for therapeutic decompression and if there is a risk of pulmonary compression, infection and malignant degeneration resection may be imperative, even in asymptomatic patients. Genetic counseling by a clinical geneticist should be offered to the parents of all patients.

■ REFERENCES

1. Palla J, Sockrider MM. Congenital lung malformations. Pediatr Ann. 2019;48(4):e169-e174.
2. Laberge JM, Flageole H, Pugash D, Khalife S, Blair G, Filiatrault D, et al. Outcome of the prenatally diagnosed congenital cystic adenomatoid lung malformation: a Canadian experience. Fetal Diagn Ther. 2001;16(3):178-86.
3. Stocker LJ, Wellesley DG, Stanton MP, Parasuraman R, Howe DT. The increasing incidence of foetal echogenic congenital lung malformations: an observational study. Prenat Diagn. 2015;35(2):148-53.
4. Berrocal T, Madrid C, Novo S, Gutiérrez J, Arjonilla A, Gómez-León N. Congenital anomalies of the tracheobronchial tree, lung, and mediastinum: embryology, radiology, and pathology. Radiographics. 2004;24(1):e17.
5. Alamo L, Gudinchet F, Reinberg O, Vial Y, Francini K, Osterheld MC, et al. Prenatal diagnosis of congenital lung malformations. Pediatr Radiol. 2012;42(3):273-83.
6. Quercia M, Panza R, Calderoni G, Di Mauro A, Laforgia N. Lung ultrasound: a new tool in the management of congenital lung malformation. Am J Perinatol. 2019;36(S 02):S99-S105.
7. Merli L, Nanni L, Curatola A, Pellegrino M, De Santis M, Silvaroli S, et al. Congenital lung malformations: a novel application for lung ultrasound? J Ultrasound. 2021;24(3):349-53.
8. Aleksandra NM. Cystic adenomatoid malformation. (2000). [online] Available from www.thefetus.net [Last accessed April, 2022].
9. Stocker JT, Madewell JE, Drake RM. Congenital cystic adenomatoid malformation of the lung. Classification and morphologic spectrum. Hum Pathol. 1977;8(2):155-71.
10. Adzick NS, Harrison MR, Crombleholme TM, Flake AW, Howell LJ. Fetal lung lesions: management and outcome. Am J Obstet Gynecol. 1998;179(4):884-9.
11. Langston C. New concepts in the pathology of congenital lung malformations. Semin Pediatr Surg. 2003;12(1):17-37.
12. Crombleholme TM, Coleman B, Hedrick H, Liechty K, Howell L, Flake AW, et al. Cystic adenomatoid malformation volume ratio predicts outcome in prenatally diagnosed cystic adenomatoid malformation of the lung. J Pediatr Surg. 2002;37(3):331-8.
13. Azizkhan RG, Crombleholme TM. Congenital cystic lung disease: contemporary antenatal and postnatal management. Pediatr Surg Int. 2008;24(6):643-57.
14. Walker L, Cohen K, Rankin J, Crabbe D. Outcome of prenatally diagnosed congenital lung anomalies in the North of England: a review of 228 cases to aid in prenatal counselling. Prenat Diagn. 2017;37(10):1001-7.
15. Duncombe GJ, Dickinson JE, Kikiros CS. Prenatal diagnosis and management of congenital cystic adenomatoid malformation of the lung. Am J Obstet Gynecol. 2002;187(4):950-4.
16. Laberge JM, Flageole H, Pugash D, Khalife S, Blair G, Filiatrault D, et al. Congenital cystic adenomatoid malformation of the lung: prognosis when diagnosed in utero. Saudi Med J. 2003;24(5 Suppl):S33.
17. Booth P, Nicolaides KH, Greenough A, Gamsu HR. Pleuro-amniotic shunting for fetal chylothorax. Early Hum Dev. 1987;15(6):365-7.
18. Nicolaides KH, Azar GB. Thoraco-amniotic shunting. Fetal Diagn Ther. 1990;5(3-4):153-64.
19. van Leeuwen K, Teitelbaum DH, Hirschl RB, Austin E, Adelman SH, Polley TZ, et al. Prenatal diagnosis of congenital cystic adenomatoid malformation and its postnatal presentation, surgical indications, and natural history. J Pediatr Surg. 1999;34(5):794-8.
20. Hall NJ, Stanton MP. Long-term outcomes of congenital lung malformations. Semin Pediatr Surg. 2017;26(5):311-6.
21. Feinberg A, Hall NJ, Williams GM, Schultz KAP, Miniati D, Hill DA, et al. Can congenital pulmonary airway malformation be distinguished from Type I pleuropulmonary blastoma based on clinical and radiological features? J Pediatr Surg. 2016;51(1):33-7.
22. Ng C, Stanwell J, Burge DM, Stanton MP. Conservative management of antenatally diagnosed cystic lung malformations. Arch Dis Child. 2014;99(5):432-7.
23. De Santis M, Masini L, Noia G, Cavaliere AF, Oliva N, Caruso A. Congenital cystic adenomatoid malformation of the lung: antenatal ultrasound findings and fetal-neonatal outcome. Fifteen years of experience. Fetal Diagn Ther. 2000;15(4):246-50.
24. Monni G, Paladini D, Ibba RM, Teodoro A, Zoppi MA, Lamberti A, et al. Prenatal ultrasound diagnosis of congenital cystic adenomatoid malformation of the lung: a report of 26 cases and review of the literature. Ultrasound Obstet Gynecol. 2000;16(2):159-62.
25. Durell J, Lakhoo K. Congenital cystic lesions of the lung. Early Hum Dev. 2014;90(12):935-9.
26. Dhingsa R, Coakley FV, Albanese CT, Filly RA, Goldstein R. Prenatal sonography and MR imaging of pulmonary sequestration. AJR Am J Roentgenol. 2003;180(2):433-7.
27. Eber E. Antenatal diagnosis of congenital thoracic malformations: early surgery, late surgery, or no surgery? Semin Respir Crit Care Med. 2007;28(3):355-66.
28. Morin L, Crombleholme TM, D'Alton ME. Prenatal diagnosis and management of fetal thoracic lesions. Semin Perinatol. 1994;18:228-53.
29. Langston C. Intralobar sequestration, revisited. Pediatr Dev Pathol. 2003;6(4):283.
30. Morville P, Malo-Ferjani L, Graesslin O, Bory JP, Harika G. Physiopathology hypotheses and treatment of pulmonary sequestration. Am J Perinatol. 2003;20(2):87-9.
31. Cannie M, Jani J, De Keyzer F, Van Kerkhove F, Meersschaert J, Lewi L, et al. Magnetic resonance imaging of the fetal lung: a pictorial essay. Eur Radiol. 2008;18(7):1364-74.
32. Biyyam DR, Chapman T, Ferguson MR, Deutsch G, Dighe MK. Congenital lung abnormalities: embryologic features, prenatal diagnosis, and postnatal radiologic-pathologic correlation. Radiographics. 2010;30(6):1721-38.
33. Daltro P, Werner H, Gasparetto TD, Domingues RC, Rodrigues L, Marchiori E, et al. Congenital chest malformations: a multimodality approach with emphasis on fetal MR imaging. Radiographics. 2010;30(2):385-95.

34. Becmeur F, Horta-Geraud P, Donato L, Sauvage P. Pulmonary sequestrations: prenatal ultrasound diagnosis, treatment, and outcome. J Pediatr Surg. 1998;33(3):492-6.

35. Rothenberg SS, Shipman K, Kay S, Kadenhe-Chiweshe A, Thirumoorthi A, Garcia A, et al. Thoracoscopic segmentectomy for congenital and acquired pulmonary disease: a case for lung-sparing surgery. J Laparoendosc Adv Surg Tech A. 2014;24(1):50-4.

36. Goldstein R. Ultrasound of the fetal thorax. In Callen PW (Ed). Ultrasonography in Obstetrics and Gynecology. Philadelphia: Saunders; 2000. pp. 426-55.

37. Stocker JT. Sequestrations of the lung. Semin Diagn Pathol. 1986;3(2):106-21.

38. Hubbard AM, Adzick NS, Crombleholme TM, Coleman BG, Howell LJ, Haselgrove JC, et al. Congenital chest lesions: diagnosis and characterization with prenatal MR imaging. Radiology. 1999;212(1):43-8.

39. Stocker JT. Cystic lung disease in infants and children. Fetal Pediatr Pathol. 2009;28(4):155-84.

40. De Catte L, De Backer T, Delhove O, Mares C. Ectopic bronchogenic cyst: sonographic findings and differential diagnosis. J Ultrasound Med. 1995;14(4):321-3.

41. Jauniaux E, Hertzkovitz R, Hall JM. First-trimester prenatal diagnosis of a thoracic cystic lesion associated with fetal skin edema. Ultrasound Obstet Gynecol. 2000;15(1):74-7.

42. Thakral CL, Maji DC, Sajwani MJ. Congenital lobar emphysema: experience with 21 cases. Pediatr Surg Int. 2001;17(2-3):88-91.

43. Demir OF, Hangul M, Kose M. Congenital lobar emphysema: diagnosis and treatment options. Int J Chron Obstruct Pulmon Dis. 2019;14:921-8.

44. Liu YP, Chen CP, Shih SL, Chen YF, Yang FS, Chen SC. Fetal cystic lung lesions: evaluation with magnetic resonance imaging. Pediatr Pulmonol. 2010;45(6):592-600.

45. Wang Y, Dai W, Sun Y, Chu X, Yang B, Zhao M. Congenital bronchial atresia: diagnosis and treatment. Int J Med Sci. 2012;9(3):207-12.

46. Louw JH. Congenital intestinal atresia and stenosis in the newborn. Observations on its pathogenesis and treatment. Ann R Coll Surg Engl. 1959;25(4):209-34.

47. Wert ES. Normal and abnormal structural development of the lung. In: Rowitch DH, Polin RA, Abman SH, Benitz WE, Fox WW (Eds). Fetal and Neonatal Physiology. Netherlands: Elsevier; 2017. pp. 627-41.

48. Schechter DC. Congenital absence or deficiency of lung tissue. The congenital subtractive bronchopneumonic malformations. Ann Thorac Surg. 1968;6(3):287-313.

49. Becker R, Novak A, Rudolph KH. A case of occipital encephalocele combined with right lung aplasia in a twin pregnancy. J Perinat Med. 1993;21(3):253-8.

50. Bromley B, Benacerraf BR. Unilateral lung hypoplasia: report of three cases. J Ultrasound Med. 1997;16(9):599-601.

51. Sanders RC (Ed). Structural Fetal Abnormalities: The Total Picture. New York: Mosby; 1996. pp. 130-2.

52. Pilu G, Nicolaides KH (Eds). Diagnosis of Fetal Abnormalities. The 18-23 Week Scan. Diploma in Fetal Medicine Series. Nashville: Parthenon Publishing; 1999. pp. 53-61.

53. Mikic AN. Pleural effusions. (2000). [online] Available from www.thefetus.net [Last accessed April, 2022].

54. Parilla BV, Tamura RK, Ginsberg NA. Association of parvovirus infection with isolated fetal effusions. Am J Perinatol. 1997;14(6):357-8.

55. Blott M, Nicolaides KH, Greenough A. Pleuroamniotic shunting for decompression of fetal pleural effusions. Obstet Gynecol. 1988;71(5):798-800.

56. Rodeck CH, Fisk NM, Fraser DI, Nicolini U. Long-term in utero drainage of fetal hydrothorax. N Engl J Med. 1988;319(17):1135-8.

57. Ahmad FK, Sherman SJ, Hagglund KH, Johnson MP, Krivchenia E. Isolated unilateral fetal pleural effusion: the role of sonographic surveillance and in utero therapy. Fetal Diagn Ther. 1996;11(6):383-9.

58. Picone O, Benachi A, Mandelbrot L, Ruano R, Dumez Y, Dommergues M. Thoracoamniotic shunting for fetal pleural effusions with hydrops. Am J Obstet Gynecol. 2004;191(6):2047-50.

59. Koike T, Minakami H, Kosuge S, Izumi A, Shiraishi H, Sato I. Severe hypoproteinemia in a fetus after pleuro-amniotic shunts with double-basket catheters for treatment of chylothorax. J Obstet Gynaecol Res. 2000;26(5):373-6.

60. Webb RD, Walkinshaw SA, Shaw NJ. Cosmetic sequelae of thoraco-amniotic shunting. Eur J Pediatr. 2000;159(1-2):133.

61. Brown R, Nicolaides K. Constriction band of the arm following insertion of a pleuro-amniotic shunt. Ultrasound Obstet Gynecol. 2000;15(5):439-40.

62. Beischer NA, Fortune DW, Macafee J. Nonimmunologic hydrops fetalis and congenital abnormalities. Obstet Gynecol. 1971;38(1):86-95.

63. Mandelbrot L, Dommergues M, Aubry MC, Mussat P, Dumez Y. Reversal of fetal distress by emergency in utero decompression of hydrothorax. Am J Obstet Gynecol. 1992;167(5):1278-83.

64. Mussat P, Dommergues M, Parat S, Mandelbrot L, de Gamarra E, Dumez Y, et al. Congenital chylothorax with hydrops: postnatal care and outcome following antenatal diagnosis. Acta Paediatr. 1995;84(7):749-55.

65. Yinon Y, Grisaru-Granovsky S, Chaddha V, Windrim R, Seaward PGR, Kelly EN, et al. Perinatal outcome following fetal chest shunt insertion for pleural effusion. Ultrasound Obstet Gynecol. 2010;36(1):58-64.

66. Achiron R, Zalel Y, Lipitz S, Hegesh J, Mazkereth R, Kuint J, et al. Fetal lung dysplasia: clinical outcome based on a new classification system. Ultrasound Obstet Gynecol. 2004;24(2):127-33.

67. Achiron R, Hegesh J, Yagel S. Fetal lung lesions: a spectrum of disease. New classification based on pathogenesis, two-dimensional and color Doppler ultrasound. Ultrasound Obstet Gynecol. 2004;24(2):107-14.

68. Mon RA, Johnson KN, Ladino-Torres M, Heider A, Mychaliska GB, Treadwell MC, et al. Diagnostic accuracy of imaging studies in congenital lung malformations. Arch Dis Child Fetal Neonatal Ed. 2019;104(4):F372-F377.

69. Hermelijn SM, Zwartjes RR, Tiddens HAWM, Cochius-den Otter SCM, Reiss IKM, Wijnen RMH, et al. Associated anomalies in congenital lung abnormalities: a 20-year experience. Neonatology. 2020;117(6):697-703.

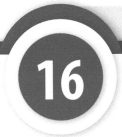

Prenatal Diagnosis of Conjoined Fetuses

Apostolos Athanasiadis, Panayiota Papasozomenou, Themistoklis Mikos, Menelaos Zafrakas

■ INTRODUCTION

Though an unusual phenomenon, conjoined fetuses have always drawn a disproportionately high degree of attention and interest from scientists and the public. This is apparently due to the intriguing processes involved in the pathogenesis of conjoined fetuses, the rare and even unique patterns of conjunction leading to complexity in management and surgical separation in individual cases, and a series of ethical questions coupled with a variety of emotional reactions and interactions between parents, relatives, and healthcare providers. In recent years, the advent of real-time ultrasound, 3D and other novel imaging techniques have made early prenatal diagnosis of conjoined fetuses possible, enabling specialists and parents to decide whether pregnancy should continue or not, and plan well in advance prenatal management, timing of delivery, and immediate and long-term postnatal management, based on future quality of life and survival issues.

■ HISTORICAL PERSPECTIVE

Fetal conjunction usually involves two fetuses in a twin pregnancy. The term "Siamese twins" is often used for conjoined twins, since the most famous case of conjoined twins surviving to adulthood in modern times were born in Siam (today's Thailand). This case was well known to the public at their time, owing to numerous photographs published in newspapers around the world. Eng and Chang Bunker were born in Thailand in 1811, grew up together, married two sisters, raised 21 children, and both died at the age of 69 years, a few hours apart from another, without ever being separated.[1] Long before this case and the invention of photography, in 1100 AD lived the Biddenden twins, who survived until the age of 34 years, probably representing the oldest well-documented case of conjoined twins surviving to adult life.[1]

Until the invention of diagnostic imaging, starting with the use of diagnostic X-rays in the early 20th century, diagnosis of conjoined twins was possible only during labor. Labor arrest was the first sign in such cases, and sacrifice of one or both fetuses was often necessary in order to accomplish delivery.[2-4] The first report of prenatal diagnosis of conjoined twins using X-rays was published in 1934, while specific radiodiagnostic criteria were first described in 1950.[2,5] Even then, however, prenatal diagnosis of conjoined twins could be missed, due to various possible factors: absence of bone connections between twins, change of twins' position in utero, and the fact that the investigator was usually not considering the possibility of conjoined twins.[2,6]

The first cases of prenatal diagnosis of conjoined twins using B-mode ultrasound were reported in the 1970's, followed by prenatal real-time ultrasonographic diagnosis shortly thereafter.[2,7-12] Since then, real-time ultrasound has been the most reliable method in establishing prenatal diagnosis of conjoined twins and in detecting associated anomalies. Moreover, recent improvements in real-time and 3D ultrasound technology—in some cases coupled with use of magnetic resonance imaging (MRI)—have made early diagnosis of conjoined fetuses in the first trimester possible,[13-18] and uncovered a "hidden mortality" of conjoined twins, because of the increase in their detection rates.[19] Furthermore, prenatal diagnosis of more complex, not previously documented cases of conjoined fetuses in triplet pregnancies has been recently made possible with real-time ultrasound: a case of conjoined triplets, i.e., three fetuses all joined together,[20] and cases of triplet pregnancies containing a pair of conjoined twins, i.e., two conjoined fetuses with a third noninvolved co-triplet comprising a triplet pregnancy.[21-23]

■ EPIDEMIOLOGY AND CLASSIFICATION

Conjoined twins have an estimated prevalence of 1 in 50,000 to 1 in 100,000 births.[24-26] In a large worldwide collaborative epidemiological study[27] which included 383 sets of conjoined twins obtained from 26,138,837 births, the prevalence was

1.47 per 100,000 births [95% confidence interval (CI): 1.32–1.62]. Incidence rates appear to be independent of maternal age, race, parity, and other demographic, genetic, and environmental factors.[24-27] Conjoined twins are generally classified according to the site at which they are joined into: (1) omphalopagus (from the Greek word "omphalos" for umbilicus), (2) thoracopagus (chest) **(Fig. 1)**, (3) cephalopagus (head), (4) ischiopagus (hip), (5) craniopagus (cranium), (6) rachipagus (spine), (7) pygopagus (rump), and (8) parapagus (side). The terms "brachius" (upper limb), "pus" (lower limb) and "cephalus" (head) and the numerals di-, tri-, and tetra- (two, three, and four respectively) are also used accordingly **(Table 1)**.[20,28] Omphalopagus and thoracopagus fetuses are joined in the trunk, but they differ in that the former have two separate hearts, while the latter share a common heart.[28] Omphalopagus are reportedly not as rare (0.5–18%) as craniopagus conjoined twins (1–5%).[2,28]

Assessment of the conjunction type is essential for the identification of shared organs and associated anomalies

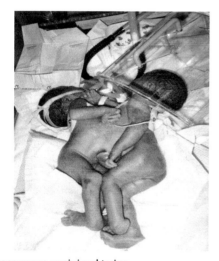

Fig. 1: Thoracopagus conjoined twins.
Source: Reprinted after author's permission from: Athanasiadis A, Mikos T, Zafrakas M, Diamanti V, Papouli M, Assimakopoulos E, et al. Prenatal management and postnatal separation of omphalopagus and craniopagus conjoined twins. Gynecol Obstet Invest. 2007; 64(1):40-3.

of conjoined fetuses. Thoracopagus twins always share a common liver, a common heart in 75% with a common pericardium in 90%, and a common gastrointestinal tract in 50% of cases. Omphalopagus and xiphopagus twins share a common liver in 81% of cases, have associated gastrointestinal tract anomalies (omphalocele, common distal ileum, and/or Meckel's diverticulum) in 33%, and congenital heart disease in 25% of cases. Pygopagus twins always share a common sacrum and coccyx, and they usually have a common rectum, bladder, and urethra. Ischiopagus twins frequently have associated anomalies of the lower spine, while the lower extremities opposite to the conjunction area are frequently rudimentary.[2] In addition, ischiopagus tetrabrachius tripus have two distinct hearts, while parapagus tetrabrachius tripus share a common heart.[2,28]

Parasites usually appear after demise of one twin possibly originally defective. The supernumerary structures (the parasite) survive and remain attached to and vascularized by the remaining usually normal twin (the autosite). The most frequent organs found in the parasite are the limbs.[28]

■ ETIOPATHOGENESIS

The etiopathogenesis of conjoined fetuses is unclear. No inherited pattern seems to exist. The inciting factor(s)—environmental, genetic, or both—leading to conjunction of fetuses are not known. Pregnancies with conjoined fetuses demonstrate a strong gender predilection: 70–95% of conjoined fetuses are female.[29] Based on this association, it has been hypothesized that the underlying molecular mechanism might be the inactivation of chromosome X. Normally, in somatic, diploid cells of female individuals one of the two X chromosomes is inactivated, and this physiologic phenomenon seems to occur randomly. Molecular analyses, however, failed to show any association between chromosome X inactivation and conjoined fetuses.[30] On the other hand, epigenetic or even genetic changes should be present at least at the interface of fetal conjunction, and this possibility could be answered by future studies. In a more recent

Type	Face	Cranium	Thorax	Heart	Abdomen	Pelvis	Spine	Arms	Legs
Cephalopagus	+	–	+	+	+	–	–	–	–
Thoracopagus	–	–	+	+	+	–	–	–	–
Omphalopagus	–	–	+		+	–	–	–	–
Ischiopagus	–	–	–	–	+	+	–	–	–
Parapagus	±	±	±	±	±	+	–	±	±
Craniopagus	–	+	–	–	–	–	–	–	–
Pygopagus	–	–	–	–	–	+	±	–	–
Rachipagus	–	–	–	–	–	±	+	–	–

TABLE 1: Classification system of conjoined twins. (Union/Fusion site)

worldwide collaborative epidemiological study[27] female predominance was confirmed, particularly for the thoracopagus type, while a significant male predominance was found in parapagus and parasitic types.

From an embryological point of view, there are two opposing theories concerning the pathogenesis of conjoined fetuses: fission versus fusion.[28,31] According to the fission theory, division of the inner cell mass between the 13th and the 15th day after fertilization results in conjoined embryos. To put things into context, it is generally accepted that division of the inner cell mass during the first 72 hours after fertilization leads to dichorionic-diamniotic, between days 4 and 8 to monochorionic-diamniotic, and between days 8 and 13 to monochorionic-monoamniotic multiple pregnancies.[32,33]

According to the fusion theory, the embryos fuse in the early embryonic period, after a short period in the first hours or days after fertilization in which they are independent from one another. This theory is supported by the fact that conjoined embryos and fetuses are united at sites where the surface ectoderm is absent or preprogrammed to become disrupted or fused.[28] A more detailed concept of the fusion theory, also referred to as the "spherical theory",[28] suggests that the monovular embryonic discs lie adjacent to one another, like floating on the surface of a sphere (the yolk sac) or in the inside of another sphere (the amniotic cavity), and gradually unite.

It has been long thought that the pathophysiological processes involved in embryonic conjunction seem to take place in the very early first trimester, in a period in which embryos are invisible with current techniques: later than the blastocyst stage, when embryos can be easily visualized with a microscope before implantation in the setting of in vitro fertilization and too early to be visualized with diagnostic ultrasound. In accordance with this view, a successful delivery of healthy dizygotic twins, which resulted from transfer of a pair of conjoined blastocysts after intracytoplasmic sperm injection (ICSI) of a pair of conjoined oocytes has been reported recently.[34] On the other hand, a reported case of conjoined twins resulting after transfer of a single eight-cell embryo with three multinuclear, even-sized blastomeres, raises the question whether the formation of multiple nuclei in the blastomeres and the development of conjoined fetuses share a common origin and common mechanisms.[35] Interestingly, at least 16 other cases of conjoined twins after assisted reproduction techniques have been reported, but information regarding the number of nuclei in blastomeres was not included in these reports.[35]

■ PRENATAL DIAGNOSIS

Prenatal diagnosis of conjoined fetuses is considered essential for further management. Parents need detailed counseling in order to decide among various management options, which include the following: (1) pregnancy continuation and scheduled neonatal surgery, (2) termination of pregnancy, and (3) multifetal pregnancy reduction or selective fetocide in cases of high-order multifetal pregnancies with a component of conjoined fetuses.[36]

Diagnosis of conjoined fetuses should be considered whenever a monochorionic, monoamniotic pregnancy is detected. Until recently, sonographic identification of distinct placentae or intervening amniotic membrane(s) was considered to be a criterion to rule out fetal conjunction.[2] However, during the last decade, at least 10 cases of diamniotic-monochorionic conjoined twins have been reported[37-46] supporting the fusion theory on the etiopathogenesis of conjoined fetuses; their detection suggests that distinct placentae and the presence of an intervening amniotic membrane should no longer be considered as criteria in order to rule out the presence of conjoined fetuses. Intriguingly, all sets of twins in these cases were conjoined in the abdominal region and in 8 out of 10 cases had conjoined bowels.[37-46] In one of these cases[37] both twins were concordant for body stalk anomaly and the presence of a single yolk sac was observed, thus leading the authors to challenge the idea that the number of yolk sacs predicts amnionicity; on the other hand these cases may represent a body stalk anomaly variant with a novel, distinct pathogenetic mechanism of conjoined twinning, similar to that leading to body stalk anomaly; according to this hypothesis, the presence of a single yolk sac suggests monoamnionicity and fission of an initial body stalk has led to formation of conjoined twins.

It has been reported that increased levels of alpha-fetoprotein are indicative of conjoined twins,[47] but data regarding specificity and sensitivity of this biochemical marker for detection of conjoined fetuses are lacking. Possible ultrasound indicators of conjoined fetuses are polyhydramnios, which is fairly common in conjoined twins occurring in 50-76%, as well as the bi-breech and face-to-face presentation of twins.[48,49] Ultrasound diagnosis of conjoined fetuses can sometimes be straightforward, particularly when fusion of fetal parts is sonographically clear. In any case, a careful approach is considered necessary in order to avoid misdiagnosis, and repeating sonographic investigations at least once is a rule that should be followed.[2]

Several cases of conjoined twins diagnosed ultrasonographically in the first trimester have been reported in the literature.[13-18] Very early sonographic diagnosis of conjoined twins appears to add minimal practical information compared with detection at the 11–14 weeks' scan. Use of 3D imaging also does not appear to improve diagnosis of conjoined fetuses **(Fig. 2)**.[36] There have been however, cases of conjoined twins reported in the literature, which were specifically diagnosed with the use of 3D ultrasound.

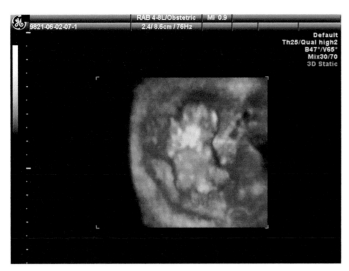

Fig. 2: First-trimester prenatal diagnosis of thoracopagus conjoined twins with three-dimensional ultrasound.

3D ultrasound appears to have advantages in differentiating between twin reversed arterial perfusion sequence and epigastric heteropagus conjoined twins.[50] Furthermore, 3D images may prove valuable during counseling, since common practice suggests that parents' perception of fetal anomalies is improved when 3D images are shown to them.[51]

The mainstay in prenatal diagnosis of conjoined twins today remains the use of 2D ultrasound enhanced by color-flow Doppler at the 11–14 week's scan. Specific sonographic features indicative of conjoined fetuses have been proposed: (1) bifid appearance of the fetal pole in the first trimester, (2) absence of separating membrane(s) between fetuses, (3) nonseparation of fetal bodies; this finding should persist and it should be always visualized at the same anatomic level, (4) detection of a variety of fetal anomalies, (5) finding more than three vessels in the umbilical cord, (6) sonographic evidence of fetal heads and bodies lying in the same plane. (7) unusual extension of the fetal spines, (8) unusual proximity of the fetal extremities, and (9) the fetuses do not change position to one another after movement or manipulation or as time passes by.[2]

On the other hand, under certain circumstances diagnosis of conjoined fetuses may be missed or separate fetuses may be misdiagnosed as conjoined, since various sonographic signs may be misleading. Occasionally, the separating membrane between monochorionic twins is hard to visualize on ultrasound, giving transiently the false impression that fetal parts are contiguous.[6] On the other hand, discordant presentation of fetuses in a multiple pregnancy does not necessarily exclude the diagnosis of conjoined fetuses, since rotation of the fetus(es) is possible, especially when the joining tissue bridge between them is small and pliable. Furthermore, in cases with extensive fetal conjunction, the sonographic appearance may mimic a singleton pregnancy, and thus attention should be given in order to identify duplication of any anatomical parts,

including the brain, heart, liver, extremities, and spine.[2] In the third trimester, the ultrasound appearance of conjoined twins can be elusive, because when one head is engaged in the pelvis and the other is found higher, conjoined twins appear to be separate.[6] Modern imaging modalities, such as 3D- and four-dimensional (4D)-ultrasound, power Doppler, and fetal rapid MRI can be used in order to support diagnosis, and exclude possible pitfalls in the sonographic diagnosis of conjoined fetuses.

The aim of the prenatal delineation of the type of fetal conjunction is to predict the immediate postnatal viability of the fetuses and viability of at least one of them after a potential surgical separation. This is important, since the overall mortality rate of conjoined twins has been reported to be as high as 28% prenatally, 54% immediately postnatally, while long-term survival rates are only about 18%.[19] Separation of omphalopagus conjoined twins is reported to have success rates of approximately 80%. In contrast, separation of craniopagus twins is unlikely without long-term seqeulae,[28] unless no neural tissue is involved.[52]

■ PRENATAL SURVEILLANCE

Accurate antenatal classification of conjoined fetuses allows early counseling of parents so that the options of pregnancy termination or near-term cesarean delivery in order to minimize maternal morbidity can be discussed. Defining prognosis prior to 24 weeks' gestation is important, since termination of pregnancy by the vaginal route is still feasible at this point.[11,53,54] 3D ultrasound enables parents to receive timely and appropriate counseling from Genetics, Maternal-Fetal Medicine, and Pediatric Surgery specialists regarding the severity of prognosis. Imaging-assisted counseling led to transition of parents' perception regarding prognosis and how serious the diagnosis was.[51] Prenatal evaluation and surveillance of conjoined fetuses includes ultrasonography, and MRI, with special attention to the fetal heart(s), preferably after 18 weeks' gestation, in order to determine the anatomy of shared organs and detect any associated anomalies.[18] Serial sonograms in the late second trimester may be necessary in order to fully assess anatomic relationships and evaluate the effects of cross-circulation, mainly polyhydramnios and hydrops.[55]

While hemodynamic analysis of the umbilical artery (UA) with color-flow Doppler does not seem to add significant information in the antenatal detection of conjoined fetuses, it seems to help in the evaluation of fetal well-being. Effective application of serial Doppler velocimetry has been recently reported in a set of thoracopagus twins: increasing UA maximum velocity led to decision for delivery at 27 weeks due to fetal distress.[56] In any case, it should be taken under consideration that the number of the umbilical cord vessels and the type of the insertion of the umbilical cord in the placental and fetal side may vary greatly in conjoined twins.[57]

According to previous reports, conjoined twins sharing a common heart will eventually succumb without surgical intervention within 3 months after delivery.[58] Prenatal cardiac evaluation of thoracopagus and omphalopagus twins allows classification of conjoined fetuses into three groups: (1) those with a single pericardium containing two normal hearts (separable conjoined twins), (2) those with fixed ventricles (inseparable conjoined twins), and (3) fetuses with conjoined atria and separate ventricles.[2,58] Conjoined six-chamber hearts are found frequently in thoracopagus twins and have never been separated successfully, while separation of twins with conjoined atria has been reported in only one case.[59] Interestingly, a case of a primigravida with a crisscross heart anomaly who was separated at birth from her thoracopagus conjoined twin and underwent a 39-week vaginal delivery without maternal or neonatal complications has been reported.[60]

Combined prenatal and postnatal echocardiography may accurately delineate cardiac fusion, intracardiac anatomy, and ventricular function in the majority of cases of fetuses joined at the thoracic level.[61] Prenatal sonographic evaluation of the fetal heart(s) can provide more valuable information than postnatal scans,[62] since the amniotic fluid is a good medium for ultrasound transmission, enhancing visualization of fetal parts. Once conjoined twins are delivered, it is difficult to place the ultrasound transducer against the small pericardial window. However, even prenatal echocardiograms may underestimate the severity of cardiac disease, as autopsy studies suggest. In particular, delineation of the relationships of the great vessels is technically demanding,[6] and severe cardiac malformations may exist even when conjoined fetuses do not share a common cardiovascular system.[6]

Associated anatomic anomalies are very common in conjoined fetuses, even in organ systems unrelated to the area of conjunction. Congenital diaphragmatic hernia, abdominal wall defect, neural tube defect, clubfoot, imperforate anus, esophageal atresia, and cystic hygroma have been repeatedly reported in conjoined fetuses. In contrast, karyotype abnormalities are virtually absent in conjoined fetuses.[19] These malformations can be indistinguishable from those encountered in singleton cases, and thus it has been postulated that certain anomalies in singletons originate in a fashion similar to that in conjoined twins.[63]

PLANNING PERINATAL AND POSTNATAL MANAGEMENT

In modern obstetrics, prenatal management of conjoined fetuses has two main objectives: (1) to maximize the potential for survival of the fetuses, and (2) to minimize maternal morbidity.[64] Sporadic reports in the literature have described successful vaginal delivery and subsequent survival of small-conjoined twins.[65] However, the method of choice for near-term delivery is cesarean section, in order to minimize maternal and neonatal birth trauma and improve neonatal survival.[6,66,67] This approach also reduces the risk of uterine atony secondary to overdistension of the uterus. The obstetrician usually plans a near-term cesarean delivery after confirmation of lung maturity. In general, it is estimated that most conjoined twins are delivered prematurely, 40% are stillborn, and 35% die within the first 24 hours after delivery.[68]

Prenatal diagnosis of conjoined fetuses today poses a great ethical dilemma: can this pregnancy have a favorable long-term outcome, leading to birth of human beings who after complex surgery will have normal physical, mental, and psychological development and an acceptable quality of life or should such a pregnancy be terminated before reaching the stage of viability? When considering continuation of pregnancy, one has to think if modern medicine should try to correct postnatally in the operating room an "error" not timely corrected by nature with a miscarriage. As long as conjoined fetuses are in a nonviable gestational age, parents' desire, after detailed counseling about treatment options and long-term outcome, is the single most important factor regarding continuation or termination of pregnancy. After this stage, however, ethical questions might be immense and emerging problems virtually impossible to be resolved. The case of Jodie and Mary, a case of conjoined twins, which gained extreme public attention some years ago, illustrates the complexity of problems arising after conjoined twins have reached the stage of viability. In this case, while medical law and ethics suggested that surgical separation was an act in favor of the twins, parents did not agree with this option.[69]

In our experience, we have encountered a unique case of conjoined triplets, the first case ever documented not only with prenatal ultrasound and MRI, but also with postnatal photography (**Figs. 3 to 8**).[20] Conjoined triplets were diagnosed in the second trimester with 2D ultrasound, followed by confirmation of diagnosis with MRI. In this particular case, parents opted for a pregnancy termination after thorough counseling regarding further management, since both parents felt that any postnatal attempt of surgical separation would have a devastating impact in at least two or all three fetuses. The conjoined triplets were delivered at 22 weeks by cesarean section, and postnatal autopsy confirmed diagnosis of tricephalus, tetrabrachius, tetrapus parapagus-thoracopagus conjoined triplets.[20]

Postnatal operative separation of conjoined twins poses great philosophical and ethical challenges, especially in cases with extensive sharing of organs and two distinguishable functioning brains.[70] Successful separation of conjoined twins depends mainly on the feasibility of surgical separation

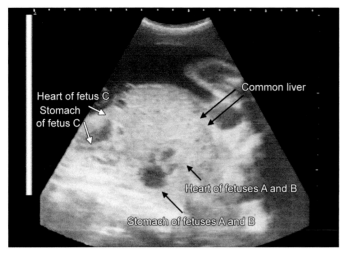

Fig. 3: Ultrasound prenatal diagnosis of conjoined triplets. A common liver, a common heart of the parapagus component, and a heart (hypolastic) of the third conjoined fetus are seen.
Source: Reprinted after author's permission from: Athanasiadis AP, Tzannatos C, Mikos T, Zafrakas M, Bontis JN. A unique case of conjoined triplets. Am J Obstet Gynecol. 2005;192(6):2084-7.

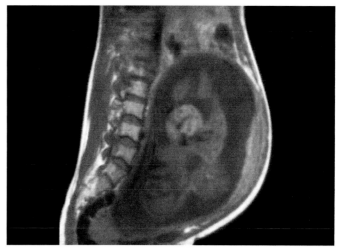

Fig. 5: Magnetic resonance imaging prenatal diagnosis of conjoined triplets.
Source: Reprinted after author's permission from: Athanasiadis AP, Tzannatos C, Mikos T, Zafrakas M, Bontis JN. A unique case of conjoined triplets. Am J Obstet Gynecol. 2005;192(6):2084-7.

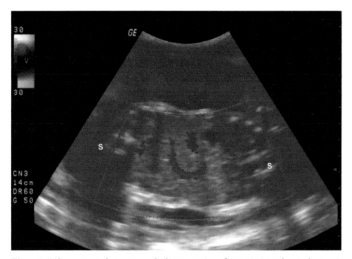

Fig. 4: Ultrasound prenatal diagnosis of conjoined triplets. A common liver and extended cardiovascular anastomoses between the conjoined fetuses are detected with the use of the color flow.
Source: Reprinted after author's permission from: Athanasiadis AP, Tzannatos C, Mikos T, Zafrakas M, Bontis JN. A unique case of conjoined triplets. Am J Obstet Gynecol. 2005;192(6):2084-7.

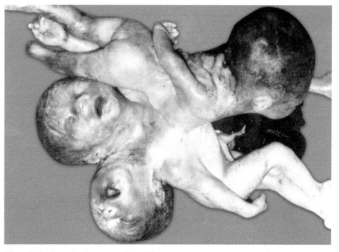

Fig. 6: A tricephalus, tetrabrachius, tetrapus, parapago-thoracopagus conjoined triplet.
Source: Reprinted after author's permission from: Athanasiadis AP, Tzannatos C, Mikos T, Zafrakas M, Bontis JN. A unique case of conjoined triplets. Am J Obstet Gynecol. 2005;192(6):2084-7.

of the common heart and or liver of the conjoined fetuses. Further management of conjoined twins surviving after delivery may fall into one of the three following scenarios: (1) those who die shortly after birth, (2) those who survive long enough until planned surgical separation is undertaken, and (3) those who may be saved by emergent separation at birth.[71] Conjoined twins undergoing planned surgical separation have a survival rate of 80–90% in most series,[72-74] compared with 30–50% survival rate in those needing emergency separation. Delayed, planned surgical separation has several advantages over emergency separation: it is associated with lower risks of anesthesia and it allows more

time to accurately reassess anatomic relationships, detect previously unrecognized congenital anomalies, and make plans to ensure adequate wound coverage.[19]

In our experience, planned postnatal surgical separation led to favorable outcomes in two cases, a case of omphalopagus and a case of craniopagus conjoined twins **(Figs. 9 to 12)**.[52] In the case of omphalopagus twins, cardiac anomalies were detected prenatally in only one of the twins, but there were no signs of shared cardiac structures, making continuation of pregnancy to a viable stage reasonable, since successful postnatal surgical separation was possible. In the case of craniopagus twins, the absence of prenatal

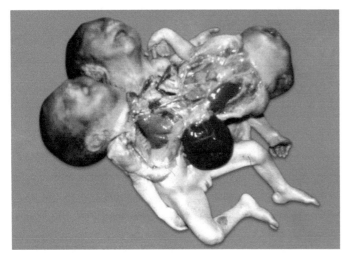

Fig. 7: A common heart and liver parapago-thoracopagus conjoined triplets.
Source: Reprinted after author's permission from: Athanasiadis AP, Tzannatos C, Mikos T, Zafrakas M, Bontis JN. A unique case of conjoined triplets. Am J Obstet Gynecol. 2005;192(6):2084-7.

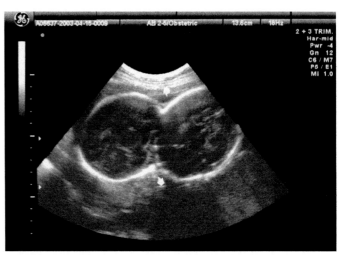

Fig. 9: Prenatal diagnosis of cephalopagus conjoined twins with two-dimensional ultrasound. The arrowheads show the level of conjunction.
Source: Reprinted after author's permission from: Athanasiadis A, Mikos T, Zafrakas M, Diamanti V, Papouli M, Assimakopoulos E, et al. Prenatal management and postnatal separation of omphalopagus and craniopagus conjoined twins. Gynecol Obstet Invest. 2007;64(1):40-3.

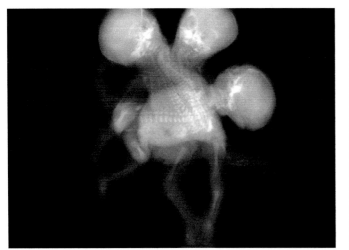

Fig. 8: Conjoined triplets. Three distinct spines and heads. A postmortem plain X-ray.
Source: Reprinted after author's permission from: Athanasiadis AP, Tzannatos C, Mikos T, Zafrakas M, Bontis JN. A unique case of conjoined triplets. Am J Obstet Gynecol. 2005;192(6):2084-7.

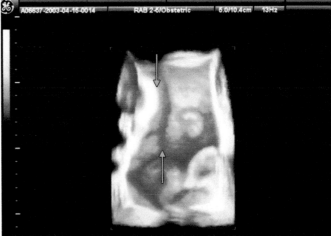

Fig. 10: Prenatal diagnosis of cephalopagus conjoined twins with three-dimensional ultrasound. The green arrows show the level of conjunction.
Source: Reprinted after author's permission from: Athanasiadis A, Mikos T, Zafrakas M, Diamanti V, Papouli M, Assimakopoulos E, et al. Prenatal management and postnatal separation of omphalopagus and craniopagus conjoined twins. Gynecol Obstet Invest. 2007;64(1):40-3.

sonographic signs of shared neural tissue showed that postnatal surgical separation might be successful as well.[52]

Detailed prenatal counseling of parents is crucial in decision-making with regard to continuation of pregnancy and planning postnatal management. An interdisciplinary medical team, involving obstetricians, neonatologists, pediatric surgeons, and anesthetists, should undertake counseling.[52] Additional consultation by radiologists may be required, if MRI or other imaging modalities are used. Psychosocial support should be always offered to parents prenatally and postnatally both prior to and after surgical separation. In special cases, additional consultation may be given by other specialists, even from specialized centers in other countries, depending on the area of conjunction, the involvement of other organ systems, and the presence of associated anomalies. In the case of craniopagus twins described above, parents received additional, prenatal consultation from a specialized neurosurgical center in Italy, and the twins were finally separated postnatally at the same center.[75] In selected cases, when the risk of neonatal demise of one or both twins is high, palliative care services should be readily available.[76]

Obstetricians play a pivotal role in coordinating meetings between parents and members of the interdisciplinary medical team.[52] Counseling should include detailed sessions

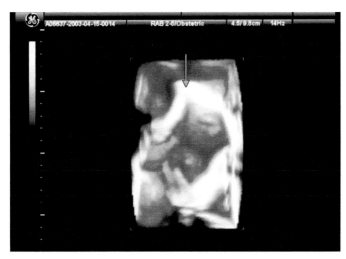

Fig. 11: Prenatal diagnosis of craniopagus conjoined twins with three-dimensional ultrasound. The green arrow shows the level of conjunction.
Source: Reprinted after author's permission from: Athanasiadis A, Mikos T, Zafrakas M, Diamanti V, Papouli M, Assimakopoulos E, et al. Prenatal management and postnatal separation of omphalopagus and craniopagus conjoined twins. Gynecol Obstet Invest. 2007;64(1):40-3.

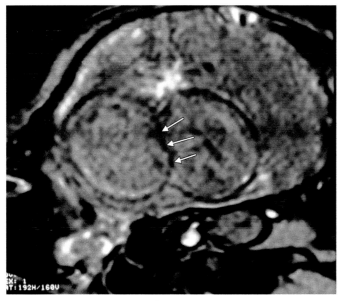

Fig. 12: Prenatal diagnosis of craniopagus conjoined twins with magnetic resonance imaging. The arrows show the level of conjunction.
Source: Reprinted after author's permission from: Athanasiadis A, Mikos T, Zafrakas M, Diamanti V, Papouli M, Assimakopoulos E, et al. Prenatal management and postnatal separation of omphalopagus and craniopagus conjoined twins. Gynecol Obstet Invest. 2007;64(1):40-3.

regarding the rarity and unclear etiology of this condition, as well as information about the anatomic structures involved in the area of conjunction, and associated or coincidental anomalies. Parents should be informed that there are no known inherited patterns or contributing environmental factors. Furthermore, adequate time should be given to parents in order to discuss the options of surgical separation, prognosis for every fetus after surgery, long-term sequelae,

cosmetic issues, and quality of life in childhood and adult life. A very important issue is to preserve privacy of the parents, in order to avoid additional psychological distress, by keeping media and unwanted visitors or even relatives in a distance. Unfortunately, conjoined gestations attract the general public attention that occasionally can evolve to malicious publicity. The media, aiming to sharp and breathtaking stories, do not hesitate to report the birth of such unusual neonates, without considering any consequences this may have on the social and the ethical integrity of the personality of the parents. A number of doctors and paramedical personnel involved in the pre- and postnatal management of the conjoined gestations are potential sources of information for journalists; apparently, it is not ethically appropriate for anyone involved in such a case to give details to the press without parental permission. Obviously, parents are going through a stressful ordeal and the increased burden of life-concerning decisions about the fetuses, makes respect from society to their privacy imperative.[52]

■ CONCLUSION

Conjoined fetuses are very rarely seen in human pregnancies. Etiopathogenesis is unclear, without any known inciting factor(s) leading to this condition. There are two opposing pathogenetic theories, supporting fission versus fusion of embryos in the early first trimester; in very rare cases of diamniotic-monochorionic conjoined twins, a distinct pathogenetic mechanism of conjoined twinning, similar to that of body stalk anomaly may exist. Prenatal diagnosis and accurate recognition of shared organs between fetuses are essential in order to decide for or against continuation of pregnancy and plan prenatal surveillance and postnatal management. Cesarean section is the preferable mode of delivery. Obstetricians play a pivotal role in prenatal counseling, and in coordinating meetings between parents and members of the interdisciplinary medical team needed in the management of such complex cases.

■ REFERENCES

1. Guttmacher AF. Biographical notes on some famous conjoined twins. Birth Defects. 1967;3:10-7.
2. van den Brand SFJJ, Nijhuis JG, van Dongen PWJ. Prenatal ultrasound diagnosis of conjoined twins. Obstet Gynecol Survey. 1994;49:656-62.
3. Harper RG, Kenigsberg K, Sia CG, Horn D, Stern D, Bongiovi V. Xiphopagus conjoined twins: a 300 year review of the obstetric, morphopathologic, neonatal, and surgical parameters. Am J Obstet Gynecol. 1980;137:617-29.
4. Melin JR. Intrapartum diagnosis of conjoined twins. Obstet Gynecol. 1967;29:50-3.
5. Gray CH, Nix HG, Wallace AJ. Thoracopagus twins: prenatal diagnosis. Radiology. 1950;54:398.
6. Barth RA, Filly RA, Goldberg J, Moore P, Silverman NH. Conjoined twins: prenatal diagnosis and assessment of associated malformations. Radiology. 1990;177:201-7.

7. Wilson RL, Cetrulo CL, Shaub MS. The prepartum diagnosis of conjoined twins by the use of diagnostic ultrasound. Am J Obstet Gynecol. 1976;126:737.

8. Fagan CJ. Antepartum diagnosis of conjoined twins by ultrasonography. Am J Roentgenol. 1977;129:921-2.

9. Morgan CL, Trought WS, Sheldon G, Barton TK. B-scan and real-time ultrasound in the antepartum diagnosis of conjoined twins and pericardial effusion. AJR Am J Roentgenol. 1978;130:578-80.

10. Wood MJ, Thompson HE, Roberson FM. Real-time ultrasound diagnosis of conjoined twins. J Clin Ultrasound. 1981;9:195-7.

11. Schmidt W, Heberling D, Kubil F. Antepartum ultrasono-graphic diagnosis of conjoined twins in early pregnancy. Am J Obstet Gynecol. 1981;139:961-3.

12. Schmidt W, Kubli F. Early diagnosis of severe congenital malformations by ultrasonography. J Perinat Med. 1982;10:233-41.

13. Skupski DW, Streltzoff J, Hutsen M, Rosenwaks Z, Cohen J, Chervenak FA. Early diagnosis of conjoined twins in triplet pregnancy after in vitro fertilization and assisted hatching. J Ultrasound Med. 1995;14:611-5.

14. Hill LM. The sonographic detection of early first-trimester conjoined twins. Prenatal Diagnosis. 1997;17:961-3.

15. Lam YH, Sin SY, Lam C, Lee CP, Tang MHY, Tse HY. Prenatal sonographic diagnosis of conjoined twins in the first trim-ester: two case reports. Ultrasound Obstet Gynecol. 1998;11:289-91.

16. Goldberg Y, Ben-Shlomo I, Weiner E, Shalev E. First trimester diagnosis of conjoined twins in a triplet pregnancy after IVF and ICSI: case report. Hum Reprod. 2000;15:1413-5.

17. Daskalakis G, Pilalis A, Tourikis I, Moulopoulos G, Karamoutzos I, Antsaklis A. First trimester diagnosis of dicephalus conjoined twins. Eur J Obstet Gynecol Reprod Biol. 2004;112:110-13.

18. Watanabe K, Ono M, Shirahashi M, Ikeda T, Yakubo K. Dicephalus parapagus conjoined twins diagnosed by first-trimester ultrasound. Case Rep Obstet Gynecol. 2016; 2016:8565193.

19. Mackenzie TC, Crombleholme TM, Johnson MP, Schnaufer L, Flake AW, Hedrick HL, et al. The natural history of prenatally diagnosed conjoined twins. J Pediatr Surg. 2002;37:303-9.

20. Athanasiadis AP, Tzannatos C, Mikos T, Zafrakas M, Bontis J. A unique case of conjoined triplets. Am J Obstet Gynecol. 2005;192(6):2084-7.

21. Tan KL, Tock EPC, Dawood MY, Ratnam SS. Conjoined twins in a triplet pregnancy. Am J Dis Child. 1971;122:455-8.

22. Sepulveda W, Munoz H, Alcalde JL. Conjoined twins in a triplet pregnancy: early prenatal diagnosis with three-dimensional ultrasound and review of the literature. Ultrasound Obstet Gynecol. 2003;22:199-204.

23. Liu H, Deng C, Hu Q, Liao H, Wang X, Yu H. Conjoined twins in dichorionic diamniotic triplet pregnancy: a report of three cases and literature review. BMC Pregnancy Childbirth. 2021; 21(1):687.

24. Hanson JW. Incidence of conjoined twining. Lancet. 1975;2:1257.

25. Edmonds LD, Layde PM. Conjoined twins in the United States, 1970-1977. Teratology. 1982;25(3):301-8.

26. Viljoen DL, Nelson MM, Beighton P. The epidemiology of conjoined twinning in Southern Africa. Clin Genet. 1983;24:15-21.

27. Mutchinick OM, Luna-Muñoz L, Amar E, Bakker MK, Clementi M, Cocchi G, et al. Conjoined twins: a worldwide collaborative epidemiological study of the International Clearinghouse for Birth Defects Surveillance and Research. Am J Med Genet C Semin Med Genet. 2011;157C(4):274-87.

28. Spencer R. Theoretical and analytical embryology of conjoined twins: part I: embryogenesis. Clin Anat. 2000; 13(1):36-53.

29. Apuzzio JJ, Ganesh V, Landau I, Pelosi M. Prenatal diagnosis of conjoined twins. Am J Obstet Gynecol. 1984;148:343-4.

30. Zeng SM, Yankowitz J, Murray JC. Conjoined twins in a monozygotic triplet pregnancy: prenatal diagnosis and X-inactivation. Teratology. 2002;66(6):278-81.

31. Steinman G. Mechanisms of twinning. V. Conjoined twins, stem cells and the calcium model. J Reprod Med. 2002;47(4):313-21.

32. Alikani M, Noyes N, Cohen J, Rosenwaks Z. Monozygotic twinning in human is associated with zona pellucida architecture. Hum Reprod. 1994;9:1318-21.

33. Edwards RG, Mettler L, Walters DE. Identical twins and in vitro fertilization. J In Vitro Fert Embryo Transf. 1986;3(2):114-7.

34. Magdi Y. Dizygotic twin from conjoined oocytes: a case report. J Assist Reprod Genet. 2020;37:1367-70.

35. Mankonen H, Seikkula J, Järvenpää T, Jokimaa V. A case of conjoined twins after a transfer of a multinuclear embryo. Clin Case Rep. 2015;3:260-5.

36. Pajkrt E, Jauniaux E. First-trimester diagnosis of conjoined twins. Prenat Diagn. 2005;25:820-6.

37. Xiang G, Wen Y, Zhang L, Tong X, Li L. Three-dimensional ultrasonographic features of diamniotic conjoined twins with body stalk anomaly. BMC Pregnancy Childbirth. 2020; 20:221.

38. Kapur RP, Jack RM, Siebert JR. Diamniotic placentation associated with omphalopagus conjoined twins: implications for a contemporary model of conjoined twinning. Am J Med Genet. 1994;52:188-95.

39. Wielgos M, Bomba-Opon D, Kociszewska-Najman B, Brawura-Biskupski-Samaha R, Kaminski A, Piotrowska A, et al. Minimally conjoined monochorionic diamniotic twins - a case report. Eur J Obstet Gynecol Reprod Biol. 2014;180: 206-7.

40. Weston PJ, Ives EJ, Honore RL, Lees GM, Sinclair DB, Schiff D. Monochorionic diamniotic minimally conjoined twins: a case report. Am J Med Genet. 1990;37:558-61.

41. Karnak I, Sanlialp I, Ekinci S, Senocak ME. Minimally conjoined omphalopagi: emphasis on embryogenesis and possibility of emergency separation. Turk J Pediatr. 2008;50(5):503-8.

42. Tihtonen K, Lagerstedt A, Kirkinen P. Diamniotic omphalopagus conjoined twins in a diamniotic pregnancy. Fetal Diagn Ther. 2009;25:343-5.

43. Costa SL, Dunn L, Pantazi S, Chitayat D, Ryan G, Keating S. A novel case of monochorionic diamniotic conjoined twins with genitourinary and gastrointestinal union. Ultrasound Obstet Gynecol. 2006;28:562-3.

44. DeStephano CC, Meena M, Brown DL, Davies NP, Brost BC. Sonographic diagnosis of conjoined diamniotic mono-chorionic twins. Am J Obstet Gynecol. 2010;203(6):e4-6.

45. Maruyama H, Inagaki T, Nakata Y, Kanazawa A, Iwasaki Y, Sasaki K, et al. Minimally conjoined omphalopagus twins with a body stalk anomaly. AJP Rep. 2015;5(2):e124-8.

46. Shah N. Monochorionic diamniotic conjoined twins: prenatal sonographic diagnosis at 8 weeks. Ultrasound Obstet Gynecol. 2019;54(5):699-700.

47. Chatterjee MS, Weiss RR, Verma UL, Tejani NA, Macri J. Prenatal diagnosis of conjoined twins. Prenat Diagn. 1983; 3:357-61.

48. Hubinont C, Pratola D, Rotschild E, Rodesch F, Schwers J. Dicephalus: unusual case of conjoined twins and its prepartum diagnosis. Am J Obstet Gynecol. 1984;149:693-4.

49. Kalchbrenner M, Weiner S, Templeton J, Losure TA. Prenatal ultrasound diagnosis of thoracopagus conjoined twins. J Clin Ultrasound. 1987;15:59-63.

50. MacKenzie AP, Stephenson CD, Funai EF, Lee MJ, Timor-Tritsch I. Three-dimensional ultrasound to differentiate epigastric heteropagus conjoined twins from a TRAP sequence. Am J Obstet Gynecol. 2004;191:1736-9.

51. Burans C, Smulian J, Rochon M, Lutte J, Hardin W. 3-dimensional ultrasound assisted counseling for conjoined twins. J Genet Couns. 2014;23(1):29-32.

52. Athanasiadis A, Mikos T, Zafrakas M, Diamanti V, Papouli M, Assimakopoulos E, et al. Prenatal management and postnatal separation of omphalopagus and craniopagus conjoined twins. Gynecol Obstet Invest. 2007;64(1):40-3.

53. Blum E, Pearlman M, Graham D. Early second-trimester sonographic diagnosis of thoracopagus twins. J Clin Ultrasound. 1986;14:207-8.

54. Scharl A, Schlensker KH, Wohlers W, Heymans L. Fruhe Ultraschall-diagnose des Thorakopagus. Z Geburtshilfe Perinatol. 1988;192:38-41.

55. Filler RM. Conjoined twins and their separation. Semin Perinatol. 1986;10:82-91.

56. Iura T, Makinoda S, Sasakura C, Hirosaki N, Inoue H, Waseda T, et al. Hemodynamic analysis of cephalothoracopagus by the color Doppler method. A comparison to normal fetuses via a longitudinal study. Fetal Diagn Ther. 2006;21:61-4.

57. Hecht C, Baumann M, Spinelli M, Trippel M, Raio L. Umbilical cord in conjoined twins: prenatal imaging and anatomopathological aspects. Ultrasound Obstet Gynecol. 2019;53:269-70.

58. Razavi-Encha F, Mulliez N, Benhaiem-Sigaux N, Gonzales M, Casasoprana A, Bloch G, et al. Cardiovascular abnormalities in thoracopagus twins: embryological interpretation and review. Early Hum Dev. 1987;15:33-44.

59. Synhorst D, Matlak M, Roan Y, Johnson D, Byrne J, McGough E. Separation of conjoined thoracopagus twins joined at the right atria. Am J Cardiol. 1979;43:662-5.

60. Rimawi BH, Krishna I, Sahu A, Badell ML. Pregnancy in a previously conjoined thoracopagus twin with a crisscross heart. Case Rep Obstet Gynecol. 2015;2015:594537.

61. Andrews RE, McMahon CJ, Yates RW, Cullen S, de Leval MR, Kiely EM, et al. Echocardiographic assessment of conjoined twins. Heart. 2006;92:382-7.

62. Sanders SP, Chin AJ, Parness IA, Benacerraf B, Greene MF, Epstein MF, et al. Prenatal diagnosis of congenital heart defects in thoracoabdominally conjoined twins. N Engl J Med. 1985;313:370-4.

63. Boer LL, Schepens-Franke AN, Winter E, Oostra RJ. Characterizing the coalescence area of conjoined twins to elucidate congenital disorders in singletons. Clin Anat. 2021;34:845-58.

64. Bianchi DW, Crombleholme TM, D'Alton ME (Eds). Fetology: Diagnosis and Management of the Fetal Patient. New-York: McGraw-Hill; 2000. pp. 892-9.

65. Gao J, Gao YF. Prenatal diagnosis of conjoined twins with real-time ultrasound. Chin Med J (Engl). 1988;101(1):58-60.

66. Vaughn TC, Powell LC. The obstetrical management of conjoined twins. Obstet Gynecol. 1979;53(3 Suppl);67S-72S.

67. Hammond DI, Okun NB, Carpenter BF, Martin DJ, Krzaniak S. Prenatal ultrasonographic diagnosis of dicephalus conjoined twins. Can Assoc Radiol J. 1991;42:357-9.

68. Sakala EP. Obstetric management of conjoined twins. Obstet Gynecol. 1986;67:21S-25S.

69. Pearn J. Bioethical issues in caring for conjoined twins and their parents. Lancet. 2001;357:1968-71.

70. Savulescu J, Persson I. Conjoined twins: philosophical problems and ethical challenges. J Med Philos. 2016;41:41-55.

71. Graivier L, Jacoby MD. Emergency separation of newborn conjoined (Siamese) twins. Tex Med. 1980;76:60-2.

72. O'Neill JA Jr, Holcomb GW 3rd, Schnaufer L, Templeton JM Jr, Bishop HC, Ross AJ 3rd, et al. Surgical experience with thirteen conjoined twins. Ann Surg. 1988;208:299-312.

73. Chiu CT, Hou SH, Lai HS, Lee PH, Lin FY, Chen WJ, et al. Separation of thoracopagus conjoined twins. A case report. J Cardiovasc Surg (Torino). 1994;35:459-62.

74. Spitz L, Kiely E. Success rate for surgery of conjoined twins. Lancet. 2000;356:1765.

75. Di Rocco C, Caldarelli M, Tamburrini G, Koutzoglou M, Massimi L, Di Rocco F, et al. Craniopagus: the Thessaloniki-Rome experience. Childs Nerv Syst. 2004;20(8-9):576-86.

76. Thomas A, Johnson K, Placencia FX. An ethically-justifiable, practical approach to decision-making surrounding conjoined-twin separation. Semin Perinatol. 2018;42:381-5.

Fetal Brain Structure and Central Nervous System Anomalies

Ritsuko K Pooh

■ INTRODUCTION

Since the brain is an organ that must be understood as a three-dimensional (3D) structure, and since the fetal skull ossifies in late pregnancy, it is difficult to depict detailed structures in the brain using conventional horizontal cross-sectional images captured by transabdominal ultrasound. However, there are large spaces such as anterior/posterior fontanelles and sagittal suture in the fetal skull. By using these spaces as a window for ultrasound, it becomes easier to observe the brain structure. Transvaginal ultrasound observation of the fetal brain began in the 1990s,[1] and the combination of fetal 3D neurosonography and transvaginal ultrasound has made it possible to observe congenital brain structural abnormalities and cortical dysgenesis in more detail. Transvaginal 3D ultrasound imaging has been reported to be effective in the evaluation of fetal brain structure.[2-7] Images of normal brain development, intracerebral vascular architecture, brain malformations, brain disorders such as intracerebral hemorrhage and stroke, and abnormalities in cortical development have gradually revealed the previously unknown development and pathology of the fetal brain. This chapter comprehensively illustrates how to observe the fetal brain using 3D ultrasound, imaging, and genetic diagnosis of brain lesions.

▌ HOW TO OBTAIN ORIENTATION BY 3D NEUROSONOGRAPHY

When the fetus is in pelvic or lateral position, the head of the fetus is located at various sites inside the uterus and neuro-imaging can be obtained by transabdominal incidence of ultrasound beam from the fontanelles or sagittal suture. In the case of a fetus in the cephalic position, the presence of the maternal pubic bone makes it difficult to approach the fetus from the top of the head with transabdominal ultrasound. Therefore, if the fetus can be externally rotated to the pelvic position or the fetal head can be manually pushed upward, it will be easier to observe the intracranial structures by the

transabdominal method. However, transvaginal ultrasound allows us to use a transvaginal probe with higher resolution than the transabdominal probe without interference from the maternal abdominal wall or placenta, allowing us to observe the brain in great detail. The difficulty with transvaginal ultrasonography is positioning the fetal head so that the anterior fontanelle or sagittal suture is located at the tip of the probe. Once the position is adjusted, the region of interest (ROI) and the angle of the scan width are determined and the automatic scan is started (**Figs. 1A and B**).

After acquiring the images, an offline analysis is performed. When observing the fetal brain with transvaginal ultrasound, unlike transabdominal ultrasound, it is difficult to align the orientation of the left and right brain hemispheres. The solution to this problem lies in the

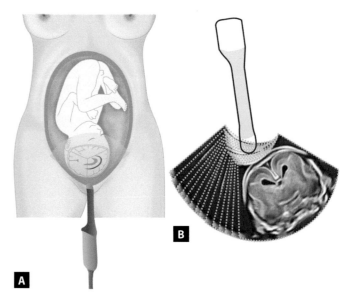

Figs. 1A and B: Illustration of transvaginal 3D neurosonography. (A) Transvaginal neurosonography. Transvaginal ultrasound can provide a very detailed view of the brain without the interference of the maternal abdominal wall or placenta; (B) Once the position is adjusted, the region of interest and the angle of scan width are determined, and the automatic scan is started.

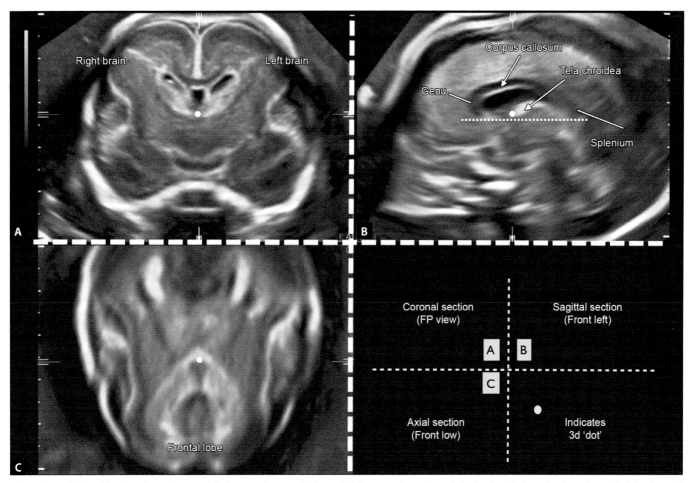

Figs. 2A to C: Fetal brain orientation on 3D three orthogonal views. (A) A coronal section of the brain; (B) A sagittal section; (C) A horizontal section. It is important to note that the anterior part of the brain should be positioned to the left of the screen in the B section. It is important to note that the brain should be rotated and adjusted so that the anterior part of the brain is positioned to the left of the screen in section B. In coronal section A, the fetal left brain is depicted on the right side of the screen and the fetal right brain is depicted on the left side of the screen.

manipulation of the 3D images. First, three orthogonal views A, B, and C are displayed. Image A shows a coronal section of the brain, B shows a sagittal section, and C shows a horizontal section. It is important to note that in B, the anterior part of the brain is located on the left side of the screen. In the coronal section A, the left side of the fetal brain is depicted on the right side of the screen, and the right side of the fetal brain is on the left side of the screen[8,9] **(Figs. 2A to C)**. By obtaining the left and right orientation of the fetus, it is possible to clearly identify which hemisphere has the asymmetric lesion. This method is currently not universal, but if you follow these rules, you can get the orientation of the brain quite easily, especially in cases with asymmetrical brain structures.

OBSERVATION IN TOMOGRAPHIC IMAGING

Similar to magnetic resonance imaging (MRI) and computed tomography (CT), tomographic ultrasound imaging (TUI) can be used to produce slice images parallel to each plane. This is a very comprehensive imaging method not only for obstetricians, but also for pediatric neurologists and pediatric

neurosurgeons. The slice width can be easily changed in TUI to view parallel slice images of the brain. Similarly, in the TUI image, the brain image itself can be moved, keeping the slice width constant, to view a series of parallel slice images. In comparison to MRI and CT in terms of offline analysis, 3D neurosonography has the advantage of being able to view a continuous cross-section of the brain with different slice widths **(Figs. 3A to D)**.

APPLICATION AND ADVANTAGES OF 3D NEUROSONOGRAPHIC IMAGE

A variety of 3D representations are available for 3D ultrasound images, including three orthogonal views, TUI, inverted image, HDlive silhouette ultrasound, thick-slice silhouette image, and volume-cutting image **(Figs. 4A to F)**. Silhouette ultrasound imaging is a recent advanced 3D technique that creates gradients in the walls of fluid-filled cavities and vascular walls where rapid changes in acoustic impedance occur.[10-17] The HDlive silhouette mode displays fluid-filled cystic structures through the outer surface structures, and in prenatal images, the image is "see-through"[15] to depict the ventricular system,

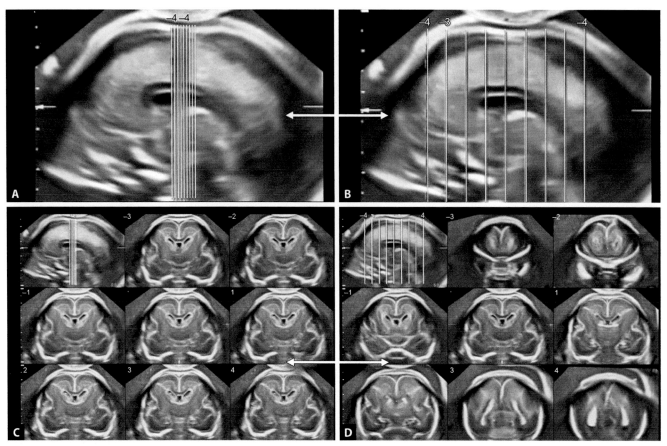

Figs. 3A to D: Tomographic ultrasound imaging with changing slice width. The slice width can be easily changed from (A) to (B) to view parallel slice images (C and D) of the brain.

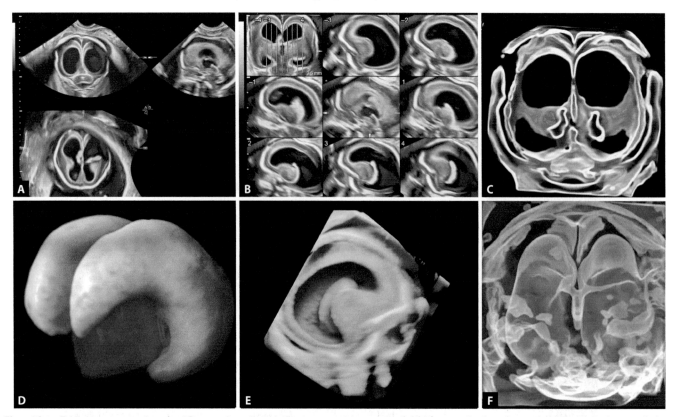

Figs. 4A to F: Various expressions by 3D neuroimaging. Various expressions are available from a single volume dataset. (A) Orthogonal view; (B) Tomographic ultrasound imaging; (C) Thick-slice silhouette image; (D) Inverted image of the enlarged ventricles; (E) Volume cutting image; (F) HDlive silhouette image.

including the lateral and third ventricles, along with the outer surface of the cranium. A thick slice silhouette image is created by cropping the volume data in a rectangular shape and rendering it using the silhouette method.

What makes 3D neurosonographic imaging so useful in clinical practice is the ability to longitudinally compare brain structures that change during pregnancy in the exact same section of the same case. Another major clinical advantage of 3D neurosonographic imaging is the ability to compare abnormal brain structures with normal brains in the exact same cut section at the exact same gestational week. The comparison between abnormal and normal is very common and useful in clinical practice.

3D ULTRASOUND INTRACRANIAL ANGIOGRAPHY

Combining transvaginal 3D ultrasonography with color Doppler and power Doppler has enabled advanced evaluation of fetal brain development and cerebral blood flow. The author reported transvaginal two-dimensional (2D) power Doppler angiography in the first trimester in 1996.[18] Since then, 3D power Doppler angiography has provided greater detail of the main cerebral arteries, dural sinuses, and fine peripheral vessels.[19,20] Another recent technology, HDlive flow, has enabled 3D visualization of blood flow and microvasculature **(Figs. 5A and B)**; the combination of HDlive silhouette and HDlive flow provides a comprehensive orientation of intracranial vascular structures and confirms the location of vascular trajectories within morphological structures.[21]

In addition, the recent advanced technology of 3D Slowflow has made it possible to visualize these vascular structures in more sophisticated 3D, and fine intracerebral vessels such as lenticular arteries and medullary veins can now be depicted even more clearly **(Figs. 6A and B)**. These innovations make it possible to easily grasp the vascular structure of the entire brain.

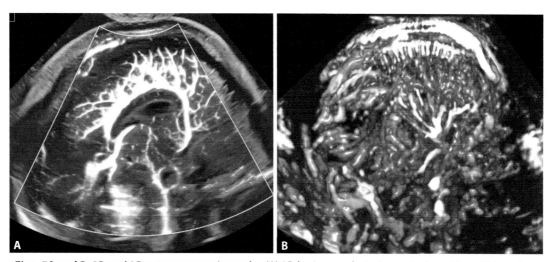

Figs. 5A and B: 2D and 3D neurosonoangiography. (A) 2D brain vascularity image in the mid-sagittal section; (B) 3D reconstructed vascular image of sagittal view.

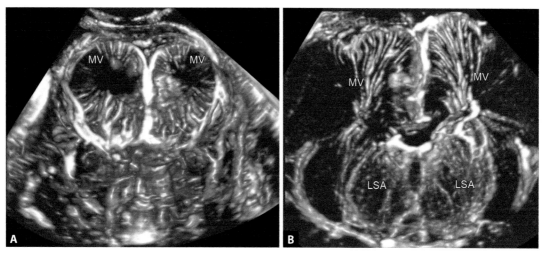

Figs. 6A and B: 3D Slowflow neurosonoangiography of medullary veins. (A) Coronal view of brain vascularity. Note the medullary veins (MV) are premature and short; (B) At 28 weeks, matured MV are demonstrated. (LSA: lenticulostriate arteries)

CRANIAL DYSRAPHISM (NEURULATION DISORDER)

The neural tube is a single tubular structure that runs from head to tail during development and is the original basis for the brain and spinal cord that make up the central nervous system. The neural tube originates from the neural plate, which has a simple flattened epithelial structure. A neural ridge is formed near the boundary between the neural plate and the epidermal ectoderm, and a neural groove is formed in the middle of the neural plate. The actin cytoskeleton, which is highly concentrated on the apical side of the neuroepithelial cells, makes up the neural plate, and contracts causing the neural plate distortion and bending of the neural plate. Later, the left and right sides of the neural plate fuse, and the neural plate finally changes from an epidermal ectoderm to a tubular structure. This developmental pattern is called primary neurulation. Meanwhile, in the caudal part of mammalian and avian embryos, neural tube formation by epithelialization of mesodermal mesenchymal cells is observed, and such a mode is called secondary neurulation.

In mice, more than 200 genes are known to cause neural tube defects (NTDs). In humans, the developmental pattern is multifactorial, polygenic, or oligogenic in etiology.[22,23] In acranial-anencephalic embryos, complete or incomplete loss of brain tissue and cranium is seen. Craniorachischisis is characterized by anencephaly with continuous spinal cord defects and exposed neural tissue. Spina bifida, such as myelomeningocele **(Figs. 7A to C)** and meningocele, is a typical NTD, and Chiari type II causes herniation of the cerebellar tonsils and medulla oblongata into the spinal canal, resulting in narrowing of the fourth ventricle and midbrain aqueduct, and consequently ventricular dilatation. In the case of enlarged ventricles associated with Chiari malformation, the enlarged ventricles have a characteristic angular or triangular shape due to intracranial negative pressure **(Fig. 8)**. The etiology of encephaloceles is not well understood. Encephalocele has been classified as an NTD. However, it has been controversial whether the encephalocele is an NTD or a postneurulation defect; Rolo et al. used mouse model experiments to show that the encephalocele is not the result of failed neural tube closure, but rather a defect in the extra surface covering of an already closed neural tube. They stated that it was due to the later collapse of the surface ectoderm covering the already closed neural tube.[24] Other etiologies of NTD include single-gene mutations, multifactorial inheritance, environmental factors, and drugs such as valproic acid. It has been thought that maternal serum alpha-fetoprotein levels are elevated in NTD. However, in skin-covered encephalocele and meningocele, maternal serum alpha-fetoprotein levels are not elevated. Therefore, neurosonography is extremely useful for detecting NTDs during pregnancy.

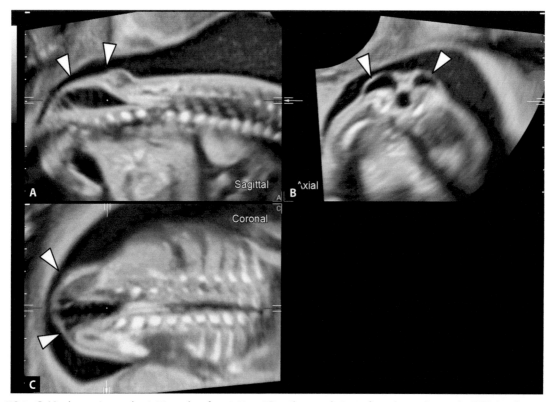

Figs. 7A to C: Myelomeningocele at 16 weeks of gestation. 3D orthogonal view of myelomeningocele. Fifth lumbar to sacral myelomeningocele is clearly demonstrated (arrowheads).

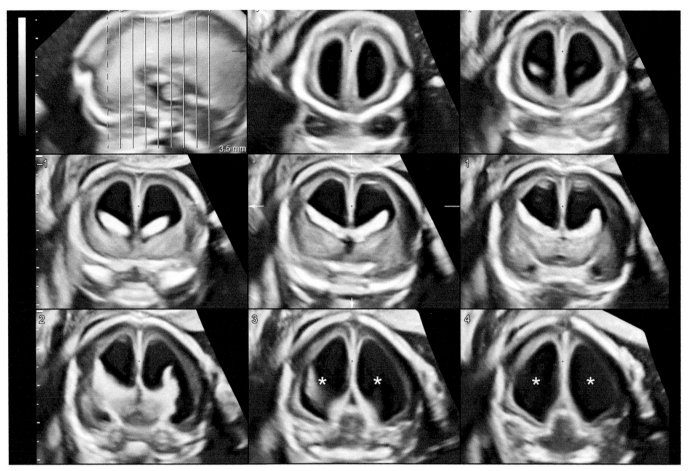

Fig. 8: Ventriculomegaly due to myelomeningocele and Chiari type II malformation. Tomographic ultrasound imaging on coronal plane. Note the triangle shape (asterisks) of the enlarged ventricles. This triangle appearance is one of the features in ventriculomegaly due to myelomeningocele and Chiari malformation.

◼ HOLOPROSENCEPHALY

The incidence of holoprosencephaly, a representative of prosencephalic disorder, is 1 out of 15,000–20,000 live births. However, it has been reported that the early incidence of aborted human embryos may be over 60 times higher than the incidence of live births.[25,26] Holoprosencephaly is mainly classified into three types: alobar, semilobar, and lobar. In 75% of holoprosencephaly cases, genetic causes have not been identified, and the rest are due to genetic factors. The most common chromosomal abnormality is trisomy 13. There are several genetic mutations that have been identified as genetic causes of holoprosencephaly, for example, *Sonic Hedgehog (SHH)* located on 7q36, *SIX3* on 2p21, *ZIC2* on 13q32, and *TGIF* on 18p11.3.[27-30] In about 22% of normal karyotypes, point mutations or pathogenic copy number changes involving these genes have been identified.[28] About 80% of cases are associated with facial abnormalities such as hypotelorism, cyclopia, arrhinia, proboscis, cleft lip, and palate due to hypoplasia of the midline of the face.[31] **Figure 9** shows semilobar holoprosencephaly at 16 weeks of gestation.

◼ AGENESIS OF THE CORPUS CALLOSUM

The corpus callosum (CC) is the most extensive fiber bundle structure in the cerebrum, connecting the left and right cerebral hemispheres, integrating sensory and motor information, and associated with higher cognition.[32] *FGF8* is an essential gene for the early forebrain patterning and formation of the commissural plate; *ZIC2, NFIA, EMX1,* and *SIX3* are genes responsible for the development of the CC, hippocampus, and anterior commissure. The final form of the CC is completed by the 20th week after conception, but axonal growth continues after birth. Although CCs are not formed during the early stages of central nervous system development, early cerebral events are essential for CC formation, including the coupling of morphogenetic gradients with the development of thalamocortical circuits,[33,34] are essential to forming the CC.

Agenesis of the corpus callosum (AOCC) is a malformation of the brain that occurs in isolation or in association with a symptomatic disease. AOCC includes complete AOCC [absence of CC completely **(Figs. 10A to D)**], partial AOCC, and hypoplastic CC with normal anterior to posterior

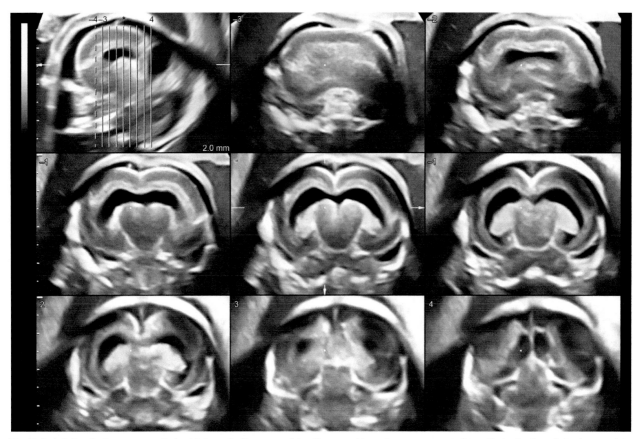

Fig. 9: Semilobar holoprosencephaly at 16 weeks. Tomographic ultrasound imaging on coronal plane. Note the fused single ventricle.

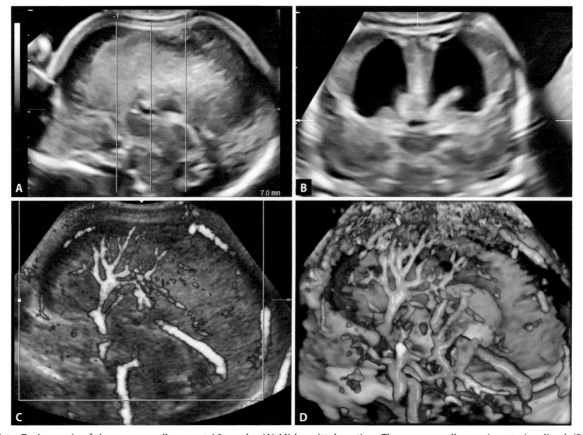

Figs. 10A to D: Agenesis of the corpus callosum at 18 weeks. (A) Mid-sagittal section. The corpus callosum is not visualized; (B) Coronal section. This particular case was associated with severe ventriculomegaly; (C) 2D sonoangiography shows the abnormal vascular direction of the pericallosal artery and its branches; (D) 3D sonoangiography provides more vascular information.

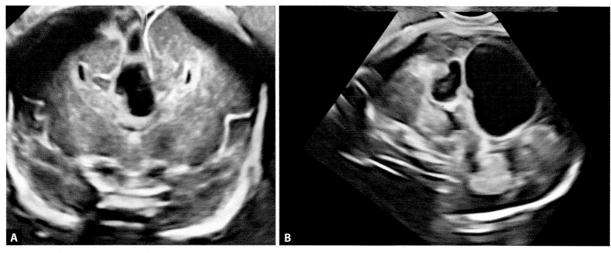

Figs. 11A and B: Interhemispheric cysts associated with agenesis of the corpus callosum at 25 weeks. (A) Coronal section; (B) Mid-sagittal section.

extent,[32] and development of the CC is deeply related to glial cell proliferation, midline patterning, CC neuron migration, specification, axon guidance, and postguidance steps.[32] 1q42-q44 deletion,[35,36] 4p16.3 deletion (Wolf–Hirschhorn syndrome),[37] 8p rearrangements,[38-40] 17p13,3 deletion (Miller–Dieker lissencephaly syndrome),[41,42] and various other copy number mutations have been implicated in CC.

Mutations in the *ARX* gene [43-46] result in X-linked lissencephaly with an AOCC and ambiguous genitalia (XLAG), and mutations in L1CAM cause L1 syndrome.[47] As an *L1CAM* (L1 cell adhesion molecule) gene is located on Xq28, the primarily male baby is affected. *L1* is an essential gene for neuronal adhesion. *L1CAM*-affected patients have severe disorders with mental retardation, lower limb spasticity, and paraplegia.

In some syndromes associated with AOCC, the causative gene has not been identified. Aicardi syndrome, which is characterized by AOCC, infantile seizures, microphthalmia, and choroidal retinal tearing such as coloboma,[48] most of the affected individuals are females with two X chromosomes, and thus the gene has not been identified, but X-linked dominantly inherited. The age-adjusted prevalence is 0.63 per 100,000 women.[49] However, males with two X chromosomes (XXY, Klinefelter syndrome) may be affected. Interhemispheric cysts **(Figs. 11A and B)** or pericallosal lipomas can be associated with AOCC.

MALFORMATIONS OF CORTICAL DEVELOPMENT

The cerebral cortex is formed by a complex dynamic process. There are three stages in the formation of the cerebral cortex.[50] The first stage is the cell proliferation stage, in which stem cells increase in the ventricular zone (VZ) and subventricular zone (SVZ) and differentiate into neurons and glial cells, as well as programmed cell apoptosis. The second is the stage of neuronal migration. Neurons migrate tangentially toward the cortical plate, via intermediate zone and subplate **(Fig. 12)**, from the ventricular surface in an inside-out mode. The third stage is the post-migrational stage.[51]

Thus, the cerebral cortex is gradually formed during the fetal period, and malformations of cortical development (MCD) is a disease completed during the fetal period. However, MCD is not often detected during the fetal period, and in most cases, it is discovered after birth by a detailed examination such as MRI due to developmental delay or epilepsy, followed by genetic testing to determine the causative factors.[52] MCD was classified into three groups according to the three developmental stages mentioned above.[52] More than 100 genes that cause MCD have been identified. However, currently, it has proved difficult to classify MCD into these three groups because MCD-related genes are involved in multiple developmental stages and growth, and migration, and postmigration tissues are thought to be genetically and functionally interdependent.[53,54]

Microcephaly is a proliferative disorder secondary to degeneration of normal growth and associated loss of nerve cells.[55] Microcephaly vera or primary microcephaly is not only a small head, but the brain itself is small, so-called microbrain, resulting in intellectual disability after birth. In microcephaly vera, there is no obvious brain malformation and the phenotype is not always uniform. There is a continuum between microcephaly with regular gyrus formation and microcephaly with other malformations,[56-58] such as microlissencephaly. Causal factors for microcephaly also include prenatal infection with cytomegalovirus (CMV), Zika virus, rubella virus, and toxoplasmosis, as well as mutations in single genes. Genes responsible for microcephaly include microcephalin (*MCPH1*),[57,59,60] *ASPM*,[61] *CDK5RAP2*,[62] *CENPJ*,[52,62,63] *STIL*,[58,63] *WDR62*,[56,58,64] and *CEP152*[65] and others. In most cases of microcephaly, it is extremely challenging to observe intracranial structures by

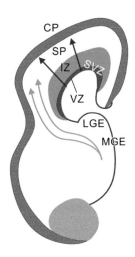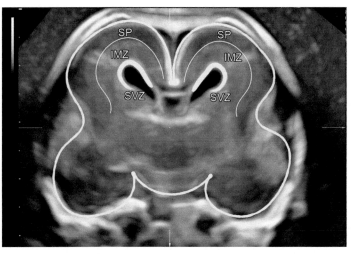

Fig. 12: Subventricular zone (SVZ), intermediate zone (IMZ), and subplate (SP). Neurosonogram demonstrates the layers of SVZ, IMZ, and SP clearly.
(CP: cortical plate; IZ: intermediate zone; LGE: lateral ganglionic eminence; MGE: medial ganglionic eminence; VZ: ventricular zone)

neurosonography through the cranial fontanelle because the cranial fontanelle and sutures are very narrow due to the microcephaly. MRI is advisable for detailed assessment of intracranial structures in cases of microcephaly.

On the surface of the brain, the brain gyri and sulci can be detected on neurosonograms after the second half of the seventh month of pregnancy. During the remainder of the fetal period and shortly after birth, further development of the gyrus continues. Neuronal migration is regulated by a series of complex chemical guidance and signals. When these signals are improper or missing, the nerve cells fail to reach the place where they should properly belong. As a result, structural abnormalities or defects can occur in any part of the intracranial structure, including the cerebral hemispheres, cerebellum, hippocampus, and brain stem. Disorders of neuronal migration include agyria, pachygyria, lissencephaly **(Figs. 13A to D)**, polygyria **(Figs. 14A and B)**, polymicrogyria, neuronal heterotopias such as periventricular nodular heterotopia **(Fig. 15)**, and band heterotopia. Developmental abnormalities in gyration often lead to seizures and neurological dysfunction from early in life; migration disorders become prominent in the cortex in late pregnancy. Toi and colleagues[66] showed a regular pattern of gyration detected by transabdominal ultrasonography. The cerebral cortex develops after 18 weeks in the second trimester of pregnancy, and the most obvious change on neuroimaging is the morphological change in the Sylvian fissure, and a link between the morphology of the Sylvian fissure and cortical dysplasia has recently been reported.[8,9,67,68] According to the development of the brain, the change in the appearance of Sylvian fissure is remarkable. Poon et al.[9] proposed the Sylvian fissure angle explaining a significant angle decrease as the gestational age progressed. Furthermore, Pooh et al.[8] showed 22 MCD cases between 18 and 30 weeks of gestation, with the delayed development of the Sylvian fissure with a wider Sylvian fissure angle

than normal cases. **Figure 16** compares Sylvian fissure appearance in the same cross sections at same gestational age between normal cases and MCD cases.

Lissencephaly is characterized as a malformation of the cerebral cortex with abnormalities in brain gyrus formation due to impaired neuronal migration. The spectrum of lissencephaly contains agyria, pachygyria, and subcortical band heterotopia. Lissencephaly has conventionally been divided into two subtypes. Type I lissencephaly was characterized by a smooth brain, while type II lissencephaly by cobblestone appearance. However, with recent rapid advances in molecular genetics, a conventional classification system became inadequate to distinguish various patterns of lissencephaly to predict the most likely causative gene mutations; a new classification based on imaging was proposed in 2017.[69] Several reports on the prenatal diagnosis of lissencephaly have been published.[66,70-75]

Conventional lissencephaly Type 1 includes Miller Dieker syndrome due to *PAFAH1B1* variant, and lissencephaly caused by doublecortin (*DCX*) variant. Cobblestone lissencephaly (Type II) includes muscle–eye–brain disease (MEB), Walker–Warburg syndrome due to *POMGnT1*,[76,77] Fukuyama syndrome due to *Fukutin*.[78-81] *ARX* gene on Xq22.13[82-85] mutation causes X-linked lissencephaly. *Reelin* gene on 7q22.1,[86-88] tubulin genes such as *TUBB2B*,[89-91] citron kinase,[92,93] ACTG1 variant,[94] and other variants cause microlissencephaly.

Polymicrogyria is the most common MCD associated with postmigration etiology. 1p36.3 deletion, 22q11.2 deletion, and copy number mutations in genes related to the mechanistic target of rapamycin (mTOR) pathway are frequently associated with polymicrogyria, hemimegalencephaly, and macrocephaly. Germline mutations affecting the PI3K/AKT/mTOR pathway have been implicated in certain inherited diseases. Defects in the tumor suppressor phosphatase tensin homolog (PTEN) cause congenital diseases such as Cowden

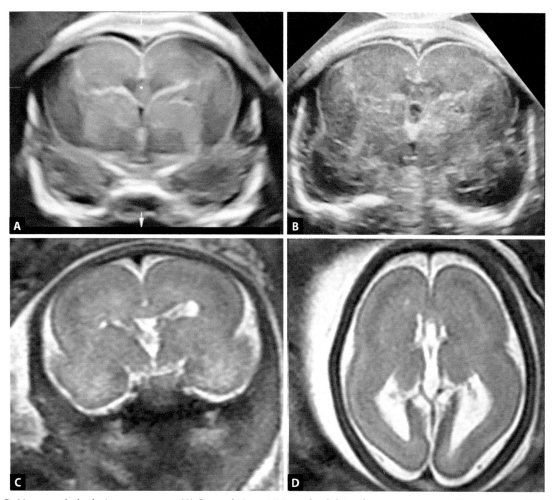

Figs. 13A to D: Lissencephaly during pregnancy. (A) Coronal view at 23 weeks. Sylvian fissures are extremely premature; (B) Coronal view at 25 weeks. 23–25 gestational weeks is a time of great change in brain morphology, but in this case there is little change; (C) Coronal MR image at 36 weeks. No gyral formation is seen. The appearance of Sylvian fissure is almost the same as in 23 weeks; (D) Axial MR image at 36 weeks.

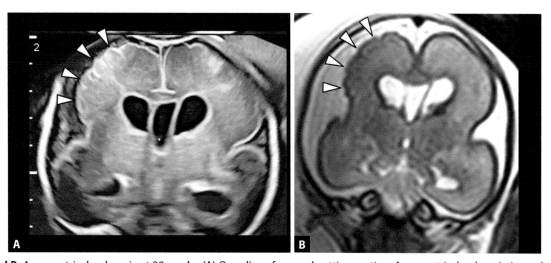

Figs. 14A and B: Asymmetrical polygyria at 28 weeks. (A) One slice of coronal cutting section. Asymmetrical polygyria (arrowheads) is seen; (B) MR image of the same case. Asymmetry, ventriculomegaly, and premature Sylvian fissure is clearly depicted by both neurosonogram and magnetic resonance imaging.

syndrome, Bannayan–Riley–Ruvalcaba syndrome, PTEN-associated Proteus syndrome, and Proteus-like syndrome. The authors recently reported a rare case of megalencephaly with cortical abnormalities caused by a PTEN mutation.[95]

Schizencephaly is characterized by congenital cerebral clefts, lined by pial-ependyma, with communication between the subarachnoid space laterally and the lateral ventricles medially. Schizencephaly occurs unilaterally in 63% and bilaterally 37%. A considerable cause is a vascular disruption during corticogenesis, genetic factors such as *WDR62* mutation, which causes schizencephaly as well as microcephaly, indicating relations between processes of proliferation and schizencephaly pathogenesis, and *COL4A1* mutation. Perisylvian bilateral polymicrogyria is also associated with schizencephaly.

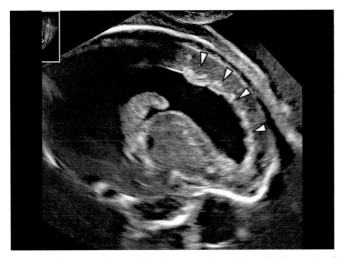

Fig. 15: Periventricular nodular heterotopia at 22 weeks. Parasagittal cutting section. Note the irregular hyperechoic nodules (arrowheads) are visualized along with a ventricular wall.

◼ VENTRICULOMEGALY

Fetal ventriculomegaly is a condition in which the ventricles of the fetal brain are enlarged, and it is the most common brain abnormality detected by prenatal ultrasound, with an incidence of about 1%.[96] There are essentially two types of ventricular dilatation: dilatation of the lateral ventricles and third ventricle due to obstruction or stenosis of the pathways of the cerebrospinal fluid (CSF) flow, resulting in increased intracranial pressure (ICP);[97] and ventricular dilatation with normal ICP due to cerebral ramus defect or cerebral dysplasia.[98] In some cases, temporary ventricular enlargement may occur and then resolve spontaneously.

The underlying etiologies of ventricular enlargement may include chromosomal abnormalities, microchromosomal abnormalities, genetic mutations, central nervous system developmental abnormalities, intracranial hemorrhage, neoplastic lesions, hypoxic brain injury, viral infections, and metabolic diseases.[99-102] The neurological prognosis of ventriculomegaly is varied and diverse, ranging from very good to severe disability. The neurological prognosis is diverse and varied, ranging from very good to severe disability. Therefore, if ventricular enlargement is suspected, detailed fetal neurosonography, systemic examination, genetic testing, testing for infections, and follow-up for ventricular enlargement are necessary.[103]

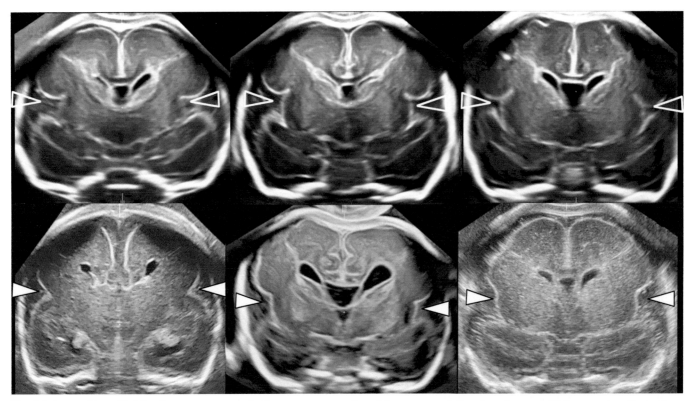

Fig. 16: Comparison of Sylvian fissure appearance in the same cross-section at the same gestational age in normal fetuses and malformations of cortical development (MCD) cases. In MCD cases (lower), Sylvian fissure (arrowheads) appearance is extremely premature, compared with normal cases (upper).

Fetal ventricular enlargement is defined as an atrial width (AW) of 10 mm or more, which was defined in 1988,[104] and remains constant regardless of the gestational age.[104-107] The AW of <10 mm has been classified as normal, 10–15 mm as mild[106] to moderate, and >15 mm as severely enlarged ventricles.[108,109] However, in 2010s, various outcomes and prognoses have been reported by systematic reviews and meta-analyses.[110-113] Hydrocephalus and ventriculomegaly are the terms that indicate the pathological condition with enlarged lateral ventricles. Hydrocephalus is mainly associated with increased ICP by occlusion or stenosis of CSF flow pathway, and neuroimaging reveals dangling choroid plexus inside the enlarged ventricles. In contrast, normal-pressure hydrocephalus (NPH) is associated with enlarged ventricles without increased ICP, with the normal appearance of choroid plexus. Hydrocephalus commonly occurs due to congenital stenosis of the cerebral aqueduct stenosis. However, secondary ventriculomegaly can occur due to vascular disease, cortical maldevelopment, intracranial tumor, or cysts, intracerebral or intraventricular hemorrhage (IVH), Chiari malformation due to myelomeningocele, encephalopathy, meningitis, and other central nervous system (CNS) abnormalities. The causal factors of hydrocephalus and ventriculomegaly vary widely, from neuronal adhesion, vesicle trafficking, dystroglycanopathies, ciliopathies, RASopathies, planar cell polarity, NTDs, lysosomal storage disorders, growth factors, Wnt signaling pathway, *PI3K/AKT/mTOR* pathway to transcription factors.[114-122]

Owing to recent advances in sequencing technologies, four genes have been well known to cause congenital hydrocephalus, *L1CAM,*[118-122] *AP1S2* (X-linked), *CCDC88C,*[115] and *MPDZ*[116] (autosomal recessive). Further, over 100 genes have been identified as the causal factors of genetic hydrocephalus or ventriculomegaly.[117]

L1CAM[118-122] located at Xq28 mediates cell–cell adhesion, the guidance of neurite outgrowth, bundling, myelination, pathfinding, long-term potentiation, neuronal cell survival, migration, and synaptogenesis. *L1CAM* gene mutation results in invariable neurological phenotypes, such as hydrocephalus, AOCC or hypoplasia, and adducted thumbs **(Figs. 17A to C)**. Because of X-linked recessive inheritance, the carrier mother's male fetus has a 50% chance of being affected.

Cerebrospinal fluid flow pathway is also affected by abnormal beating or asynchronism of the ependymal cilia which is lining the ventricular system. Therefore, ciliopathies such as Bardet–Biedl syndrome (*CEP290*),[123,124] Meckel syndromes (*MKS1, TMEM67* [125-127]), and Joubert syndromes (*TMEM216*,[128,129] *CC2D2A*[130]) are often associated with ventriculomegaly **(Figs. 18A to C)**.

Muscular dystrophies is associated with the aberrant glycosylation of α-dystroglycan and collectively termed dystroglycanopathies.[131] Dystroglycanopathies are often associated with brain and ocular pathology. In cases of dystroglycanopathy, disorder of neuronal cell migration results in cortical maldevelopment and subsequent ventricular enlargement. Walker–Warburg syndrome (*POMT1, PONT2,* and *B3GALNT2*), MEB disease (*POMGnT1*), and Fukuyama congenital muscular dystrophy (*FKTN*) are representative dystroglycanopathies.

PI3K/AKT/mTOR pathway-related genes are identified in several other overgrowth syndromes.[132] The megalencephaly-capillary malformation-polymicrogyria syndrome (MCAP) and megalencephaly-polymicrogyria-polydactyly-hydrocephalus syndrome (MPPH) are classified in the spectrum of megalencephaly-associated syndromes.[132] In megalencephaly-associated syndromes, the mechanism of ventriculomegaly is that megalencephaly induces polymicrogyria and cerebellar overgrowth, which leads to oppression of the posterior fossa and cerebellar tonsillar herniation, which eventually obstructs CSF flow. However, as Chiari malformation does not always exist, CSF flow obstruction may occur within the overgrown brain.

Mutations of growth factors related to genes such as *FGFR3* can lead to skeletal dysplasia (thanatophoric dysplasia) with enlarged ventricles associated with overgrown and hyperconvoluted posterior temporal lobe[133] **(Figs. 19A to E)**.

The term isolated ventriculomegaly is often used when no other structural abnormalities have been notified prenatally. However, in many cases of "isolated prenatally" ventriculomegaly, extra-CNS abnormalities or single-gene mutations may be found after birth. Chromosomal microarrays, exome sequencing, genome sequencing, and viral antibody analysis are recommended to elucidate causal genetic factors. In addition, a longitudinal observation is quite important because spontaneous resolution of ventriculomegaly during pregnancy is occasionally seen in some of the mid-gestational isolated ventriculomegaly cases **(Figs. 20A and B)**.

■ IN UTERO BRAIN INJURY AND DAMAGE

In cases of neonatal encephalopathy and cerebral palsy, "is the timing of the causative event prenatal, intrapartum, or postpartum?" is a point to be discussed because it involves medical, social, legal, and ethical issues. Brain damage may be associated with prenatal events such as cerebral hemorrhage, encephalopathy, and migration disorder. It is not always possible to identify when the event occurred. In the case of monozygotic twins, the timing of the encephalopathy may be speculated, such as selective intrauterine fetal death (sIUFD) **(Figs. 21A and B)** or medical intervention for twin-to-twin transfusion syndrome or twin reversed arterial perfusion (TRAP) sequence **(Fig. 22)**. However, it is difficult to ascertain prenatal evidence of in

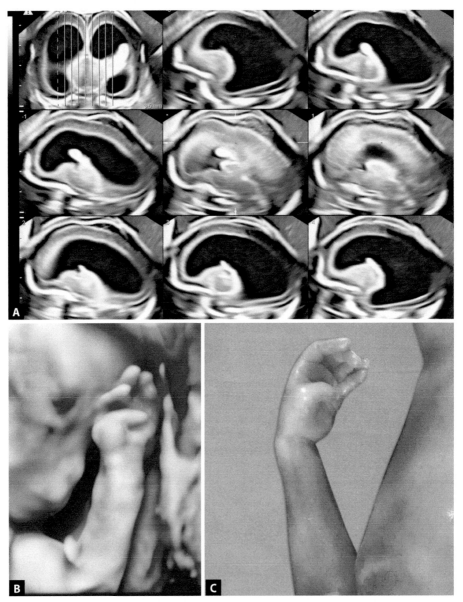

Figs. 17A to C: L1 syndrome at 21 weeks. (A) Tomographic ultrasound image in the sagittal section. Severe ventriculomegaly is seen; (B) 3D image of fetal hand. The adducted thumb is clearly visualized; (C) The adducted thumb of aborted fetus.

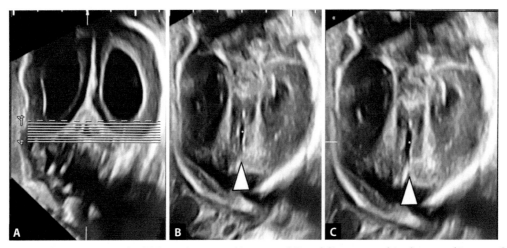

Figs. 18A to C: Joubert syndrome at 27 weeks. (A) Posterior coronal image and (B and C) tomographic ultrasound images. Cerebellar vermian defects are seen, with a slit-like space (arrowhead) continuing from between the bilateral cerebellar hemispheres to the center of the brainstem.

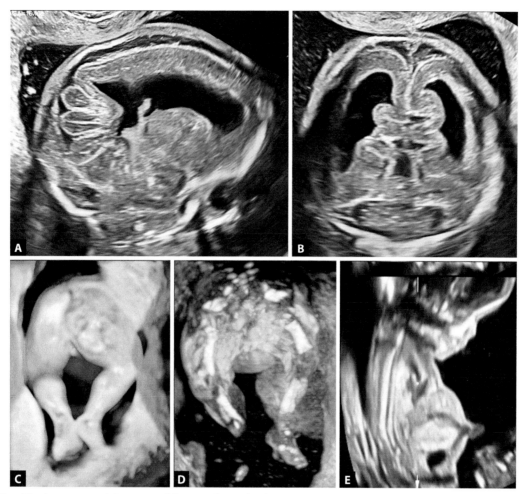

Figs. 19A to E: Focal brain overgrowth in a case of thanatophoric dysplasia at 16 weeks. Hyperconvoluted posterior-temporal lobe: (A and B) Indicates a focal brain overgrowth due to *FGFR3* mutation; (C and D) Show surface appearance and bones of fetal legs respectively; (E) Shows fetal narrow chest. In this case, mutation site was confirmed in c.1948A>A/G, p.K650E.

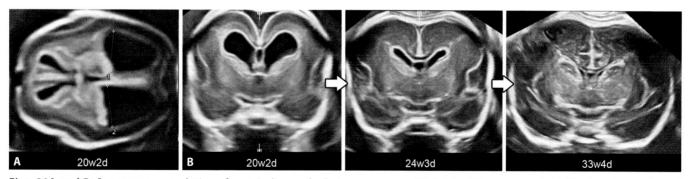

Figs. 20A and B: Spontaneous resolution of ventriculomegaly during pregnancy. (A) Axial cutting section of fetal brain at 20 weeks and 2 days. The atrial width was measured to be 15 mm bilaterally; (B) Coronal images at 20, 24, and 33 weeks. Spontaneous resolution of ventriculomegaly was seen during pregnancy. This case has favorable outcome and prognosis after birth for 3 years.

utero brain damage that can cause postnatal neurological disorders. Neurosonography and neuro-MRI are reliable modalities for detecting prenatal brain injury. However, in full-term infants with normal biparietal diameter (BPD) without ventricular enlargement and a reassuring pattern observed on fetal heart rate monitoring at birth, brain damage is not suspected, and later on, brain damage from the fetal period may be suspected based on symptoms such as cerebral palsy. In such cases, brain damage may have

existed before birth, but the timing of the cause is unknown after birth.

Fetal intracranial bleeding is a rare condition and has been called a fetal stroke after 2004[134-136] and other various descriptions were used in published reports, such as fetal cerebrovascular disorder, or perinatal brain injury.[137] It was reported that fetal stroke is an event between 14th week and labor onset and cited an incidence of about 17–35 of 100,000 live births, or 0.5–1.0/1,000 pregnancies. A series of stillbirth

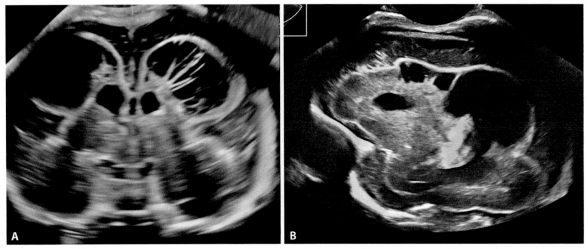

Figs. 21A and B: Destructive brain damage at 28 weeks after selective intrauterine fetal death of monochorionic diamniotic cotwin. (A) Anterior coronal image of fetal brain. Note the destructive brain damage is clearly demonstrated; (B) Parasagittal image. Most of the brain parenchyma was lost.

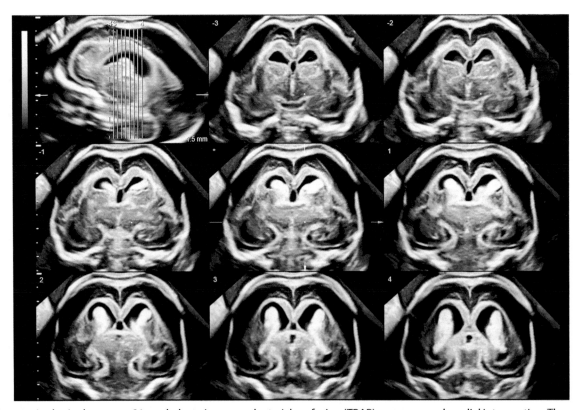

Fig. 22: Destructive brain damage at 21 weeks by twin reversed arterial perfusion (TRAP) sequence and medial intervention. The case of TRAP sequence with monochorionic diamniotic acardiac twin circulated by the living cotwin. Radiofrequency ablation was performed at 17 weeks to stop the circulation of acardiac twin. At 21 weeks, destructive brain damage was demonstrated.

autopsies report in 1985 revealed 6% with the evidence of fetal intracranial hemorrhage.[138]

Intracranial hemorrhage in the fetus can have a variety of causes, including idiopathic, fetal blood pressure changes, fetal hemorrhage, umbilical abnormalities, placental abnormalities, fetal infections, single-gene mutations, and trauma.[139] Possible causes include alloimmune and idiopathic thrombocytopenia, von Willebrand disease, abuse of illicit drugs (cocaine) and certain medications (warfarin), congenital factor X and V deficiencies, twin-to-twin transfusions, vascular disease, intracranial tumors, and sIUFD in monochorionic twins. Several reports described *COL4A1* and *COL42A* gene mutations strongly related to perinatal cerebral bleeding and porencephaly[140-146] **(Figs. 23A and B)**. Fetal neuroimaging demonstrates hyperechoic lined ventricular wall shown

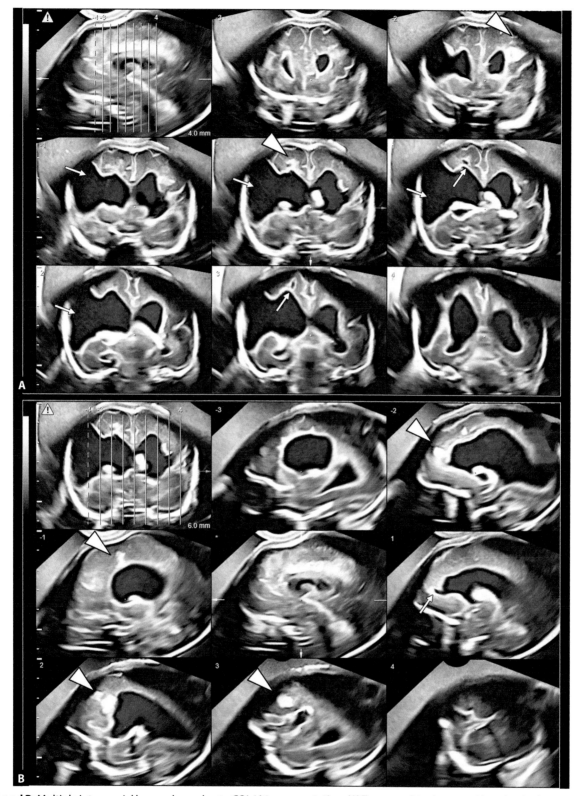

Figs. 23A and B: Multiple intracranial hemorrhage due to *COL4A1* gene mutation. (A) Tomographic ultrasound imaging in the coronal section; (B) Tomographic ultrasound imaging in the sagittal section. Hyperechoic lesions (arrowheads) indicate new hemorrhaging sites, and the arrows indicate the site of posthemorrhagic foramen encephalopathy. Amniocentesis revealed *COL4A1* gene mutation.

in **Figure 24**, avascular intracranial mass, parenchymal echogenicity, porencephalic cysts, hyperechoic acute clot adherent to choroid plexus, hyperechoic nodular ependyma, and increased periventricular white matter echogenicity is demonstrated in cases with intracerebral hemorrhage. Secondary ventricular dilatation is often seen due to stenosis or occlusion of the foramen of Monro by thrombosis.

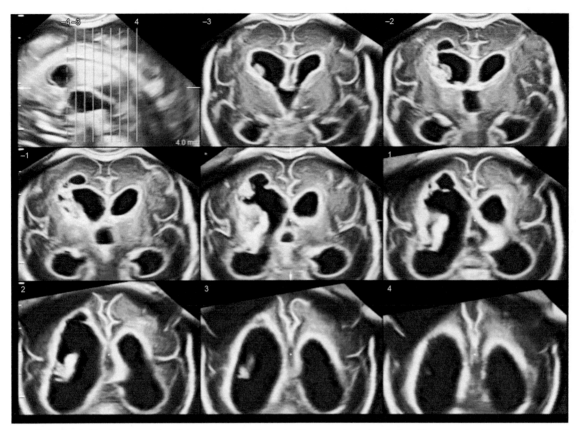

Fig. 24: Porencephaly due to focal intracerebral hemorrhage at 28 weeks. Porencephaly due to focal intracerebral hemorrhage and subsequent ventriculomegaly and intraventricular hemorrhage due to intraventricular perforation, indicating the intraventricular hemorrhage is the secondary finding. Note that the hyperechoic lined ventricular wall is seen.

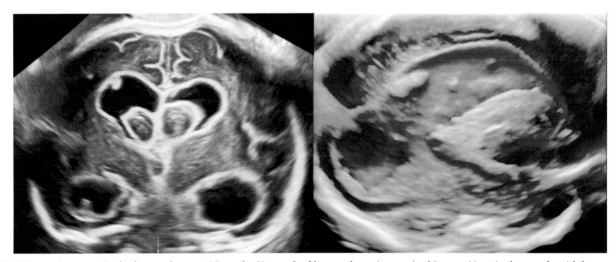

Fig. 25: Primary intraventricular hemorrhage at 32 weeks. No cerebral hemorrhage is seen in this case. Ventriculomegaly with hyperechoic lined ventricular wall, intraventricular clots, and choroid plexus bleeding was suspected.

Primary IVH **(Fig. 25)** is defined, when intraventricular events such as choroid plexus tumor or bleeding are obvious. The incidence of primary IVH is approximately 30%, and the rest 70% is secondary IVH. The most common cause of secondary IVH is intraparenchymal hemorrhage in the periventricular area extending into the ventricular system as shown in **Figure 26**. The IVH grading system in the infant was first reported by Papile et al.[147] Grade I is isolated to the periventricular (subependymal) germinal matrix, Grade II implies IVH (10–50%) without ventricular dilatation, Grade III is IVH (>50% or with ventriculomegaly), and Grade IV is with parenchymal hemorrhage or periventricular hemorrhagic infarction.

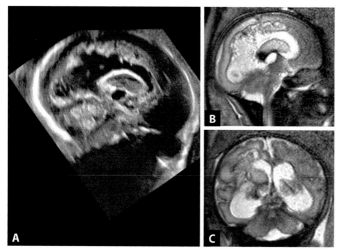

Figs. 26A to C: Periventricular intraparenchymal massive hemorrhage at 32 weeks. (A) Neurosonographic image in the sagittal section. Porencephalic lesion due to massive hemorrhage fused with ventricles, causing secondary intraventricular hemorrhage; (B) MR sagittal image; (C) MR coronal image.

CONCLUSION

As introduced in this chapter, fetal 3D neurosonography provides information on the orientation of the fetal brain, brain development during pregnancy, the exact location of brain lesions, and the inner structure of the lesions. In pediatric neurology, the relationship between cortical dysplasia and developmental abnormalities or intractable epilepsy is currently being discussed. In addition, molecular genetic techniques have revealed many genetic variants associated with brain morphological abnormalities that cause developmental delay, learning disabilities, epilepsy, and mental retardation, and the field of fetal neurology has been established.

Detailed neuroimaging is now available for diagnosis of the central nervous system, and genetic tests such as chromosomal microarrays, exome sequencing, and genome sequencing add information on genetic causative factors. The combination of detailed neurosonography and molecular genetics has established a new interdisciplinary field of fetal neurology called "neurosonogenetics,"[4] which will enable accurate perinatal management and care in the future.

REFERENCES

1. Timor-Tritsch IE, Monteagudo A. Tansvaginal fetal neurosonography: standardization of the planes and sections by anatomic landmarks. Ultrasound Obstet Gynecol. 1996;8(1):42-7.
2. Timor-Tritsch IE, Monteagudo A, Mayberry P. Three-dimensional ultrasound evaluation of the fetal brain: the three horn view. Ultrasound Obstet Gynecol. 2000;16(4):302-6.
3. Pooh RK. Contribution of transvaginal high-resolution ultrasound in fetal neurology. Donald School J Ultrasound Obstet Gynecol. 2011;5(2):93-9.
4. Pooh RK. Recent fetal neurology: from neurosonography to neurosonogenetics. Donald School J Ultrasound Obstet Gynecol. 2021;15(3):229-39.
5. Monteagudo A, Timor-Tritsch IE, Mayberry P. Three-dimensional transvaginal neurosonography of the fetal brain: "Navigating" in the volume scan. Ultrasound Obstet Gynecol. 2000;16(4):307-13.
6. Pooh RK, Kurjak A. 3D and 4D sonography and magnetic resonance in the assessment of normal and abnormal CNS development: alternative or complementary. J Perinat Med. 2011;39(1):3-13.
7. Pooh RK. Neuroimaging. 2012:45-53. [Published online]
8. Pooh RK, Machida M, Nakamura T, Uenishi K, Chiyo H, Itoh K, et al. Increased Sylvian fissure angle as early sonographic sign of malformation of cortical development. Ultrasound Obstet Gynecol. 2019;54(2):199-206.
9. Poon LC, Sahota DS, Chaemsaithong P, Nakamura T, Machida M, Naruse K, et al. Transvaginal three-dimensional ultrasound assessment of Sylvian fissures at 18-30 weeks' gestation. Ultrasound Obstet Gynecol. 2019;54(2):190-8.
10. Pooh RK, Kurjak A. Three-dimensional ultrasound in detection of fetal anomalies. Donald School J Ultrasound Obstet Gynecol. 2016;10(3):214-34.
11. Pooh RK. Three-dimensional evaluation of the fetal brain. Donald School J Ultrasound Obstet Gynecol. 2017;11(4):268-75.
12. Pooh RK. Fetal brain imaging. Ultrasound Med Biol. 2017;43(Suppl 1):S132.
13. Pooh RK. 13-week pulmonary sonoangiogram by 3D HDlive flow. Donald School J Ultrasound Obstet Gynecol. 2015;9(4):355-6.
14. Pooh RK, Kurjak A. Novel application of three-dimensional HDlive imaging in prenatal diagnosis from the first trimester. Journal of Perinatal Medicine. 2014. DOI: 10.1515/jpm-2014-0157.
15. Pooh RK. 'See-through fashion' in prenatal diagnostic imaging. Donald School J Ultrasound Obstet Gynecol. 2015;9(2):111.
16. Pooh RK. Fetal central nervous system: new insights with ultrasound. Int J Gynecol Obstet. 2018. doi:10.1002/ijgo.12584 LK.
17. Pooh RK. Recent advances in 3D ultrasound, silhouette ultrasound, and sonoangiogram in fetal neurology. Donald School J Ultrasound Obstet Gynecol. 2016;10(2):193-200.
18. Pooh RK, Aono T. Transvaginal power Doppler angiography of the fetal brain. Ultrasound Obstet Gynecol. 1996;8(6):417-21.
19. Pooh RK. The role of issmaging detection of congenital defects in the era of PGT-A and NIPT. J Perinat Med. 2019;47(eA):92.
20. Pooh RK, Pooh K. Transvaginal 3D and Doppler ultra-sonography of the fetal brain. Semin Perinatol. 2001;25(1):38-43.
21. Pooh RK. 20-week brain vascularity by transvaginal 3D HDlive flow. Donald School J Ultrasound Obstet Gynecol. 2016;10(3):203-4.
22. Copp AJ, Greene NDE. Genetics and development of neural tube defects. J Pathol. 2010;220(2):217-30.
23. Greene NDE, Copp AJ. Development of the vertebrate central nervous system: formation of the neural tube. Prenat Diagn. 2009;29(4):303-11.

24. Rolo A, Galea GL, Savery D, Greene NDE, Andrew J. Novel mouse model of encephalocele: post-neurulation origin and relationship to open neural tube defects. Dis Model Mech. 2019;12(11):dmm040683.

25. Cohen MM Jr. Perspectives on holoprosencephaly: Part I. Epidemiology, genetics, and syndromology. Teratology. 1989;40(3):211-35.

26. Matsunaga E, Shiota K. Holoprosencephaly in human embryos: epidemiologic studies of 150 cases. Teratology. 1977;16(3):261-72.

27. Cohen MM Jr. Holoprosencephaly: clinical, anatomic, and molecular dimensions. Birth Defects Res Part A Clin Mol Teratol. 2006;76(9):658-73.

28. Roessler E, Muenke M. The molecular genetics of holo-prosencephaly. Am J Med Genet C Semin Med Genet. 2010; 154C(1):52-61.

29. Robbins DJ, Nybakken KE, Kobayashi R, Sisson JC, Bishop JM, Thérond PP. Hedgehog elicits signal transduction by means of a large complex containing the kinesin-related protein costal2. Cell. 1997;90(2):225-34.

30. Robbins DJ, Fei DL, Riobo NA. The hedgehog signal transduction network. Sci Signal. 2012;5(246):re6.

31. Blaas HGK. Holoprosencephaly. In: D'Alton M, Feltovich H, Gratacos E, Odibo A, Platt L, Tutschek B (Eds). Obstetric Imaging: Fetal Diagnosis and Care, 2nd edition. Netherlands: Elsevier; 2017.

32. Edwards TJ, Sherr EH, Barkovich AJ, Richards LJ. Clinical, genetic and imaging findings identify new causes for corpus callosum development syndromes. Brain. 2014;137: 1579-613.

33. O'Leary DDM, Chou SJ, Sahara S. Area patterning of the mammalian cortex. Neuron. 2007;56(2):252-69.

34. Hoerder-Suabedissen A, Hayashi S, Upton L, Nolan Z, Casas-Torremocha D, Grant E, et al. Subset of cortical layer 6b neurons selectively innervates higher order thalamic nuclei in mice. Cereb Cortex. 2018;28(5):1882-97.

35. Puthuran MJ, Rowland-Hill CA, Simpson J, Pairaudeau PW, Mabbott JL, Morris SM, et al. Chromosome 1q42 deletion and agenesis of the corpus callosum. Am J Med Genet A. 2005;138(1):68-9.

36. Filges I, Röthlisberger B, Boesch N, Weber P, Wenzel F, Huber AR, et al. Interstitial deletion 1q42 in a patient with agenesis of corpus callosum: phenotype-genotype comparison to the 1q41q42 microdeletion suggests a contiguous 1q4 syndrome. Am J Med Genet A. 2010;152A(4):987-93.

37. Righini A, Ciosci R, Selicorni A, Bianchini E, Parazzini C, Zollino M, et al. Brain magnetic resonance imaging in Wolf-Hirschhorn syndrome. Neuropediatrics. 2007;38(1):25-8.

38. O'Driscoll MC, Black GCM, Clayton-Smith J, Sherr EH, Dobyns WB. Identification of genomic loci contributing to agenesis of the corpus callosum. Am J Med Genet A. 2010; 152A(9):2145-59.

39. Heide S, Keren B, de Villemeur TB, Chantot-Bastaraud S, Depienne C, Nava C, et al. Copy number variations found in patients with a corpus callosum abnormality and intellectual disability. J Pediatr. 2017;185:160-6.e1.

40. Schell-Apacik CC, Wagner K, Bihler M, Ertl-Wagner B, Heinrich U, Klopocki E, et al. Agenesis and dysgenesis of the corpus callosum: clinical, genetic and neuroimaging findings in a series of 41 patients. Am J Med Genet A. 2008;146A(19):2501-11.

41. Chen CP, Chang TY, Guo WY, Wu PC, Wang LK, Chern SR, et al. Chromosome 17p13.3 deletion syndrome: aCGH characterization, prenatal findings and diagnosis, and literature review. Gene. 2013;532(1):152-9.

42. Chen CP, Chien SC. Prenatal sonographic features of Miller-Dieker syndrome. J Med Ultrasound. 2010;18(4):147-52.

43. Kitamura K, Yanazawa M, Sugiyama N, Miura H, Iizuka-Kogo A, Kusaka M, et al. Mutation of ARX causes abnormal development of forebrain and testes in mice and X-linked lissencephaly with abnormal genitalia in humans. Nat Genet. 2002;32(3):359-69.

44. Kato M, Das S, Petras K, Kitamura K, Morohashi KI, Abuelo DN, et al. Mutations of ARX are associated with striking pleiotropy and consistent genotype-phenotype correlation. Hum Mutat. 2004;23(2):147-59.

45. Dobyns WB, Berry-Kravis E, Havernick NJ, Holden KR, Viskochil D. X-linked lissencephaly with absent corpus callosum and ambiguous genitalia. Am J Med Genet. 1999;86(4):331-7.

46. Bonneau D, Toutain A, Laquerrière A, Marret S, Saugier-Veber P, Barthez MA, et al. X-linked lissencephaly with absent corpus callosum and ambiguous genitalia (XLAG): clinical, magnetic resonance imaging, and neuropathological findings. Ann Neurol. 2002;51(3):340-9.

47. Fransen E, Vits L, Van Camp G, Willems PJ. The clinical spectrum of mutations in L1, a neuronal cell adhesion molecule. Am J Med Genet. 1996;64(1):73-7.

48. Aicardi J. Aicardi syndrome. Brain Dev. 2005;27(3):164-71.

49. Lund C, Bjørnvold M, Tuft M, Kostov H, Røsby O, Selmer KK. Aicardi syndrome: an epidemiologic and clinical study in Norway. Pediatr Neurol. 2015;52(2):182-6.e3.

50. Parrini E, Conti V, Dobyns WB, Guerrini R. Genetic basis of brain malformations. Mol Syndromol. 2016;7(4):220-33.

51. Guerrini R, Dobyns WB. Malformations of cortical development: clinical features and genetic causes. Lancet Neurol. 2014;13(7):710-26.

52. Desikan RS, Barkovich AJ. Malformations of cortical development. Ann Neurol. 2016;80(6):797-810.

53. Barkovich J. Complication begets clarification in classification. Brain. 2013;136(2):368-70.

54. Severino M, Geraldo AF, Utz N, Tortora D, Pogledic I, Klonowski W, et al. Definitions and classification of malformations of cortical development: practical guidelines. Brain. 2020;143(10):2874-94.

55. Gilmore EC, Walsh CA. Genetic causes of microcephaly and lessons for neuronal development. Wiley Interdiscip Rev Dev Biol. 2013;2(4):461-78.

56. Yu TW, Mochida GH, Tischfield DJ, Sgaier SK, Flores-Sarnat L, Sergi CM, et al. Mutations in WDR62, encoding a centrosome-associated protein, cause microcephaly with simplified gyri and abnormal cortical architecture. Nat Genet. 2010;42(11):1015-20.

57. Jackson AP, Eastwood H, Bell SM, Adu J, Toomes C, Carr IM, et al. Identification of microcephalin, a protein implicated in determining the size of the human brain. Am J Hum Genet. 2002;71(1):136-42.

58. Nicholas AK, Khurshid M, Désir J, Carvalho OP, Cox JJ, Thornton G, et al. WDR62 is associated with the spindle

pole and is mutated in human microcephaly. Nat Genet. 2010;42(11):1010-4.

59. Trimborn M, Bell SM, Felix C, Rashid Y, Jafri H, Griffiths PD, et al. Mutations in microcephalin cause aberrant regulation of chromosome condensation. Am J Hum Genet. 2004;75(2):261-6.

60. Brunk K, Vernay B, Griffith E, Reynolds NL, Strutt D, Ingham PW, et al. Microcephalin coordinates mitosis in the syncytial Drosophila embryo. J Cell Sci. 2007;120(Pt 20):3578-88.

61. Bond J, Roberts E, Mochida GH, Hampshire DJ, Scott S, Askham JM, et al. ASPM is a major determinant of cerebral cortical size. Nat Genet. 2002;32(2):316-20.

62. Bond J, Roberts E, Springell K, Lizarraga SB, Scott S, Higgins J, et al. A centrosomal mechanism involving CDK5RAP2 and CENPJ controls brain size. Nat Genet. 2005;37(4):353-5.

63. Kumar A, Girimaji SC, Duvvari MR, Blanton SH. Mutations in STIL, encoding a pericentriolar and centrosomal protein, cause primary microcephaly. Am J Hum Genet. 2009;84(2):286-90.

64. Bilgüvar K, Öztürk AK, Louvi A, Kwan KY, Choi M, Tatli B, et al. Whole-exome sequencing identifies recessive WDR62 mutations in severe brain malformations. Nature. 2010;467(7312):207-10.

65. Guernsey DL, Jiang H, Hussin J, Arnold M, Bouyakdan K, Perry S, et al. Mutations in centrosomal protein CEP152 in primary microcephaly families linked to MCPH4. Am J Hum Genet. 2010;87(1):40-51.

66. Toi A, Lister WS, Fong KW. How early are fetal cerebral sulci visible at prenatal ultrasound and what is the normal pattern of early fetal sulcal development? Ultrasound Obstet Gynecol. 2004;24(7):706-15.

67. Namburete AIL, Stebbing RV, Kemp B, Yaqub M, Papageorghiou AT, Alison Noble J. Learning-based prediction of gestational age from ultrasound images of the fetal brain. Med Image Anal. 2015;21(1):72-86.

68. Chen X, Li SL, Luo GY, Norwitz ER, Ouyang SY, Wen HX, et al. Ultrasonographic characteristics of cortical sulcus development in the human fetus between 18 and 41 weeks of gestation. Chin Med J (Engl). 2017;130(8):920-8.

69. Di Donato N, Chiari S, Mirzaa GM, Aldinger K, Parrini E, Olds C, et al. Lissencephaly: expanded imaging and clinical classification. Am J Med Genet A. 2017;173(6):1473-88.

70. Pooh RK. Fetal neuroimaging of neural migration disorder. Ultrasound Clin. 2008;3(4):541-52.

71. McGahan JP, Grix A, Gerscovich EO. Prenatal diagnosis of lissencephaly: Miller-Dieker syndrome. J Clin Ultrasound. 1994;22(9):560-3.

72. Greco P, Resta M, Vimercati A, Dicuonzo F, Loverro G, Vicino M, et al. Antenatal diagnosis of isolated lissencephaly by ultrasound and magnetic resonance imaging. Ultrasound Obstet Gynecol. 1998;12(4):276-9.

73. Kojima K, Suzuki Y, Seki K, Yamamoto T, Sato T, Tanaka T, et al. Prenatal diagnosis of lissencephaly (type II) by ultrasound and fast magnetic resonance imaging. Fetal Diagn Ther. 2002;17(1):34-6.

74. Fong KW, Ghai S, Toi A, Blaser S, Winsor EJT, Chitayat D. Prenatal ultrasound findings of lissencephaly associated with Miller-Dieker syndrome and comparison with pre- and postnatal magnetic resonance imaging. Ultrasound Obstet Gynecol. 2004;24(7):716-23.

75. Gha S, Fong KW, Toi A, Chitayat D, Pantazi S, Blaser S. Prenatal US and MR imaging findings of lissencephaly: review of fetal cerebral sulcal development. Radiographics. 2006;26(2):389-405.

76. Yoshida A, Kobayashi K, Manya H, Taniguchi K, Kano H, Mizuno M, et al. Muscular dystrophy and neuronal migration disorder caused by mutations in a glycosyltransferase, POMGnT1. Dev Cell. 2001;1(5):717-24.

77. Hehr U, Uyanik G, Gross C, Walter MC, Bohring A, Cohen M, et al. Novel POMGnT1 mutations define broader phenotypic spectrum of muscle-eye-brain disease. Neurogenetics. 2007;8(4):279-88.

78. Godfrey C, Clement E, Mein R, Brockington M, Smith J, Talim B, et al. Refining genotype phenotype correlations in muscular dystrophies with defective glycosylation of dystroglycan. Brain. 2007;130(Pt 10):2725-35.

79. Kobayashi K, Nakahori Y, Miyake M, Matsumura K, Kondo-Iida E, Nomura Y, et al. An ancient retrotransposal insertion causes Fukuyama-type congenital muscular dystrophy. Nature. 1998;394(6691):388-92.

80. Toda T, Kobayashi K, Kondo-Iida E, Sasaki J, Nakamura Y. The Fukuyama congenital muscular dystrophy story. Neuromuscul Disord. 2000;10(3):153-9.

81. Takeda S, Kondo M, Sasaki J, Kurahashi H, Kano H, Arai K, et al. Fukutin is required for maintenance of muscle integrity, cortical histiogenesis and normal eye development. Hum Mol Genet. 2003;12(12):1449-59.

82. Friocourt G, Kanatani S, Tabata H, Yozu M, Takahashi T, Antypa M, et al. Cell-autonomous roles of ARX in cell proliferation and neuronal migration during corticogenesis. J Neurosci. 2008;28(22):5794-805.

83. Friocourt G, Poirier K, Rakić S, Parnavelas JG, Chelly J. The role of ARX in cortical development. Eur J Neurosci. 2006;23(4):869-76.

84. Sherr EH. The ARX story (epilepsy, mental retardation, autism, and cerebral malformations): one gene leads to many phenotypes. Curr Opin Pediatr. 2003;15(6):567-71.

85. Colasante G, Simonet JC, Calogero R, Crispi S, Sessa A, Cho G, et al. ARX regulates cortical intermediate progenitor cell expansion and upper layer neuron formation through repression of Cdkn1c. Cereb Cortex. 2015;25(2):322-35.

86. Folsom TD, Fatemi SH. The involvement of Reelin in neurodevelopmental disorders. Neuropharmacology. 2013;68:122-35.

87. Tissir F, Goffinet AM. Reelin and brain development. Nat Rev Neurosci. 2003;4(6):496-505.

88. Chen Y, Beffert U, Ertunc M, Tang TS, Kavalali ET, Bezprozvanny I, et al. Reelin modulates NMDA receptor activity in cortical neurons. J Neurosci. 2005;25(36):8209-16.

89. Kato M. Genotype-phenotype correlation in neuronal migration disorders and cortical dysplasias. Front Neurosci. 2015;9:181.

90. Fallet-Bianco C, Laquerrière A, Poirier K, Razavi F, Guimiot F, Dias P, et al. Mutations in tubulin genes are frequent causes of various foetal malformations of cortical development including microlissencephaly. Acta Neuropathol Commun. 2014;2:69.

91. Laquerriere A, Gonzales M, Saillour Y, Cavallin M, Joyē N, Quēlin C, et al. De novo TUBB2B mutation causes fetal akinesia deformation sequence with microlissencephaly:

an unusual presentation of tubulinopathy. Eur J Med Genet. 2016;59(4):249-56.

92. Harding BN, Moccia A, Drunat S, Soukarieh O, Tubeuf H, Chitty LS, et al. Mutations in citron kinase cause recessive microlissencephaly with multinucleated neurons. Am J Hum Genet. 2016;99(2):511-20.

93. Barkovich AJ, Ferriero DM, Barr RM, Gressens P, Dobyns WB, Truwit CL, et al. Microlissencephaly: a heterogeneous malformation of cortical development. Neuropediatrics. 1998;29(3):113-9.

94. Poirier K, Martinovic J, Laquerrière A, Cavallin M, Fallet-Bianco C, Desguerre I, et al. Rare ACTG1 variants in fetal microlissencephaly. Eur J Med Genet. 2015;58(8):416-8.

95. Pooh RK, Machida M, Imoto I, Arai EN, Ohashi H, Takeda M, et al. Fetal megalencephaly with cortical dysplasia at 18 gestational weeks related to paternal UPD mosaicism with PTEN mutation. Genes (Basel). 2021;12(3):358.

96. Salomon LJ, Bernard JP, Ville Y. Reference ranges for fetal ventricular width: a non-normal approach. Ultrasound Obstet Gynecol. 2007;30(1):61-6.

97. Heaphy-Henault KJ, Guimaraes CV, Mehollin-Ray AR, Cassady CI, Zhang W, Desai NK, et al. Congenital aqueductal stenosis: findings at fetal MRI that accurately predict a postnatal diagnosis. AJNR Am J Neuroradiol. 2018;39(5):942-8.

98. Norton ME, Fox NS, Monteagudo A, Kuller JA, Craigo S; Society for Maternal-Fetal Medicine (SMFM). Fetal ventriculomegaly. Am J Obstet Gynecol. 2020;223(6):B30-B33.

99. Huang RN, Chen JY, Pan H, Liu QQ. Correlation between mild fetal ventriculomegaly, chromosomal abnormalities, and copy number variations. J Matern Neonatal Med. 2020;1-9.

100. Etchegaray A, Juarez-Peñalva S, Petracchi F, Igarzabal L. Prenatal genetic considerations in congenital ventriculomegaly and hydrocephalus. Childs Nerv Syst. 2020;36(8):1645-60.

101. Putbrese B, Kennedy A. Findings and differential diagnosis of fetal intracranial haemorrhage and fetal ischaemic brain injury: what is the role of fetal MRI? Br J Radiol. 2017; 90(1070):20160253.

102. Melchiorre K, Bhide A, Gika AD, Pilu G, Papageorghiou AT. Counseling in isolated mild fetal ventriculomegaly. Ultrasound Obstet Gynecol. 2009;34(2):212-24.

103. Fox NS, Monteagudo A, Kuller JA, Craigo S, Norton ME; Society for Maternal-Fetal Medicine (SMFM). Mild fetal ventriculomegaly: diagnosis, evaluation, and management. Am J Obstet Gynecol. 2018;219(1):B2-B9.

104. Cardoza JD, Goldstein RB, Filly RA. Exclusion of fetal ventriculomegaly with a single measurement: the width of the lateral ventricular atrium. Radiology. 1988;169(3):711-4.

105. Almog B, Gamzu R, Achiron R, Fainaru O, Zalel Y. Fetal lateral ventricular width: what should be its upper limit? J Ultrasound Med. 2003;22(1):39-43.

106. Malinger G, Paladini D, Haratz KK, Monteagudo A, Pilu GL, Timor-Tritsch IE. ISUOG Practice Guidelines (updated): sonographic examination of the fetal central nervous system. Part 1: performance of screening examination and indications for targeted neurosonography. Ultrasound Obstet Gynecol. 2020;56(3):476-84.

107. Cardoza D, Filly A, Goldstein B. Exclusion of fetal ventriculomegaly with a single measurement: the width of the lateral ventricular atrium. J Diagnostic Med Sonogr. 1989;5(2):82-3.

108. Gaglioti P, Danelon D, Bontempo S, Mombrò M, Cardaropoli S, Todros T. Fetal cerebral ventriculomegaly: outcome in 176 cases. Ultrasound Obstet Gynecol. 2005;25(4):372-7.

109. Chu N, Zhang Y, Yan Y, Ren Y, Wang L, Zhang B. Fetal ventriculomegaly: pregnancy outcomes and follow-ups in ten years. Biosci Trends. 2016;10(2):125-32.

110. Pagani G, Thilaganathan B, Prefumo F. Neurodevelopmental outcome in isolated mild fetal ventriculomegaly: systematic review and meta-analysis. Ultrasound Obstet Gynecol. 2014;44(3):254-60.

111. Scelsa B, Rustico M, Righini A, Parazzini C, Balestriero MA, Introvini P, et al. Mild ventriculomegaly from fetal consultation to neurodevelopmental assessment: a single center experience and review of the literature. Eur J Paediatr Neurol. 2018;22(6):919-28.

112. Carta S, Kealin Agten A, Belcaro C, Bhide A. Outcome of fetuses with prenatal diagnosis of isolated severe bilateral ventriculomegaly: systematic review and meta-analysis. Ultrasound Obstet Gynecol. 2018;52(2):165-73.

113. Hannon T, Tennant PWG, Rankin J, Robson SC. Epidemiology, natural history, progression, and postnatal outcome of severe fetal ventriculomegaly. Obstet Gynecol. 2012;120(6):1345-53.

114. Shaheen R, Sebai MA, Patel N, Ewida N, Kurdi W, Altweijri I, et al. The genetic landscape of familial congenital hydrocephalus. Ann Neurol. 2017;81(6):890-7.

115. Ekici AB, Hilfinger D, Jatzwauk M, Thiel CT, Wenzel D, Lorenz I, et al. Disturbed Wnt signalling due to a mutation in CCDC88C causes an autosomal recessive non-syndromic hydrocephalus with medial diverticulum. Mol Syndromol. 2010;1(3):99-112.

116. Al-Dosari MS, Al-Owain M, Tulbah M, Kurdi W, Adly N, Al-Hemidan A, et al. Mutation in MPDZ causes severe congenital hydrocephalus. J Med Genet. 2013;50(1):54-8.

117. Kousi M, Katsanis N. The genetic basis of hydrocephalus. Annu Rev Neurosci. 2016;39:409-35.

118. Yamasaki M, Thompson P, Lemmon V. CRASH syndrome: mutations in L1CAM correlate with severity of the disease. Neuropediatrics. 1997;28(3):175-8.

119. Itoh K, Fushiki S. The role of L1cam in murine corticogenesis, and the pathogenesis of hydrocephalus. Pathol Int. 2015;65(2):58-66.

120. Takahashi S, Makita Y, Okamoto N, Miyamoto A, Oki J. L1CAM mutation in a Japanese family with X-linked hydrocephalus: a study for genetic counseling. Brain Dev. 1997;19(8):559-62.

121. Jouet M, Rosenthal A, Armstrong G, MacFarlane J, Stevenson R, Paterson J, et al. X-linked spastic paraplegia (SPG1), MASA syndrome and X-linked hydrocephalus result from mutations in the L1 gene. Nat Genet. 1994;7(3):402-7.

122. Adle-Biassette H, Saugier-Veber P, Fallet-Bianco C, Delezoide AL, Razavi F, Drouot N, et al. Neuropathological review of 138 cases genetically tested for X-linked hydrocephalus: evidence for closely related clinical entities of unknown molecular bases. Acta Neuropathol. 2013;126(3):427-42.

123. Rachel RA, Yamamoto EA, Dewanjee MK, May-Simera HL, Sergeev YV, Hackett AN, et al. CEP290 alleles in mice disrupt tissue-specific cilia biogenesis and recapitulate features of syndromic ciliopathies. Hum Mol Genet. 2015;24(13):3775-91.

124. Manzini MC, Walsh CA. The genetics of brain malformations. In: Kevin J Mitchell (Ed). The Genetics of Neurodevelopmental Disorders. Hoboken: Wiley Blackwell; 2015.

125. Iannicelli M, Brancati F, Mougou-Zerelli S, Mazzotta A, Thomas S, Elkhartoufi N, et al. Novel TMEM67 mutations and genotype-phenotype correlates in meckelin-related ciliopathies. Hum Mutat. 2010;31(5):E1319-31.

126. Abdelhamed ZA, Natarajan S, Wheway G, Inglehearn CF, Toomes C, Johnson CA, et al. The Meckel-Gruber syndrome protein TMEM67 controls basal body positioning and epithelial branching morphogenesis in mice via the non-canonical Wnt pathway. Dis Model Mech. 2015;8(6): 527-41.

127. Leightner AC, Hommerding CJ, Peng Y, Salisbury JL, Gainullin VG, Czarnecki PG, et al. The Meckel syndrome protein meckelin (TMEM67) is a key regulator of cilia function but is not required for tissue planar polarity. Hum Mol Genet. 2013;22(10):2024-40.

128. Valente EM, Logan CV, Mougou-Zerelli S, Lee JH, Silhavy JL, Brancati F, et al. Mutations in TMEM216 perturb ciliogenesis and cause Joubert, Meckel and related syndromes. (Letter) Nature Genet. 2010;42:619-25.

129. Edvardson S, Shaag A, Zenvirt S, Erlich Y, Hannon GJ, Shanske AL, et al. Joubert syndrome 2 (JBTS2) in Ashkenazi Jews is associated with a TMEM216 mutation. Am J Hum Genet. 2010;86:93-7.

130. Xiao D, Lv C, Zhang Z, Wu M, Zheng X, Yang L, et al. Novel CC2D2A compound heterozygous mutations cause Joubert syndrome. Mol Med Rep. 2017;15(1):305-8.

131. Johnson K, Bertoli M, Phillips L, Töpf A, Van den Bergh P, Vissing J, et al. Detection of variants in dystroglycanopathy-associated genes through the application of targeted whole-exome sequencing analysis to a large cohort of patients with unexplained limb-girdle muscle weakness. Skelet Muscle. 2018;8(1):23.

132. Mirzaa GM, Rivière JB, Dobyns WB. Megalencephaly syndromes and activating mutations in the PI3K-AKT pathway: MPPH and MCAP. Am J Med Genet C Semin Med Genet. 2013;163C(2):122-30.

133. Itoh K, Pooh R, Kanemura Y, Yamasaki M, Fushiki S. Brain malformation with loss of normal FGFR3 expression in thanatophoric dysplasia type I. Neuropathology. 2013; 33(6): 663-6.

134. Özduman K, Pober BR, Barnes P, Copel JA, Ogle EA, Duncan CC, et al. Fetal stroke. Pediatr Neurol. 2004;30(3):151-62.

135. Elchalal U, Yagel S, Gomori JM, Porat S, Beni-Adani L, Yanai N, et al. Fetal intracranial hemorrhage (fetal stroke): does grade matter? Ultrasound Obstet Gynecol. 2005;26(3):233-43.

136. Huang YF, Chen WC, Tseng JJ, Ho ESC, Chou MM. Fetal intracranial hemorrhage (fetal stroke): report of four antenatally diagnosed cases and review of the literature. Taiwan J Obstet Gynecol. 2006;45(2):135-41.

137. Dicuonzo F, Palma M, Fiume M, Scarpello R, Lefons V, Maghenzani M, et al. Cerebrovascular disorders in the prenatal period. J Child Neurol. 2008;23(11):1260-6.

138. Sims ME, Turkel SB, Halterman G, Paul RH. Brain injury and intrauterine death. Am J Obstet Gynecol. 1985;151(6):721-3.

139. Kutuk MS, Yikilmaz A, Ozgun MT, Dolanbay M, Canpolat M, Uludag S, et al. Prenatal diagnosis and postnatal outcome of fetal intracranial hemorrhage. Childs Nerv Syst. 2014;30(3):411-8.

140. Shannon P, Hum C, Parks T, Schauer GM, Chitayat D, Chong K, et al. Brain and placental pathology in fetal COL4A1 related disease. Pediatr Dev Pathol. 2021;24(3):175-86.

141. Itai T, Miyatake S, Taguri M, Nozaki F, Ohta M, Osaka H, et al. Prenatal clinical manifestations in individuals with COL4A1/2 variants. J Med Genet. 2021;58(8):505-13.

142. Nakamura Y, Okanishi T, Yamada H, Okazaki T, Hosoda C, Itai T, et al. Progressive cerebral atrophies in three children with COL4A1 mutations. Brain Dev. 2021;43(10):1033-8.

143. Smigiel R, Cabala M, Jakubiak A, Kodera H, Sasiadek MJ, Matsumoto N, et al. Novel COL4A1 mutation in an infant with severe dysmorphic syndrome with schizencephaly, periventricular calcifications, and cataract resembling congenital infection. Birth Defects Res A Clin Mol Teratol. 2016;106(4):304-7.

145. Watanabe J, Okamoto K, Ohashi T, Natsumeda M, Hasegawa H, Oishi M, et al. Malignant hyperthermia and cerebral venous sinus thrombosis after ventriculoperitoneal shunt in infant with schizencephaly and COL4A1 mutation. World Neurosurg. 2019;127:446-50.

146. ERRATA: Intracranial hemorrhage and tortuosity of veins detected on susceptibility-weighted imaging of a child with a type IV collagen α1 mutation and schizencephaly. Magn Reson Med Sci. 2015;14(4):373.

147. Papile LA, Burstein J, Burstein R, Koffler H. Incidence and evolution of subependymal and intraventricular hemorrhage: a study of infants with birth weights less than 1,500 gm. J Pediatr. 1978;92(4):529-34.

Embryonal/Fetal Anomalies in the First Half of Pregnancy

Ritsuko K Pooh

■ INTRODUCTION

Recent innovations in assisted reproductive technology (ART), the observation of dead embryos by experimental magnetic resonance (MR) microscopy,[1,2] computer graphics, and other advanced technologies have provided amazing insights into the beginning of human life. Sonoembryology was first reported in 1990 by Timor-Tritsch et al.[3] after the introduction of transvaginal ultrasonography with high frequency probes into obstetrics. The combination of the transvaginal approach and three-dimensional (3D) ultrasound was introduced as "3D sonoembryology"[4,5] and began to provide more accurate information about the natural history of embryo–fetal development and fetal abnormalities. The latest in 3D technology, such as HDlive, silhouette imaging, HDflow angiography, and Slowflow technology, further elaborate the sophisticated sonoembryology.[5]

Three-dimensional sonoembryology is approaching modern high-tech embryology, but it has not yet been able to clearly show the internal organs of the embryo like MR embryo microscopy.[1,2,6] However, the major advantage of sonoembryology, which is not present in human embryology, is the "in vivo depiction of the embryo with living blood circulation." Human embryology is based on well-preserved dead embryos, and 3D ultrasound embryo culture has the potential to make new discoveries of live embryos and fetuses in utero. In addition, most of the congenital abnormalities are caused by the developmental process being disturbed at an early stage. Therefore, by observing live embryos and fetuses from the early stages using sonoembryology, many developmental abnormalities can be detected at an early stage.

Furthermore, with the development of molecular genetics, it has become clear that many genetic mutations are involved in these developmental disorders. Therefore, dysmorphology has come to the point where it cannot be discussed without genetic verification, and a new field of sonogenetics has been established.

In this chapter, we will show many examples of cases in which dysmorphological findings were detected by 3D sonography, and genetic abnormalities were explored by cytogenetics and molecular genetics techniques.

▌ VISUALIZATION OF NORMAL MORPHOLOGY IN THE FIRST TRIMESTER

The anatomy of the central nervous system develops rapidly during early fetal life. 3D sonography with transvaginal ultrasound using a high-resolution probe allows imaging of the embryonic brain structures. The early embryonic central nervous system is divided into three parts (**Fig. 1**): (1) Forebrain (prosencephalon); (2) Midbrain (mesencephalon); and (3) Hindbrain (rhombencephalon). The forebrain

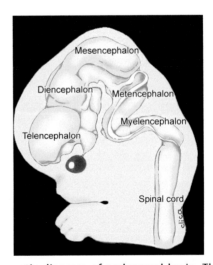

Fig. 1: Schematic diagram of embryonal brain. The forebrain (prosencephalon) includes the telencephalon containing cerebral hemispheres and diencephalon containing thalamus, hypothalamus, epithalamus, and subthalamus. The midbrain (mesencephalon) is the most rostral part of the brainstem and located above the pons, and adjoined rostrally to the thalamus. The hindbrain (rhombencephalon) is the posterior of the three primary divisions includes metencephalon containing pons and cerebellum and myelencephalon containing medulla oblongata.

(prosencephalon) includes the telencephalon containing cerebral hemispheres and diencephalon containing thalamus, hypothalamus, epithalamus, and subthalamus. The midbrain (mesencephalon) is the most rostral part of the brainstem, and locates above the pons, and adjoins to the thalamus rostrally.

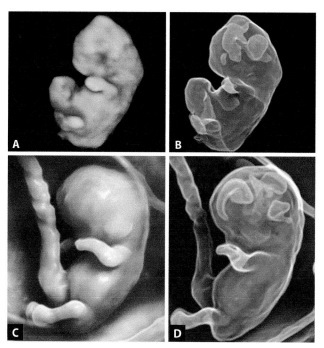

Figs. 2A to D: Embryo to fetus by HDlive imaging and HDlive silhouette mode. (A) Embryo with crown–rump length (CRL) 19.3 mm compatible to the beginning of 8th gestational week; (B) HDlive silhouette images from the same volume datasets as the left; (C) Fetus with CRL 23.9 mm compatible to 9th gestational week; (D) HDlive silhouette images from the same volume datasets as the left. Note that the rapid development of three primary brain divisions of forebrain, midbrain, and hindbrain is well demonstrated.

The hindbrain (rhombencephalon) is the posterior part of the three initial divisions, which includes metencephalon containing pons and cerebellum and myelencephalon containing medulla oblongata. Blaas et al. first visualized the brain cavity by 3D imaging[7] in 1995 and then in 1998 sensationally demonstrated early human brain vesicles in different colors and measured their volumes by 3D scanning embryos ranged between 9.3 and 39 mm, and performed postprocessing procedure.[8] Thereafter, embryonic brain structure was demonstrated by advancing 3D technology of inversion-rendering mode,[9,10] and sonoembryology has become more sophisticated and objective. Advancing imaging techniques allow the definition of in vivo anatomy including visualization of the embryonic features that could not be characterized in fixed specimens.[11] 3D images of embryos were generated using the high-frequency transvaginal transducer. By using the advanced technology of HDlive silhouette imaging, outer surface as well as inner brain structure is clearly depicted **(Figs. 2 and 3)**. HDlive silhouette imaging further enabled us to visualize the lens and vitreous body in tiny fetal eyes **(Figs. 4A and B)**. The utilization of postprocessing algorithms such as maximum mode can be used to demonstrate the fetal skeleton. Chaoui et al. reported clear 3D images for the identification of an abnormally wide metopic suture in the second trimester of pregnancy.[12] However, rapid ossification of the craniofacial bones occurs during the first trimester of pregnancy. As described above, HDlive silhouette algorithm creates a gradient at organ boundaries, where an abrupt change of the acoustic impedance exists within tissues. Therefore, silhouette mode can depict not only cystic structure but also hyperechoic structure such as bones. **Figures 5A and B** show HDlive image of fetal head and HDlive silhouette images extracting early cranial bones such as frontal, parietal,

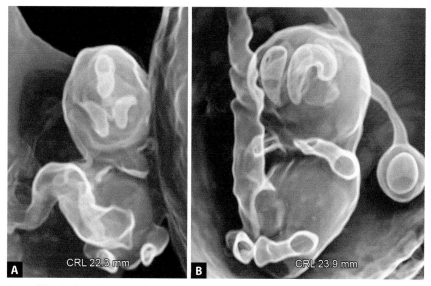

Figs. 3A and B: Frontal view of brain development by HDlive silhouette. (A) Fetus with crown–rump length (CRL) 22.3 mm. Bilateral telencephalon (forebrain) and midbrain are well demonstrated; (B) Frontal-oblique view. Rapid development of early brain is comprehensively depicted. Note the rapid growth of the telencephalon.

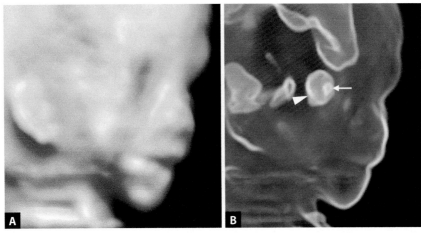

Figs. 4A and B: Eye of 13-week normal fetus by HDlive silhouette imaging. (A) HDlive image of fetal face; (B) Same image with HDlive silhouette as left. Lens (arrow) and vitreous body (arrowhead) are well demonstrated with facial surface.

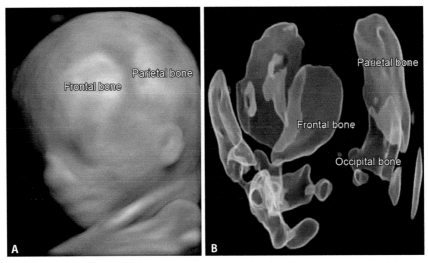

Figs. 5A and B: Cranial bones of 13-week normal fetus with HDlive silhouette. (A) HDlive image of fetal head. Frontal bone and parietal bone are demonstrated through thin skin; (B) Same image with HDlive silhouette as left. Cranial bones (frontal bone, parietal bone, and occipital bone) and facial bones are extracted.

and occipital bones from the same volume dataset. Silhouette imaging can visualize fetal vertebrae and ribs from the first trimester **(Fig. 6)**.

The development of the embryonic circulation became visualized by 3D power Doppler imaging technology.[13] In 1993 and 1994, color Doppler detection and assessment of brain vessels in the early fetus using a transvaginal approach was reported.[14,15] Clear visualization by transvaginal power Doppler of the common carotid arteries, internal and external carotid arteries, middle cerebral arteries at 12 weeks of gestation was reported in 1996.[16] Current sonoangiography technology such as HDflow and Slowflow can demonstrate the intracorporeal vascular structure **(Figs. 7A and B)**, and the cervicocranial vascular hemodynamic structure comprehensively from the first trimester **(Fig. 8)**. Intracardiac flow dynamics **(Figs. 9A and B)** can also be demonstrated.

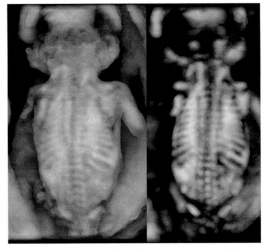

Fig. 6: Vertebrae and ribs of 12-week normal fetus by 3D HDlive silhouette image.

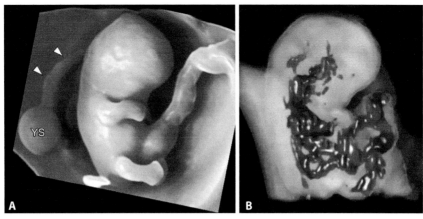

Figs. 7A and B: 3D Slowflow sonoangiography of a normal fetus with crown–rump length 25.1 mm at 9 weeks. (A) HDlive image of the fetus with umbilical cord, yolk sac (YS), and YS stalk (arrowheads); (B) Slowflow HD 3D image of the same fetus. Intracorporeal vascularity, vessels toward the brain, and umbilical cord vessels are clearly seen.

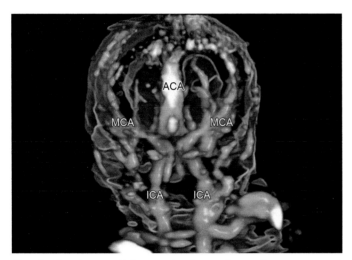

Fig. 8: Cervicocranial vascular hemodynamic structure at 13 weeks of gestation.
(ACA: anterior cerebral artery; ICA: internal carotid artery; MCA: middle cerebral artery)

ANOMALIES BEFORE 11 WEEKS

The yolk sac (YS) forms primarily at around 3 weeks of the menstrual age. Following the formation of the extraembryonic coelom, and the YS is secondarily formed. Thereafter, the YS begins to degenerate and rapidly stop functioning. In the fifth week of pregnancy, a white ring-shaped YS is visualized by sonography in the gestational sac. In the middle of the fifth week, a small embryo can be seen adjacent to the YS, and an embryonal heartbeat can be observed. The YS is usually 2–5 mm in diameter, but a large YS[17] **(Figs. 10A and B)** may associated with ominous pregnant outcome such as a miscarriage, autosomal aneuploidy, or congenital anomaly.

Close observation of small embryos before 11th gestational week by advanced 3D technology allows us to make diagnoses of various abnormalities. For example, an abnormal midbrain cavity at 10 weeks of gestation can be visualized as shown in **Figures 11A and B**.

Holoprosencephaly, a typical brain midline anomaly, can be detected in a fetus with crown–rump length (CRL) 26.2 mm **(Figs. 12A to D)** and CRL 29.9 mm **(Figs. 13A to C)**, which are associated with aneuploidy.

FETAL ANOMALIES BETWEEN 11 AND 13 WEEKS

The 11–13-week ultrasound scan includes a combination of nuchal translucency (NT) measurement, presence or absence of nasal bone (NB), tricuspid regurgitation (TR), and pulsatility index (PI) of ductus venous blood flow, or a combination of NT measurement and maternal serum pregnancy-associated plasma protein A (PAPP-A), and free beta-human chorionic gonadotrophin (β–hCG) in maternal serum has been used to screen for aneuploidy, mainly Down syndrome, trisomy 18 and 13.[18] However, ultrasonography at 11–13 weeks has enabled further anomaly scans, and the association of dysmorphology with microchromosomal abnormalities and genetic mutations[19] other than trisomy can be determined by using molecular genetic techniques.

Anomaly scan is based on two-dimensional (2D) ultrasound, but the additional 3D ultrasound makes the diagnostics even more objective and comprehensible. For instance, increased NT and NB defects are commonly used in screening for Down syndrome, but the facial features characteristic of Down syndrome appear from early pregnancy **(Figs. 14A and B)**. In the case of trisomy 18, in addition to micrognathia and low-set ears, wrist contracture and finger malarrangement can be observed from early on **(Figs. 15A to C)**. Although holoprosencephaly can be diagnosed before 11 weeks as described above, fused ventricles and fused choroid plexus are more prominently depicted on the 11–13-week scan **(Figs. 16 and 17)**. **Figures 18A to C** show Meckel–Gruber syndrome (MGS) at 12 weeks of gestation, with excencephaly, polycystic kidneys, and polydactyly. In the case of cardiac abnormalities, spatiotemporal image correlation (STIC) imaging[19] using

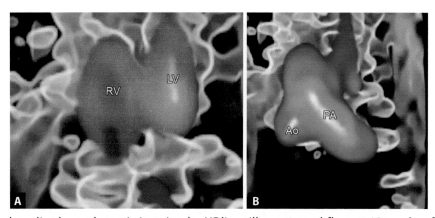

Figs. 9A and B: Normal cardiac hemodynamic imaging by HDlive silhouette and flow at 12 weeks of gestation. (A) Cardiac angiostructure. Intraventricular flows of right ventricles (RV) and left ventricles (LV) are visible; (B) Crossing of great arteries are well demonstrated.
(Ao: aorta; PA: pulmonary artery)

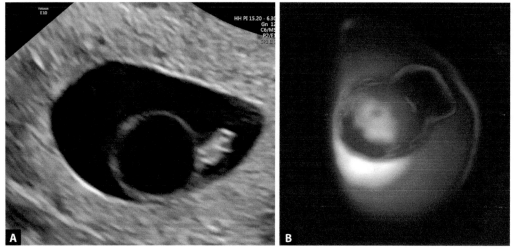

Figs. 10A and B: Large yolk sac (YS) at 7 weeks. (A) 2D image of large YS and embryo. The size of the embryo was 4.8 mm, equivalent to the size of a 6-week embryo; (B) 3D HDlive silhouette image. The embryo died 1 week later and karyotyping result was 47,XX,+22.

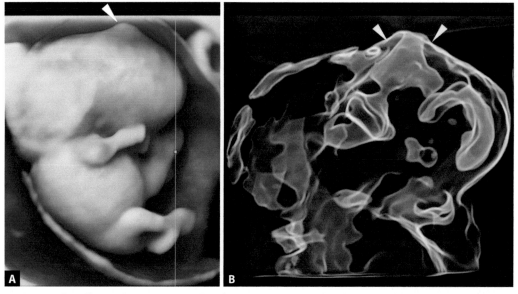

Figs. 11A and B: Abnormal midbrain cavity at 10 weeks of gestation. (A) 3D HDlive image of the fetus. Note the prominent top of the fetal head (arrowhead) due to abnormal midbrain; (B) HDlive silhouette image of the fetal head. Abnormal prominent midbrain (arrowheads) is depicted between forebrain and hindbrain. This fetus died in utero 1 week later.

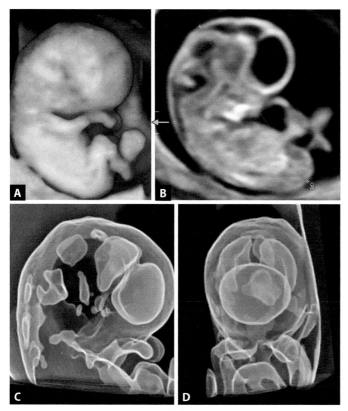

Figs. 12A to D: Early stage of holoprosencephaly in a fetus with crown–rump length 26.2 mm. (A) 3D HDlive image of the fetus. The fetal size was –3.7 SD despite the in vitro fertilization pregnancy. Note that the head is large for the size of the fetus' body; (B) Mid-sagittal section of the fetus. Note the enlarged forebrain; (C) Lateral view of the fetal head; (D) Frontal view of the fetal head. The fused telencephalon indicates the early stage of holoprosencephaly. This fetus's karyotyping resulted in triploidy (69,XXX).

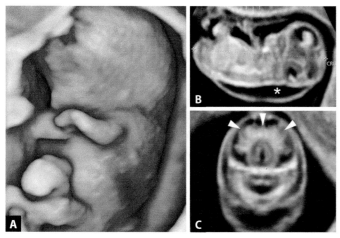

Figs. 13A to C: Trisomy 18 in a fetus with crown–rump length 29.9 mm at 9 weeks. (A) 3D HDlive image. Note the wrist contracture at this very early stage; (B) Mid-sagittal image. Increased nuchal translucency (asterisk) is demonstrated; (C) Fused choroid plexus (arrowheads) indicates early holoprosencephaly.

four-dimensional (4D) ultrasound has made it possible to display intracardiac circulatory dynamics from early pregnancy **(Fig. 19)**.

It has been well documented in pediatrics and genetics that low-set ears are associated with various genetic abnormalities and congenital anomalies. Various congenital syndromes affecting the face result from defects in the first and second branchial arches,[20] and disorders of the first and second gill arches typically result in a combination of inadequate migration and insufficient formation of the facial mesenchyme, resulting in low-set ears and micrognathia.

There have been only a few reports of low-set ears in the fetus during the first trimester of pregnancy.[21,22] The normal position of the external ear is on the imaginary line between the orbit and the back of the head, even in early pregnancy, but low-set ears below the imaginary line have occasionally been observed and have been strongly associated with congenital genetic abnormalities such as autosomal trisomy, Treacher Collins syndrome, Smith–Lemli–Opitz syndrome, Rubinstein–Taybi syndrome, Beckwith–Wiedemann syndrome, and others. **Figure 20** demonstrates low-set ears of three major trisomy cases. Micrognathia has been described as a single structural abnormality, as a feature of a chromosomal abnormality, one of syndromic features, or as a genetic abnormality.[23] Evaluation of facial features, jaw development, and mandibular size by 3D ultrasonography in the second and third trimesters of pregnancy has been reported.[23] Thereafter, prenatal detection of micrognathia in Pierre Robin sequence (PRS) was reported[20] and the evaluation, correlation between inferior facial angle and jaw index were reported.[24] The etiology of PRS may be different from branchial arch defect. PRS is associated with micrognathia, glossoptosis, and cleft soft palate in most cases. At approximately 7th–10th gestational week, the mandible begins to grow rapidly and the tongue begins to come down between the palates. If the mandible does not grow properly, the tongue can prevent the palate from closing, resulting in a cleft palate. Also, if the lower jaw is small or misaligned, the tongue will be positioned at the back of the mouth, making it hard for a newborn to breathe. This "sequential process" is the reason why PRS is classified as a sequence.[25] Micrognathia caused by disorders of the first and second branchial arches is accompanied by low-set ears, whereas PRS is not accompanied by low-set ears. This difference in the morphology of micrognathia due to etiology is obvious from the first trimester **(Figs. 21A and B)**.

About 65% of cleft lip and palate are demonstrated and diagnosed in the second trimester and 99% of cleft lip only in the second and third trimesters.[26] However, recent advances in transvaginal 3D ultrasonography have made it possible to obtain accurate and informative diagnostic images of cleft lip and palate even in the first trimester of pregnancy, if conditions are favorable **(Figs. 22 and 23)**. In addition, tomographic ultrasound imaging (TUI) can confirm cleft palate and provide an early diagnosis of cleft palate, as shown in **Figure 24**.

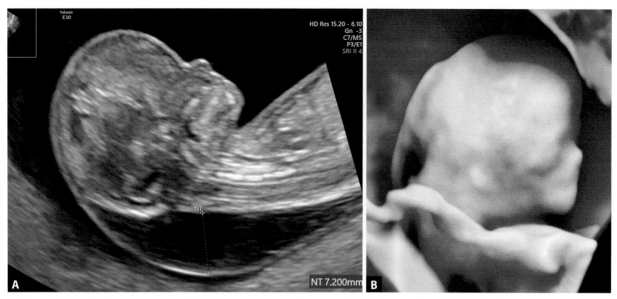

Figs. 14A and B: Typical appearances of Down syndrome at 12 weeks. (A) Mid-sagittal section of the fetus. Note the nasal bone defect and increased nuchal translucency; (B) HDlive image of typical Down face with flat face and low-set ear.

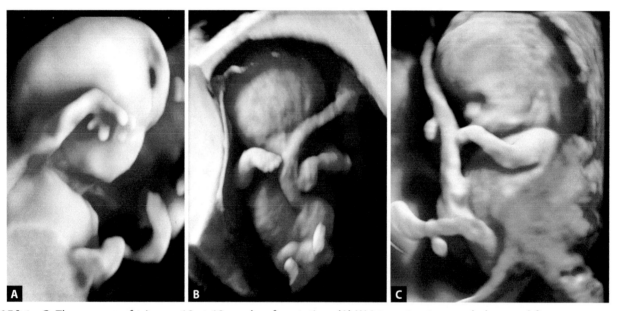

Figs. 15A to C: Three cases of trisomy 18 at 12 weeks of gestation. (A) Wrist contracture and abnormal finger arrangement with contracture is demonstrated; (B) Bilateral wrist contracture; (C) Wrist contracture, low-set ear and small omphalocele indicate trisomy 18.

Spina bifida such as myelomeningocele and myeloschisis can be visualized by sonography in the first trimester **(Figs. 25A to C)**. However, it is not always possible to delineate the back of the fetus. For early screening of spina bifida, intracranial translucency (IT) **(Figs. 26A and B)** indicating the fourth ventricle was proposed as an ultrasound marker for spina bifida in the first trimester by Chaoui et al.[27-29] The presence of IT is a simple screening item for early detection of spina bifida. Another sign of spina bifida in the first trimester is the "crash sign"[30] as posterior displacement of the mesencephalon and deformation against the occipital bone.

Omphalocele is associated with structural malformations and chromosomal abnormalities in 45 or 35%[31,32] of fetuses, respectively, and 3D demonstration of omphalocele was published in 2002.[33] Advanced 3D HDlive demonstrates the contents of ectopic abdominal organs by creating shadows as shown in **Figures 27A and B**.

HDflow imaging demonstrates vascular abnormalities such as excessive coiling cord **(Figs. 28A and B)** and absent ductus venosus in a case of 45,X **(Figs. 29A and B)**. Thus, by combining HDflow and silhouette mode, the exact location of blood vessels inside the organ can be highlighted and shown. Simultaneous visualization of both structure and

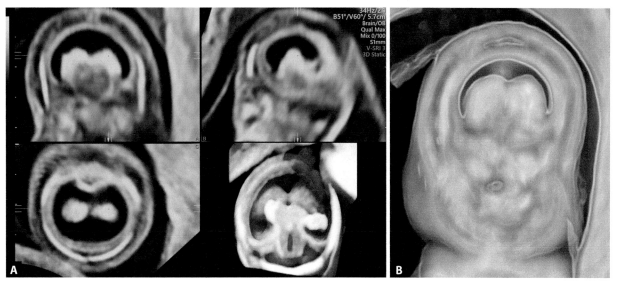

Figs. 16A and B: Holoprosencephaly (Alobar type) at 12 weeks. (A) The three orthogonal view of fused ventricle and volume cutting image showing intracranial structure; (B) Volume cutting HDlive silhouette image of the brain. Karyotyping result was trisomy 13.

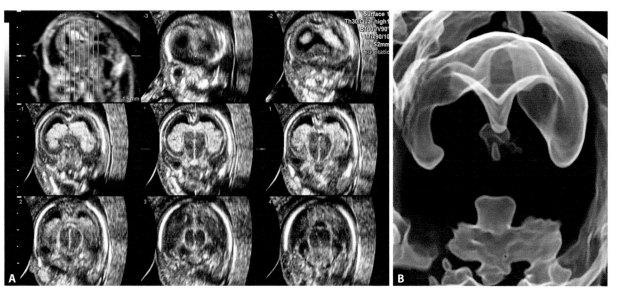

Figs. 17A and B: Holoprosencephaly (semilobar type) at 13 weeks of gestation. (A) Tomographic ultrasound image shows fused choroid plexus in fused lateral ventricle; (B) HDlive silhouette image of the fused ventricle.

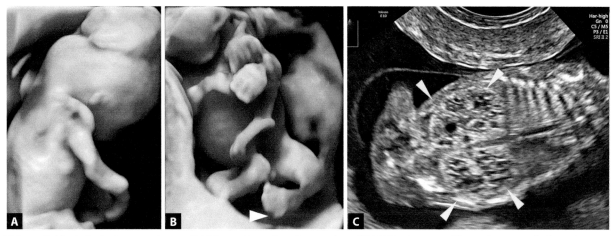

Figs. 18A to C: Meckel–Gruber syndrome (MGS) at 12 weeks of gestation. (A) HDlive image of fetus. Excencephaly is demonstrated; (B) Polydactyly (arrowhead) is demonstrated by HDlive mode; (C) 2D image of fetal kidneys. Multiple cysts are visualized (arrowheads) in bilateral kidneys. MGS is autosomal recessive genetic syndrome therefore incident is one out of four in the next pregnancy.

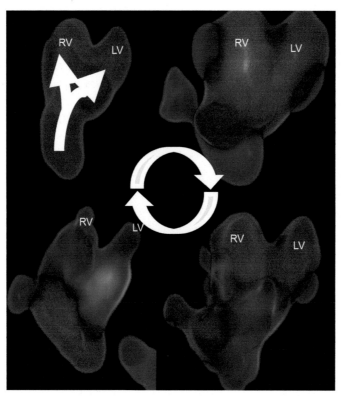

Fig. 19: Atrioventricular (AV) septal defect at 11 weeks. Sequential images of HD flow silhouette imaging are shown. Note the blood flow through the common AV valve (arrows) toward bilateral ventricles. (LV: left ventricle; RV: right ventricle)

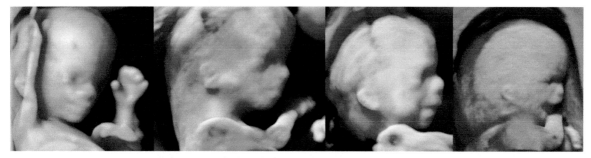

Fig. 20: Different facial expressions of normal, trisomy fetuses at 12 weeks. From the left, faces of normal karyotype, trisomy 21, trisomy 18, and trisomy 13, respectively. Note that all trisomies had low-set ears and micrognathia. However, facial expression is different.

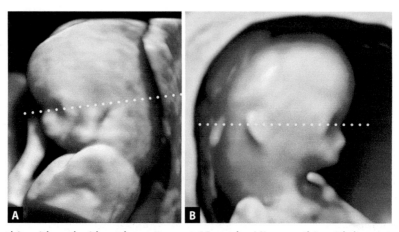

Figs. 21A and B: Micrognathia with and without low-set ear at 12 weeks. Micrognathia with low-set ear (left) and micrognathia with normal ear position (right). (A) A case of trisomy 18. Micrognathia is associated with low-set ear (arrowhead) because of maldevelopment of branchial arch; (B) A case of Pierre Robin sequence, associated with micrognathia but normal external ear position. Pierre Robin sequence is associated with micrognathia due to abnormal development of the mandible, but the position of the external ear is usually normal.

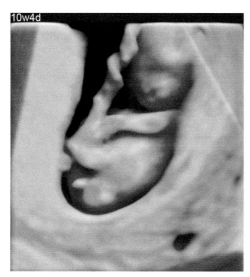

Fig. 22: Cleft lip at 10 weeks.

vascularity is quite comprehensive and may add further clinical information of vascularization.[5,21,34]

Sonographic detection of skeletal dysplasia in the first trimester is challenging. However, achondrogenesis, the most obvious type of dwarfism, can be clearly visualized even in the first trimester **(Fig. 30)**.

Clubfoot or talipes can occur as an isolated finding or one component of syndromes or sequences. However, only 5% of congenital hand anomalies occur as part of a recognized syndrome.[5] Overlapping fingers, wrist contracture (*see* **Figs. 15A to C**), and forearm deformities are often associated with a chromosomal abnormality such as trisomy 18. Sirenomelia in the first trimester have been reported[35,36] and **Figure 31** shows the comprehensive 3D HDlive image of sirenomelia at 12 weeks. Finger abnormalities such as polydactyly, oligodactyly, split hand, and syndactyly, are detectable from

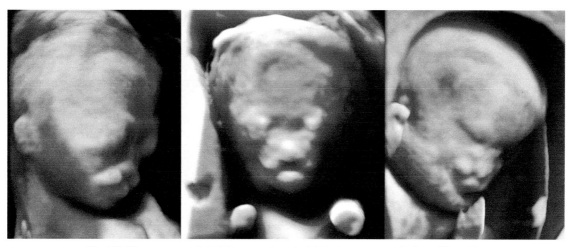

Fig. 23: Three cases of cleft lip associated with holoprosencephaly at 12 weeks.

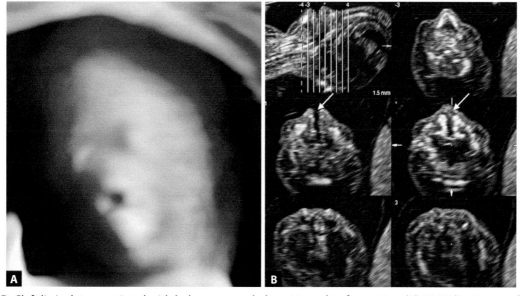

Figs. 24A and B: Cleft lip/palate associated with holoprosencephaly at 12 weeks of gestation. (A) 3D HDlive image of fetal face. Cleft lip is demonstrated; (B) Tomographic ultrasound image. Outer surface opening of cleft lip and inner structure of cleft palate (arrows) are well demonstrated.

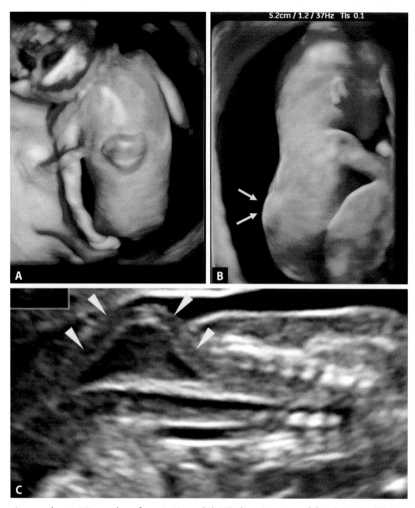

Figs. 25A to C: Myelomeningocele at 12 weeks of gestation. (A) HD live image of fetal back; (B) Lateral view. Arrows indicate protrusion of myelomeningocele; (C) Sagittal section image. Ectopic spinal cord from spinal canal is well demonstrated (arrowheads).

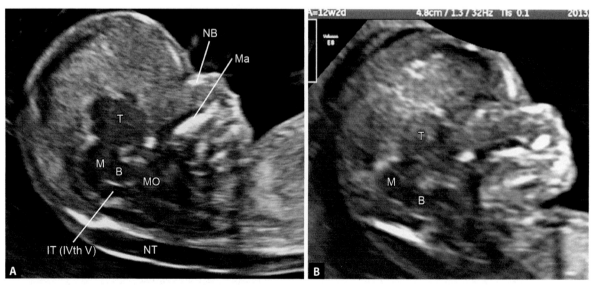

Figs. 26A and B: Mid-sagittal section of (A) normal fetus and (B) a case of spina bifida. Nuchal translucency and intracranial translucency (IT) are visible. In a case of spina bifida, IT disappears due to Chiari type II malformation. Disappearance of IT is useful for screening of spina bifida.
(B: brainstem; IVth V: fourth ventricle; Ma: maxilla; M: midbrain; MO: medulla oblongata; NB: nasal bone; NT: nuchal translucency; T: thalamus)

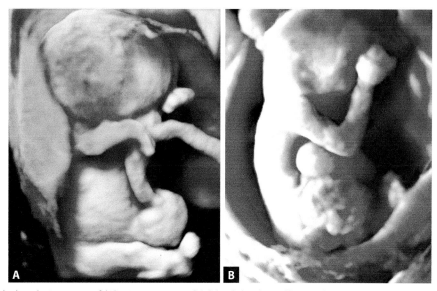

Figs. 27A and B: Omphalocele in cases of (A) trisomy 18 and (B) limb body wall complex at 12 and 13 weeks, respectively. Note the contents of ectopic organs such as liver and bowel (B) are well demonstrated by HDlive imaging.

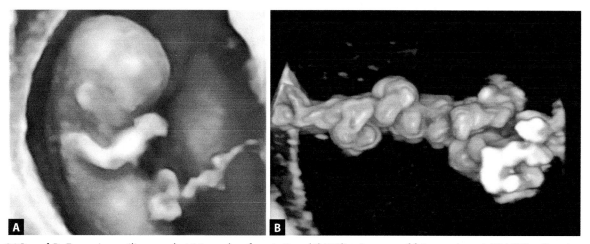

Figs. 28A and B: Excessive coiling cord at 12 weeks of gestation. (A) HDlive images of fetus and cord; (B) HDlive flow image of excessive coiling cord. Note the high pitch of coils. This fetus died in utero 5 days later.

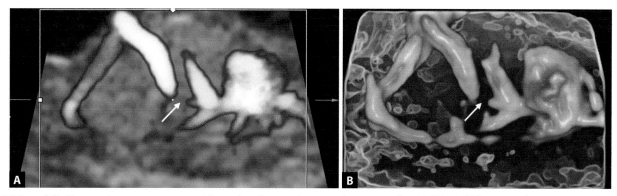

Figs. 29A and B: Absent ductus venosus at 11 weeks of gestation seen in a case of 45,X. (A) 2D bidirectional power Doppler image; (B) 3D HDlive flow image. Arrows indicate the original location of ductus venosus. Absent ductus venosus is occasionally seen in cases of Turner syndrome.

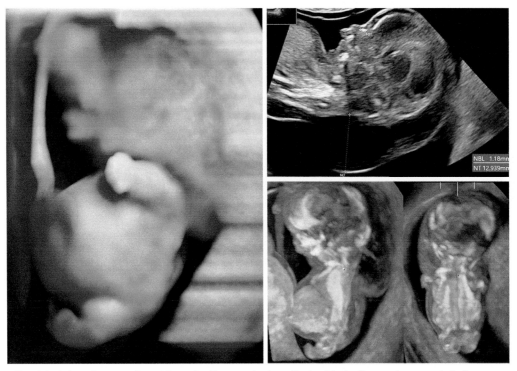

Fig. 30: Achondrogenesis at 12 weeks. Extremely short limbs, big belly are characteristic features of achondrogenesis from early pregnancy.

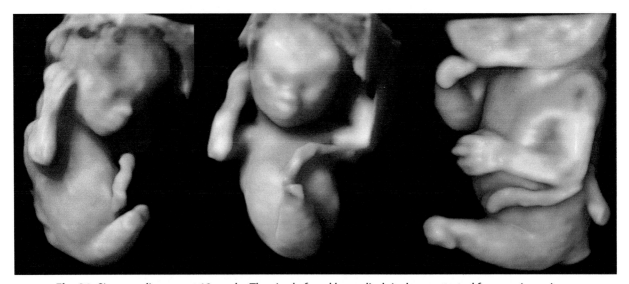

Fig. 31: Sirenomelia apus at 12 weeks. The single fused lower limb is demonstrated from various views.

the late first trimester with high resolution by advanced 3D imaging as shown in **Figures 32A to D**.

Conjoined twins, known as Siamese twins,[37] are twins fused in utero and consequently also at birth. The incidence of conjoined twins is 1 in 50,000-200,000.[38] Chen CP et al. reviewed 75 cases of conjoined twins diagnosed in the first trimester.[39] **Figures 33A and B** show the cephalopagus conjoined twins and their brain structure at 13 weeks, and **Figures 34A and B** show the thoracopagus conjoined twins at 12 weeks.

FETAL ANOMALIES BETWEEN 14 AND 20 WEEKS

Although it was mentioned above that many morphological abnormalities can now be objectively detected by 13 weeks gestation, the fetus is small and detectable cases are still limited. Of course, considering the time required for the parents to decide whether to terminate the pregnancy, for counseling, and for the process of identifying genetic factors in the amniotic fluid test, an accurate diagnosis as

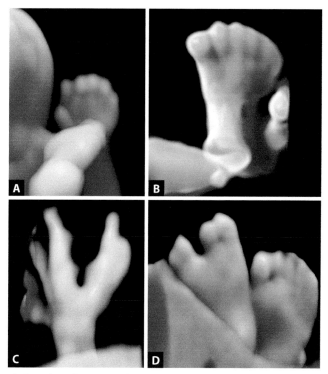

Figs. 32A to D: Polydactyly and oligodactyly with cleft hand/foot at 12 weeks. (A) Polydactyly fingers; (B) Polydactyly toes; (C) Cleft hand with oligodactyly; (D) Cleft foot with oligodactyly.

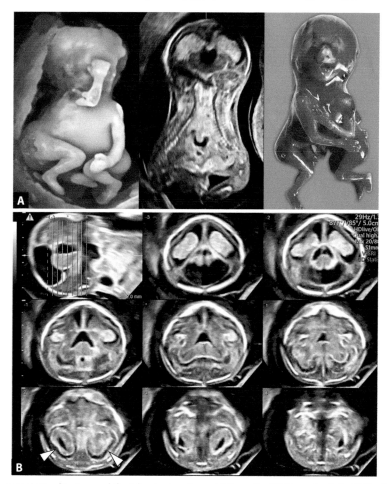

Figs. 33A and B: Cephalopagus conjoined twins and their brain structure at 13 weeks. (A) From the left, HDlive image, coronal cutting section, and aborted fetuses of the cephalopagus twins. Note that they share brain, face, chest, and partial abdomen; (B) Tomographic ultrasound imaging of coronal planes. They share one pair of cerebri and the brainstem, but two cerebelli were visualized (arrowheads).

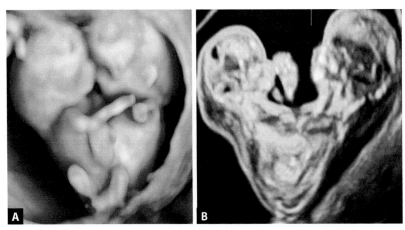

Figs. 34A and B: Thoracopagus conjoined twins at 12 weeks. (A) HDlive image of thoracopagus twins; (B) Sagittal cutting section image. Note that they share the heart and liver.

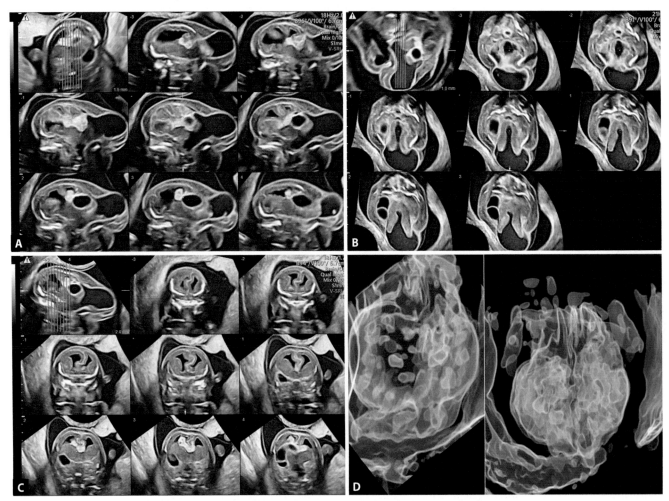

Figs. 35A to D: Meckel–Gruber syndrome at 15 weeks. (A) Tomographic ultrasound imaging (TUI) sagittal section images; (B) TUI coronal section images. Note the abnormal brain structure with irregular ventricular walls and encephalocele; (C) TUI axial section images; (D) HDlive silhouette images of bilateral huge polycystic kidneys. Other findings such as lower polydactyly, upper syndactyly, wrist contracture, micrognathia, and low-set ears were demonstrated. Exome sequencing resulted in *TCTN2* gene mutation by compound heterozygous inheritance.

early as possible is desirable. From the 14th to 20th week of pregnancy, many fetal morphological abnormalities can be visualized with 3D ultrasound in greater detail than at 11th-13th week. **Figures 35A to D** demonstrates the detailed brain structure and polycystic kidneys in a

case of MGS due to *TCTN2* gene mutation, which is one of ciliopathies. Other dysmorphological structures diagnosed at 14–20 weeks are shown, such as cleft lip/alveolar/palate **(Figs. 36A to C)**, clubfoot **(Fig. 37)**, thanatophoric dysplasia due to *FGFR3* mutation **(Figs. 38A and B)**, abnormal face

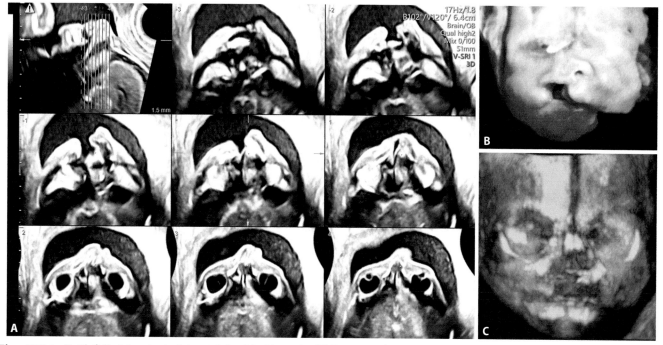

Figs. 36A to C: Cleft lip/alveolar/palate at right side 19 weeks. (A) Tomographic ultrasound imaging axial images of lip, alveolar, and palate; (B) HDlive image of the face (frontal view); (C) Skeletal image of the face.

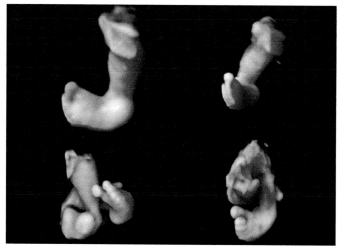

Fig. 37: HDlive images of clubfoot from various angles at 18 weeks.

and contracted fingers in a case of Stickler syndrome due to *COL2A1* mutation **(Figs. 39A to C)**, and Cornelia de Lange syndrome due to *NIPBL* mutation **(Figs. 40A and B)**. Filges et al. reported that in 73.8% of case series, the diagnosis of multiple congenital contractures was missed prenatally. The general contracture as shown in **Figure 41** can be detected. Careful observation of contractures, joint positioning, the quality of fetal movements, and bone growth in the first or early second trimester will be helpful in a field of clinical practice. In addition, longitudinal observations can be quite useful. For example, **Figures 42A and B** show a case of Costello syndrome due to *HRAS* gene mutation, where a normal unclenched hand is observed at 13 weeks, but

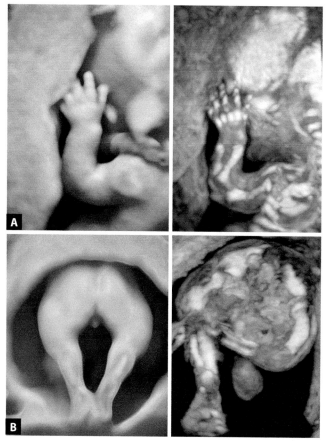

Figs. 38A and B: Thanatophoric dysplasia type I at 16 weeks. (A) Shows the surface and skeletal modes of a short arm; (B) Shows the lower extremities. Note the bent femur and humerus. In this case, a pathological variant (missense mutation) was found in exon 7 of the *FGFR3* gene.

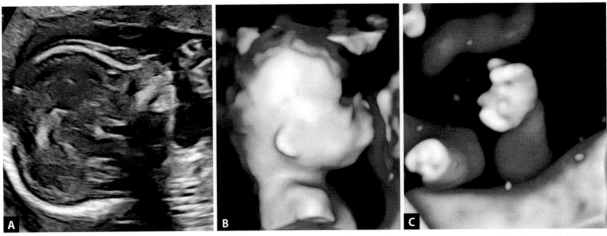

Figs. 39A to C: Stickler syndrome at 18 weeks. (A) 2D sagittal image. Note the micrognathia and prenasal thickness; (B) HDlive image of the face. Low-set ear and micrognathia are visualized; (C) HDlive image of the clenched hand with overlapping fingers. Exome sequencing resulted in de novo *COL2A1* gene mutation.

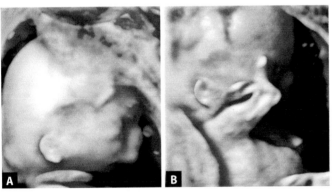

Figs. 40A and B: Cornelia de Lange syndrome at 15 weeks. (A) HDlive image of the face. Note the agnathia and low-set ear; (B) HDlive image of the upper extremity. Note the short limb with hypoplastic forearm, sprit hand, and oligodactyly. Exome sequencing resulted in *NIPBL* mutation.

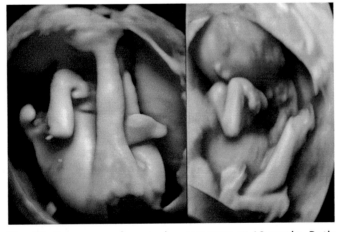

Fig. 41: Two cases of general contracture at 18 weeks. Both images show general contracture. The left case had *SCN3A* gene mutation and the right case had negative result of exome sequencing.

an abnormal clenched hand is seen at 20 weeks. Thus, neurological findings that are not present in early pregnancy may be added in mid-pregnancy or later.

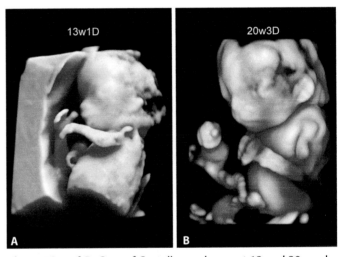

Figs. 42A and B: Case of Costello syndrome at 13 and 20 weeks. Normal appearance of hands at 13 weeks (A) changed to clenched hands with contracture at 20 weeks (B). Exome sequencing resulted in *HRAS* mutation.

■ CONCLUSION

As described in this chapter, detailed fetal morphology has become diagnosable from the first trimester to the early second trimester. Further improvements in imaging techniques and molecular genetics will allow for earlier and more accurate diagnosis.

■ REFERENCES

1. Pooh RK, Kurjak A. 3D and 4D sonography and magnetic resonance in the assessment of normal and abnormal CNS development: alternative or complementary. J Perinat Med. 2011;39(1):3-13.
2. Pooh RK, Shiota K, Kurjak A. Imaging of the human embryo with magnetic resonance imaging microscopy and high-resolution transvaginal 3-dimensional sonography: human embryology in the 21st century. Am J Obstet Gynecol. 2011; 204(1):77.e1-16.

3. Timor-Tritsch I, Peisner D, Raju S. Sonoembryology: an organ-oriented approach using a high-frequency vaginal probe. J Clin Ultrasound. 1990;18(4):286-98.

4. Pooh RK, Kurjak A. 3D/4D sonography moved prenatal diagnosis of fetal anomalies from the second to the first trimester of pregnancy. J Matern Fetal Neonatal Med. 2012;25(5):433-55.

5. Pooh RK. Sonoembryology by 3D HDlive silhouette ultrasound: what is added by the "see-through fashion"? J Perinat Med. 2016;44(2):139-48.

6. Yamada S, Uwabe C, Nakatsu-Komatsu T, Minekura Y, Iwakura M, Motoki T, et al. Graphic and movie illustrations of human prenatal development and their application to embryological education based on the human embryo specimens in the Kyoto collection. Dev Dyn. 2006;235(2):468-77.

7. Blaas HG, Eik-Nes SH, Kiserud T, Berg S, Angelsen B, Olstad B. Three-dimensional imaging of the brain cavities in human embryos. Ultrasound Obstet Gynecol. 1995;5(4):228-32.

8. Blaas HG, Eik-Nes SH, Berg S, Torp H. In-vivo three-dimensional ultrasound reconstructions of embryos and early fetuses. Lancet. 1998;352(9135):1182-6.

9. Hata T, Dai SY, Kanenishi K, Tanaka H. Three-dimensional volume-rendered imaging of embryonic brain vesicles using inversion mode. J Obstet Gynaecol Res. 2009;35(2):258-61.

10. Mi SK, Jeanty P, Turner C, Benoit B. Three-dimensional sonographic evaluations of embryonic brain development. J Ultrasound Med. 2008;27(1):119-24.

11. Pooh RK. Neurosonoembryology by three-dimensional ultrasound. Semin Fetal Neonatal Med. 2012;17(5):261-8.

12. Chaoui R, Levaillant JM, Benoit B, Faro C, Wegrzyn P, Nicolaides KH. Three-dimensional sonographic description of abnormal metopic suture in second- and third-trimester fetuses. Ultrasound Obstet Gynecol. 2005;26(7):761-4.

13. Kurjak A, Pooh RK, Merce LT, Carrera JM, Salihagic-Kadic A, Andonotopo W. Structural and functional early human development assessed by three-dimensional and four-dimensional sonography. Fertil Steril. 2005;84(5):1285-99.

14. Kurjak A, Zudenigo D, Predanic M, Kupesic S. Recent advances in the Doppler study of early fetomaternal circulation. J Perinat Med. 1993;21(6):419-39.

15. Kurjak A, Schulman H, Predanic A, Predanic M, Kupesic S, Zalud I. Fetal choroid plexus vascularization assessed by color flow ultrasonography. J Ultrasound Med. 1994;13:841-4.

16. Pooh RK, Aono T. Transvaginal power Doppler angiography of the fetal brain. Ultrasound Obstet Gynecol. 1996;8(6):417-21.

17. Moradan S, Forouzeshfar M. Are abnormal yolk sac characteristics important factors in abortion rates? Int J Fertil Steril. 2012;6(2):127-30.

18. Nicolaides KH, Wright D, Poon LC, Syngelaki A, Gil MM. First-trimester contingent screening for trisomy 21 by biomarkers and maternal blood cell-free DNA testing. Ultrasound Obstet Gynecol. 2013;42(1):41-50.

19. Pooh RK, Machida M, Nakamura T, Matsuzawa N, Chiyo H. Early sonographic findings for suspecting de novo single-gene mutation. Donald School J Ultrasound Obstet Gynecol. 2020;14(2):125-30.

20. Teoh M, Meagher S. First-trimester diagnosis of micrognathia as a presentation of Pierre Robin syndrome. Ultrasound Obstet Gynecol. 2003;21(6):616-8.

21. Pooh RK, Kurjak A. Novel application of three-dimensional HDlive imaging in prenatal diagnosis from the first trimester. J Perinat Med. 2015;43(2):147-58.

22. Paladini D. Fetal micrognathia: almost always an ominous finding. Ultrasound Obstet Gynecol. 2010;35(4):377-84.

23. Tsai MY, Lan KC, Ou CY, Chen JH, Chang SY, Hsu TY. Assessment of the facial features and chin development of fetuses with use of serial three-dimensional sonography and the mandibular size monogram in a Chinese population. Am J Obstet Gynecol. 2004;190(2):541-6.

24. Colasante G, Simonet JC, Calogero R, Crispi S, Sessa A, Cho G, et al. ARX regulates cortical intermediate progenitor cell expansion and upper layer neuron formation through repression of Cdkn1c. Cereb Cortex. 2015;25(2):322-35.

25. Bütow KW, Hoogendijk CF, Zwahlen RA. Pierre Robin sequence: appearances and 25 years of experience with an innovative treatment protocol. J Pediatr Surg. 2009;44(11):2112-8.

26. Syngelaki A, Hammami A, Bower S, Zidere V, Akolekar R, Nicolaides KH. Diagnosis of fetal non-chromosomal abnormalities on routine ultrasound examination at 11-13 weeks' gestation. Ultrasound Obstet Gynecol. 2019;54(4): 468-76.

27. Chaoui R, Benoit B, Mitkowska-Wozniak H, Heling KS, Nicolaides KH. Assessment of intracranial translucency (IT) in the detection of spina bifida at the 11-13-week scan. Ultrasound Obstet Gynecol. 2009;34(3):249-52.

28. Chaoui R, Nicolaides KH. From nuchal translucency to intracranial translucency: towards the early detection of spina bifida. Ultrasound Obstet Gynecol. 2010;35(2):133-8.

29. Karl K, Heling KS, Chaoui R. Fluid area measurements in the posterior fossa at 11-13 weeks in normal fetuses and fetuses with open spina bifida. Fetal Diagn Ther. 2015;37(4):289-93.

30. Ushakov F, Sacco A, Andreeva E, Tudorache S, Everett T, David AL, et al. Crash sign: new first-trimester sonographic marker of spina bifida. Ultrasound Obstet Gynecol. 2019;54(6):740-5.

31. Nicolaides KH, Snijders R, Cheng HH, Cosden C. Fetal gastrointestinal and abdominal wall defects: associated malformations and chromosomal abnormalities. Fetal Diagn Ther. 1992;7:102-15.

32. Lindham S. Omphalocele and gastroschisis in Sweden 1965-1976. Acta Paediatr Scand. 1981;70(1):55-60.

33. Anandakumar C, Badruddin MN, Chua TM, Wong YC, Chia D. First-trimester prenatal diagnosis of omphalocele using three-dimensional ultrasonography. Ultrasound Obstet Gynecol. 2002;20(6):635-6.

34. Pooh RK. A new field of 'fetal sono-ophthalmology' by 3D HDlive silhouette and flow. Donald School J Ultrasound Obstet Gynecol. 2015;9(3):221-2.

35. Clemente C, Farina M, Cianci A, Iraci Sareri M. Sirenomelia with oligodactylia: early ultrasonographic and hysteroscopic embryoscopic diagnosis during the first trimester of gestation. Fetal Diagn Ther. 2010;28(1):43-5.

36. Carbillon L, Seince N, Largillière C, Bucourt M, Uzan M. First-trimester diagnosis of sirenomelia: a case report. Fetal Diagn Ther. 2001;16(5):284-8.

37. Mian A, Gabra NI, Sharma T, Topale N, Gielecki J, Tubbs RS, et al. Conjoined twins: from conception to separation, a review. Clin Anat. 2017;30(3):385-96.

38. De Ugarte D, Boechat M, Shaw W, Laks H, Williams H, Atkinson JB. Parasitic omphalopagus complicated by omphalocele and congenital heart disease. J Pediatr Surg. 2002;37(9):1357-8.

39. Chen CP, Hsu CY, Su JW, Chen HEC, Hsieh AHR, Hsieh AHJ, et al. Conjoined twins detected in the first trimester: a review. Taiwan J Obstet Gynecol. 2011;50(4):424-31.

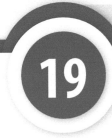

CHAPTER

19

Gastrointestinal Tract and Internal Abdominal Wall

Fernando Bonilla-Musoles, Luiz Eduardo Machado

■ INTRODUCTION

These are infrequent malformations. Their global incidence is estimated to be below 3–6 cases in every 1,000 newborns, although it is probably higher, since many of them are part of very severe polymalformative syndromes, with a high incidence of intrauterine death even in early stages of pregnancy. These occurrences are the fourth or fifth most frequent malformations; furthermore, it is remarkable that their interest in the ultrasound field since 10% of the polyhydramnios are associated with upper digestive atresias, and another 10% with lower digestive atresias.[1,2]

Colon atresia is responsible of 5–10% of all the intestinal atresias; anal atresia is the most frequent type, the incidence is around 1 every 5,000 live births.

Many other intestinal fetal disorders have been described by ultrasound including small intestines or anorectal atresia, Hirschsprung disease, megacolon with anourethral atresia, and distended and descended colon, which is associated with Johanson–Blizzard syndrome.

Although in the past years, the approach to the diagnosis was based in radiological procedures, especially the injection of contrast in the amniotic fluid so that the fetus would swallow it and fill in the digestive system with such contrast, nowadays these procedures have been substituted by ultrasound with which most of these defects can be diagnosed.

It is frequent that an inexperienced ultrasound technician might doubt to differentiate physiological findings (swallowing, gastrointestinal fluid formation, peristaltic, meconium accumulation, urine production) from pathological occurrences.

It is also important to diagnose the possible malformations in other organs and systems that can be related to these defects and therefore, will determine the neonatal prognosis.

These well-known anomalies are diagnosed through two-dimensional (2D) ultrasound explorations, many of them even in the first trimester, but three dimensional (3D) and four dimensional (4D) mean a remarkable advance in a better definition of the defect, as many reports are already available.[1,2]

■ EMBRYOLOGY

During the 6th week of pregnancy, the endoderm lining epithelium of the primitive gut proliferates and obliterates the lumen. In the two following weeks, it vacuolizes and suffers a recanalization.

Stenosis or colon duplication results from the incomplete recanalization that will produce an intestinal obstruction. Rotation or abnormal fixation of the gut loops results on a variety of malformations, including the compression or intestinal volvulus.

■ BASES FOR DIAGNOSIS

A complete gastrointestinal tract examination must include:
- Visualization of the stomach, starting at week 9, in the upper left quadrant of the abdomen.
- Visualization of the small and large intestines starting at the 16th week, checking the appearance of the peristaltic (in the 16th week) and the progressive maturation of the loops with their austras and meconium accumulation.
- Visualization of the gallbladder, liver, and their blood supply.
- Checking the integrity of the anterior abdominal wall.
- Checking the integrity of the diaphragm.
- Checking the umbilical cord insertion.
- Differentiating the possible anomalies from those that occur in other organs, especially kidneys, suprarenal, bladder, and ovaries.

The observation of abnormal images in these structures will allow diagnose of the most common abdominal wall or/ and gastrointestinal tract defects (**Box 1**).

The sensibility of 2D ultrasound for these malformations is estimated to be between 46 and 86%.[3]

ESOPHAGEAL ATRESIA

It is a sporadic anomaly which incidence is estimated to be 2–12 cases in every 10,000 live births and is associated in 90% of the cases to a tracheoesophageal (TE) fistula.

Both situations are the result of a failure in the division of the anterior primitive gut, in the formation of the trachea up front and the esophagus behind that normally takes place between week 3 and 5, and is completed in week 8.

Classification has been made in:[4]
- Esophageal atresia without TE fistula
- Proximal esophageal atresia with proximal TE fistula
- Proximal esophageal atresia with distal TE fistula **(Fig. 1)**

BOX 1: Abdominal defects.

- Esophageal atresia
- Situs inversus
- Ascites and anasarca
- Diaphragmatic defects
- *Abdominal wall defects:*
  - Omphalocele
  - Gastroschisis
  - Cantrell pentalogy
  - *Exstrophy:*
    - Bladder
    - Cloaca
  - Ectopia cordis
  - Limb-body wall complex
  - Body stalk complex
- *Intestinal atresia:*
  - Duodenal
  - Intestinal
  - Cloacal
- *Miscellaneous:*
  - Umbilical cord herniation
  - Liver calcifications
  - Meconium peritonitis liver calcifications
  - Meconium peritonitis

- Proximal esophageal atresia with both proximal and distal TE fistulas
- TE fistula without esophageal atresia.

The most common is the third type (80%), followed by the first type (8%).

It is associated in 3–4% of the cases to chromosomal anomalies.

The *first diagnostic approach* can be made observing a polyhydramnios and in successive ultrasound examinations a gastric chamber cannot be seen **(Fig. 2)**.

Also, very occasionally, it has been observed a distended esophagus above the atresia and amniotic fluid regurgitation after the fetus has swallowed it. But these are exceptional findings.

Also, the failure of visualization of the gastric chamber is not very valuable because of two reasons:
1. The gastric chamber produces gastric juices that allow its visualization.
2. When there is a fistula associated to the chamber, it is also filled up.

Therefore, in <10% of the cases a prenatal diagnosis can be securely established.

Up to 50–70% of the cases affected by this condition are also associated with cardiovascular (29%) and gastrointestinal (28%) malformations, such as intestinal malrotation, anorectal atresia, duodenal and annular pancreas.

This anomaly is also part of the VATER syndrome: *V*ertebral or inter *V*entricular septum defects, *A*nal atresia, *T*racheoesophageal fistula, *E*sophageal atresia, *R*adial dysplasia and *R*enal anomalies, and single-artery umbilical cord.

The prognosis, with or without a TE fistula, will depend on the associated malformations. Consequently, a morphologic and karyotype in amniotic fluid must be always performed

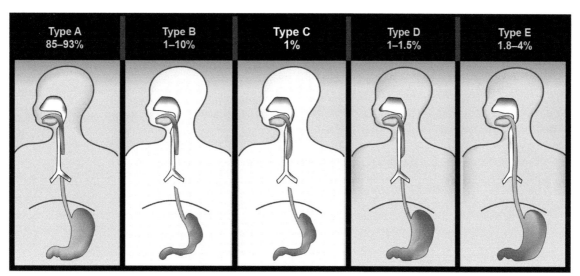

Fig. 1: Classification of esophageal atresia fistula.

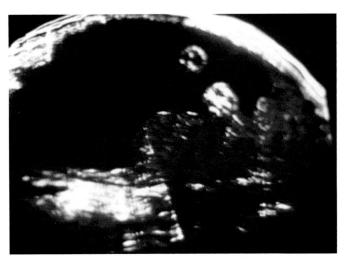

Fig. 2: Esophageal atresia. Polyhydramnios.

after reaching a prenatal diagnosis of an esophageal atresia based on ultrasound.

SITUS INVERSUS

Thoracic and abdominal organs are in the opposite side than usual (situs inversus totalis). A partial variant is known in which only the thoracic organs are abnormally located in the other side (situs inversus partialis).

The incidence is estimated to be 1–2 cases in every 10,000 live births. Rarely, the thoracic organs are normally placed when the abdominal organs are in reversal position. The situs partialis variant is classified in asplenic syndrome (both at the right side) or polysplanic (both at the left side).

The so frequent association between the heart and the spleen, both developed in the sixth week suggests that an unknown factor might exist and might affect before or during the formation of these organs.

In the asplenic variant, the spleen does not exist, both lungs are trilobulated and the liver is centered and symmetric. There is an intestinal malrotation and the stomach can be in either side or even in the center.

In the polysplenic variant, generally there are two spleens and a variable number of some other spleens of smaller size, the liver and stomach can be either on the left or on the right side, and a superior bilateral cava vein can be seen.

A first diagnosis can be made when reversal abdominal organs and heart anomalies are observed through ultrasound **(Fig. 3)**.

The most frequently anomalies associated with situs inversus are the complex heart malformations that are present in 90% of the asplenic and in 70% of the polysplenic syndrome.

Also, the genitourinary tract malformations and the neural tube defects are frequent in the situs inversus partialis variant and the association of these with the situs inversus totalis variant is rare. The prognosis is very poor since 90%

of the newborns affected by this condition die from the associated malformations.

ASCITES AND ANASARCA

The ascites or hydrops fetalis occurs in 1 case in every 1,500–4,000 newborns. It is a relatively frequent finding always secondarily to severe obstetric problems; therefore, it is considered a challenge to the diagnostic skills for any ultrasound technician or obstetrician.

Differentiation

Ascites: An accumulation of fluid in the abdominal cavity.

Anasarca: Generalized edema with accumulation of fluid in subcutaneous connective tissue all throughout the body. It is generally an advanced stage of the ascites, and sometimes it is associated with a pleural and pericardial effusion, etc. **(Figs. 4 to 6)**.

There are many causes that can provoke this fluid retention, starting with immunologic causes, in which the Rh-sensibilization is the most common, infections, or metabolic disorders such as diabetes, anemia, or hypo-proteinemia, up to numerous anomalies and malformations.

Hydrops fetalis in an ultrasound examination is characterized by an abdominal distension with a very thin wall, a variable increase of the intraperitoneal fluid, reduced echoes from intestinal masses since they are compressed by the fluid and usually displaced against the vertebral column or toward one of the sides, and gut loops also compressed, but sometimes partially visible floating in the ascetic fluid **(Fig. 6)**.

The presence of ascites fluid facilitates the identification of abdominal organs, which are also better defined **(Fig. 6)**.

When the edema surrounds and is extended throughout the whole fetal body, it can be called anasarca or generalized hydrops fetalis or Ballantyne syndrome.

The presence of hydrops indicates a serious danger to the fetus that is probably in a much compromised situation, most likely terminal **(Box 2)**.

In 50–70% of the cases, there is a coexisting polyhydramnios and usually is very accentuated. It is essential to have a closer approach as possible to the etiology of the ascites, in order to start any feasible treatment and to determine the fetal prognosis.

Hydrops fetalis can appear as an isolated occurrence or associated to other findings such as hydrothorax, pericarditis, hernias, hepatosplenomegaly or an increase of the thickness, and hyperechogenicity of the placenta.

- *Ascites or fetal-isolated anasarca:* This form of fetal ascites is generally associated to the abdominal lymphatic system anomalies. Ultrasound-guided paracentesis will show the typical lymphocytosis.

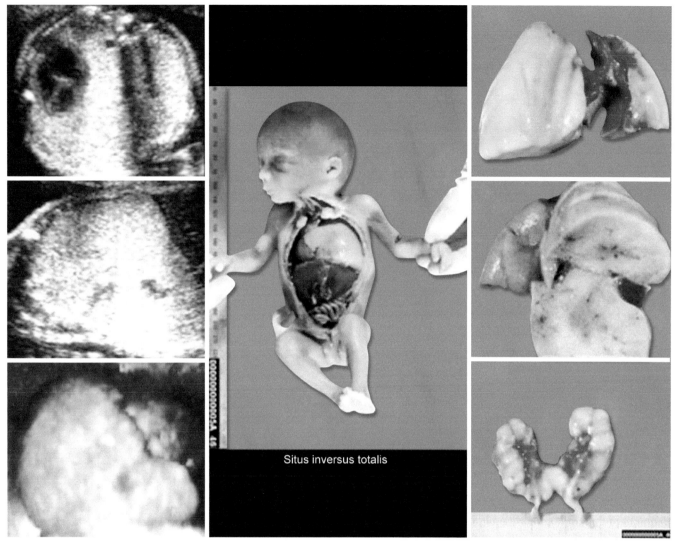

Fig. 3: Situs inversus in week 24. Dextrocardia and intestinal malrotation (above left and central picture). Policystuc kidney (below right). Left pulmonary hipoplasia (above right). Cystic adenoma in the right lung (above left). Liver on the right side (midle right).

In case that the hydrops fetalis is associated to heartbeat disorders, a supraventricular tachycardia, or a cardiopathy must be suspected.

- *Fetal ascites associated to other ultrasound anomalies:* If the hydrops fetalis is associated with other anomalies such as hydrothorax, pericarditis, hernia, hepatosplenomegaly or an increase of the thickness, homogeneity, hyperechogenicity, or irregularity in the placenta, it is thinkable that it is a nonimmune hydrops fetalis. In these cases, there could be a multiple etiology. The obstetrician must consider several causes such as anomalies, or malformations, cardiac, urinary, pulmonary, polymalformative syndromes, chromosomal syndromes, fetal infections, or other metabolic or hematological diseases that can affect the fetus.

The finding of a hydrops fetalis requires a very systematic examination of the fetus and the placenta; also a color Doppler and echocardiography evaluation should be performed in order to find out the cardiac and hemodynamic situation of the fetus.

Also some maternal screening should be performed to rule out any metabolism pathology or other infections.

It is important to obtain fetal blood and ascites fluid from the fetus so that fetal anemia, chromosomopathies, hypoproteinemias, bacterial or virus related infections, and thalassemia could be ruled out.

Finally, regardless of how much effort was put to reach a diagnosis, hydrops fetalis in 30% of the cases will still be considered "idiopathic."

■ DIAPHRAGMATIC DEFECTS

A diaphragmatic hernia is a defect that appears between the 9th and 10th week, and is due to a failure in the closure of the peritoneal pleura, that allows the entrance or the herniation of abdominal organs, especially of gut loops inside the thoracic cavity. It is estimated an incidence of

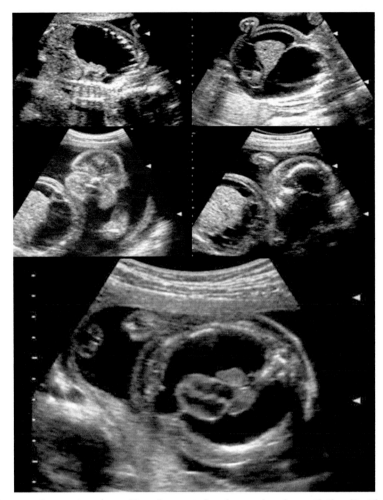

Fig. 4: Generalized fetal edema, ascites, and anasarca. The edema can be observed underneath the skin. The ascites can be found in the central images. The anasarca with pleural effusion can be seen in the top and bottom images.

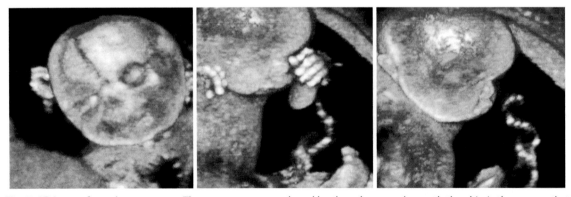

Fig. 5: 3D image from the same case. The transparency produced by the edema underneath the skin is the reason that these type of fetuses are called "glass baby."

1 every 3,000/5,000 live births, although the real incidence is, with no doubt, higher since many of these fetuses die in the uterus.

The prognosis is very poor since the origin of this malformation occurs very early, the defect is substantial, there are other associated malformations, and can produce pulmonary hypoplasia.

The etiology of this malformation is unknown, although its origin could be sporadic or familial, some of the cases have been related to the use of drugs such as anticonvulsants, quinine, thalidomide, and others.

The pathogenesis can occur by a double mechanism:
1. Delay in the diaphragm fusion
2. Primary defect in the development of the diaphragm

Classification depends on the location of:
- Diaphragmatic hernia (Bochdalek and Morgagni)
- Septum transversum defects—consist on a defect of the central tendon.

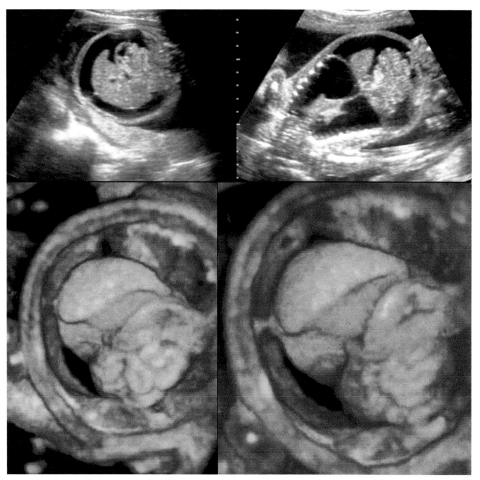

Fig. 6: 2D and 3D ultrasound images of the ascites. The 3D image shows the hepatic ligamentum teres and the gut loops immersed in the ascites fluid. Thanks to it we can obtain these spectacular images, where we can see the interior of the abdomen, the gut loops, and liver.

> **BOX 2:** Causes of fetal ascites.
> - Diseases in the mother
> - Abnormalities in the placenta
> - Fetal diseases or anomalies
> - Umbilical cord anomalies

- *Hiatal hernia*—occurs through a congenitally large esophageal orifice.
- Eventration of the diaphragm
- Agenesis of the diaphragm

The most common diaphragmatic hernia is *Bochdalek*, which is caused by a posterolateral defect that can be located either on the left side (80%), or on the right side (15%), or even on both sides (5%).

Stomach, spleen, and colon are the most frequently herniated organs. Pancreas and liver herniations are less frequent. When the defect takes place on the right side, herniation of the liver and gallbladder occurs.

Usually, it does not have a peritoneal sac (10%) **(Fig. 7)**.

Morgagni hernia: It is produced by a parasternal defect located on the anterior portion of the diaphragm between the costal and sternum origin of the muscle.

It is relatively infrequent (1–2% of all hernias), and even though it can be bilateral, it generally affects the right side.

The foramen is usually small, and it can only contain the liver although sometimes the stomach, small and large intestines can herniate. If only the liver herniates, it would be almost impossible to diagnose this malformation by ultrasound, since the ultrasound appearance of liver and lungs is almost identical.

A peritoneal sac is always present.

Hiatus hernia: Similar to those that occur in adults, is a simple defect of the area close to the juncture of the esophagus through which the gastric cavity can penetrate into the thoracic cavity. Generally appears as a single cyst **(Figs. 8 to 10)**.

Eventration: Displacement of abdominal contents toward the thoracic cavity, due to the development of a weak diaphragm, reduced practically to a simple and thin aponeurotic layer that has no muscle fibers. It means 5% of all the diaphragmatic defects, and most frequently affects the right side.

After the observation of several organs especially stomach or loops, and also the heart that is usually displaced toward the right side, ultrasound diagnosis is established **(Figs. 7 to 10)**.

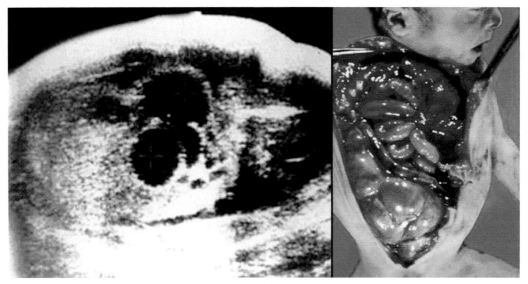

Fig. 7: Bochdalek herniation.

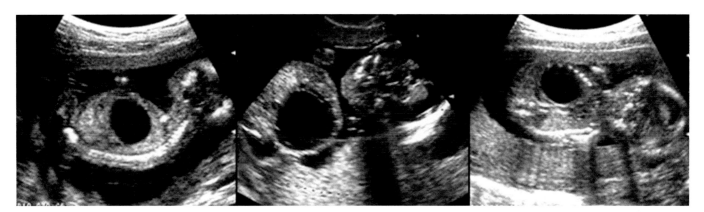

Fig. 8: Hiatal herniation.

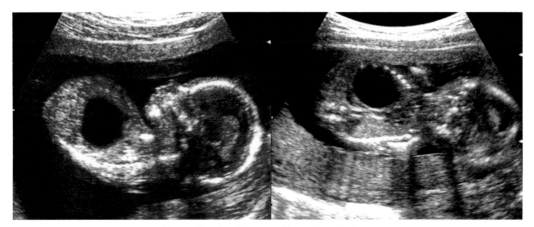

Fig. 9: Another images of hiatal herniation.

If peristaltic movements of the loops are detected, a differential diagnosis can be made with those thoracic pathologies that present similar cystic images such as pulmonary adenomatosis, bronchogenic, and mediastinal cysts.

During the ultrasound examination, the absence of gastric cavity in the abdomen must be always searched, which is usually accompanied by polyhydramnion and a decrease in the fetal abdominal circumference.

It is commonly associated with anomalies and defects of the central nervous system (CNS) (25–75%), cardiac, omphalocele, cleft lip, and carriers of chromosomal malformations (trisomy 21, 18, and 13).

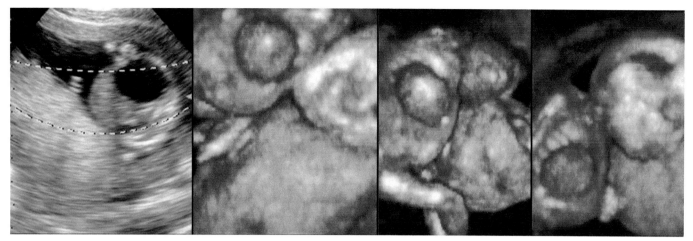

Fig. 10: 3D-4D of a hiatal herniation.

CLASSIFICATION OF ABDOMINAL ANOMALIES INCLUDING ABDOMINAL WALL DEFECTS

Classification of abdominal anomalies including abdominal wall defects has been shown in **Figure 11**.

Duodenal Atresia

This sporadic condition, caused by an atresia or stenosis has an incidence of 1 in every 10,000 newborns.

At week 5 the lumen of the duodenum is obliterated by the proliferation of the epithelium. The path of the lumen is usually restored by week 11, and failure of vacuolization may lead to stenosis or atresia.

Familial inheritance has been suggested by an autosomal recessive pattern.

Etiology: Some causes have been argued—

- *Vascular:* A vascular accident or interruption of the lumen by a diaphragm or membrane may cause ischemia of a segment of bowel.
- *Drugs:* Exposure to thalidomide between the fourth and sixth weeks, may cause atresia, during a critical time for development.
- An annular pancreas is an associated finding (20%); and whereas some believe that this is another feature of an abnormal development, others think that abnormal development of the pancreas may be the cause of the obstruction.

Prenatal diagnosis is based on demonstration of the characteristic "double bubble" appearance of the dilated stomach and proximal duodenum, commonly associated with polyhydramnion **(Figs. 12A and B)**.

However, obstruction due to a central web may result in only a "single bubble" representing the fluid-filled stomach.

Approximately 50% of fetuses have associated malformations such as skeletal defects (vertebral and rib anomalies, sacral agenesis, radial abnormalities, talipes), gastrointestinal abnormalities (esophageal atresia, TE fistula, intestinal malrotation, Meckel's diverticulum, anorectal atresia), cardiovascular malformations (endocardial cushion defects and ventricular septal defects), and renal defects.

Also chromosomal anomalies have been observed quite commonly (trisomy 21, 29%).

The overall mortality is high (36%), and it is mainly due to the associated abnormalities. Prenatal diagnosis may reduce morbidity associated with diagnostic delay.

BOWEL OBSTRUCTION

Small bowel atresia and stenosis occur in 2–3 in every 10,000 newborns. They are sporadic, although familial cases have been described, particularly with the type IV variety.

The most common sites of atresia are the distal ileum (36%), proximal jejunum (31%), distal jejunum (20%), and proximal ileum (13%). Intestinal obstruction at any level may lead to proximal bowel dilation and on rare occasions even to perforation.

Intestinal atresia is more common than stenosis and is usually multiple. There are four types of small bowel atresia:
1. Mucosal diaphragm (20%)
2. Blind ends of intestine joined by a fibrous band (32%)
3. Blind ends of intestine not connected by a fibrous band (48%)
4. Absence of a large portion of the small bowel with a typical apple peel configuration of small bowel along the mesenteric artery.

Small bowel atresia is thought to result from vascular accidents, although volvulus or intussusception may lead to vascular impairment at a later stage. Type IV atresia probably is due to occlusion of a branch of the superior mesenteric artery.

Diagnosis: Jejunal and ileal obstructions are seen as multiple fluid-filled loops of bowel **(Fig. 13)**.

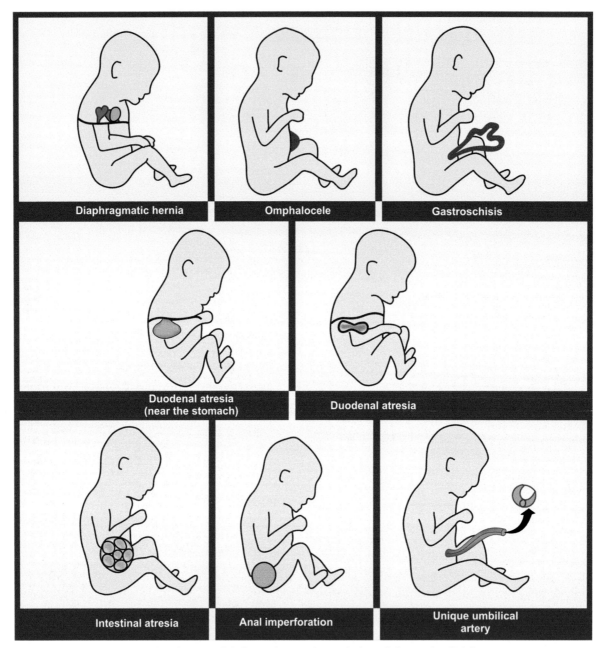

Fig. 11: Classification of abdominal anomalies including abdominal wall defects.

The abdomen may be significantly distended, and active peristalsis may be observed. If bowel perforation occurs, transient ascites, meconium peritonitis, and meconium pseudocysts may ensue.

Another presentation of small bowel obstruction is hyperechogenicity in the fetal abdomen. Polyhydramnion is usually also observed and occurs more frequently with proximal obstructions.

Similar bowel appearances and polyhydramnion may be found in fetuses with Hirschsprung disease and the megacystis-microcolon-intestinal hypoperistalsis syndrome. Occasionally, calcified intraluminal meconium in the fetal pelvis is seen and suggests a diagnosis of anorectal atresia.

The prognosis is related to the gestational age at delivery, the presence of associated anomalies, and the site of obstruction.

■ ANORECTAL ATRESIA

Anorectal atresia, with an incidence of 2 in every 10,000 live births, results from abnormal division of the cloaca during the ninth week of development.

Ultrasonically, it is characterized by a cystic tumor, frequently with irregular contour and a gray sonic content **(Fig. 14)**.

Additional abnormalities are found in 44% of cases, including malrotation, imperforate anus, meconium peritonitis and ileus, omphalocele or gastroschisis (20%), cardiovascular, and other gastrointestinal and chromosomal anomalies (7%).

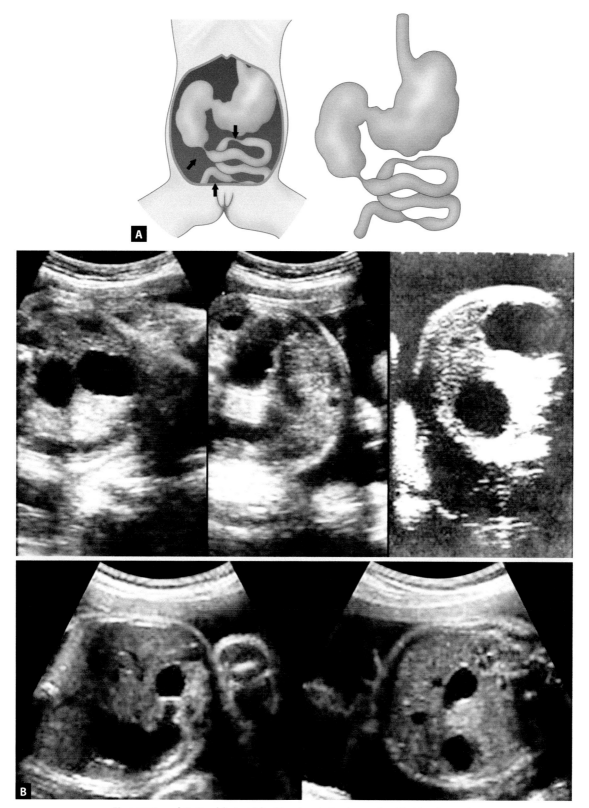

Figs. 12A and B: Double bubble. Duodenal atresia proximal to the stomach.

■ ABDOMINAL WALL DEFECTS

Umbilical Herniation

It should not be considered as an abdominal wall defect, since it is only a simple abnormal insertion of the umbilical cord in the navel without further significance.

It is a broad insertion of the umbilical cord on the abdominal wall that produces a skin-covered wide opening of the umbilicus **(Fig. 15)**. The cosmetic prognosis is excellent since the gap eventually approximates and closes up along the years. It also can be treated with surgical repair.

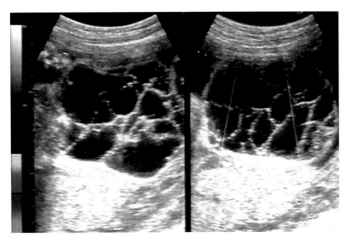

Fig. 13: Ileal atresia, characterized by multiple cystic intestinal dilations.

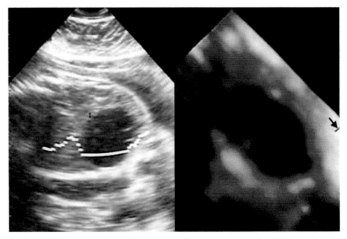

Fig. 14: Anal imperforation. These pictures have to be differentiated from ovarian cysts, distended urine bladder, and kidney cysts.

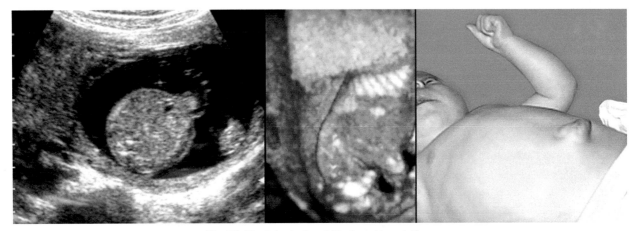

Fig. 15: Physiological umbilical cord herniation.

Omphalocele or Exomphalos

It consists of an abdominal ventral wall defect, due to a defect in the closure of both lateral folds characterized by herniation of some of the intestinal loops, liver, or both, through the defect located in the base of the umbilical insertion.

A fine limiting membrane, nearly transparent and very similar to the amnion or peritoneum, through which the herniated abdominal structures can be seen in the newborn, coats the whole herniation **(Fig. 16)**.

The umbilical cord is always inserted and fully conserved in the herniated sac apex **(Figs. 17 to 19)**, where the vessels arrive, which can be clearly studied with 2D or 3D color Doppler.

The most common herniated organs are the gut loops, stomach and depending on the hernial opening sac size, the liver and exceptionally, the heart (i.e., pentalogy of Cantrell).

The incidence of this anomaly is 1–3 in every 10,000 newborns. Nevertheless, it should be higher especially because the carriers of trisomy 18 die and the pregnancy is early interrupted. The prevalence is 30% in the second trimester and only 15% at birth, which shows the high mortality rate during pregnancy.

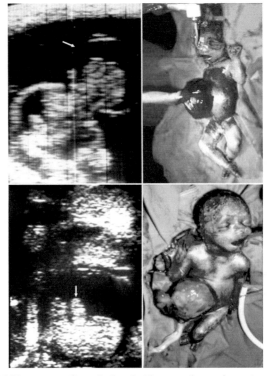

Fig. 16: Two cases of omphalocele. The one above shows intestines and the one in the bottom shows the liver in the herniation.

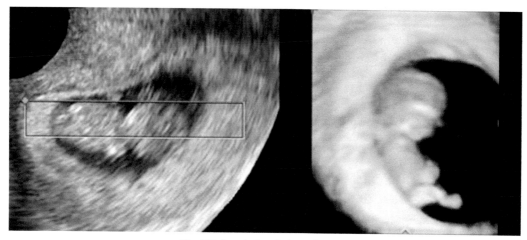

Fig. 17: Omphalocele in 11th week.

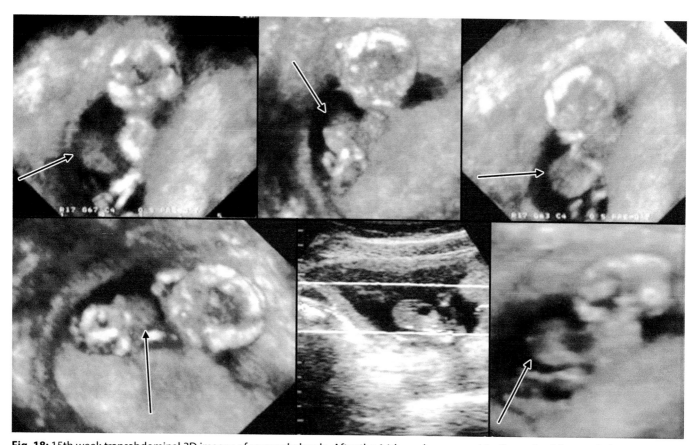

Fig. 18: 15th week transabdominal 3D images of an omphalocele. After the 14th week, sonographic diagnosis of the omphalocele is usually not a problem, since some other indirect signs (besides the own tumor), systematically associated with this disorder are detectable **(Figs. 19 and 20).**

Independent of the size and herniated organs, prognosis is poor, because it is usually associated with chromosomal pathologies and other malformations.

As mentioned, basically the herniated organs are gut loops, and in our experience, 2D is superior to 3D for detection of the contents within the omphalocele **(Figs. 17 to 20).**

Early diagnosis can be made based on ultrasound from the end of the first trimester, through either vaginal or abdominal ultrasound **(Fig. 17).**

The content of the omphalocele marks the probability of the association with chromosomal pathologies. When the gut loops are herniated, the risk of aneuploidy is higher than when it is the liver the only herniated organ.

Diagnosis is based on the evidence of an adjacent mass in direct contact with the abdominal wall generally sonoluscent, due to the herniated organs and surrounded by a thin membrane, much thinner than the abdominal wall, which forms the herniation sac. This characteristic of

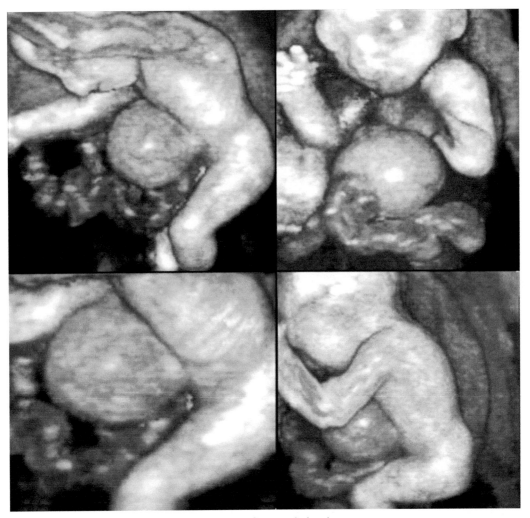

Fig. 19: 3D of an omphalocele.

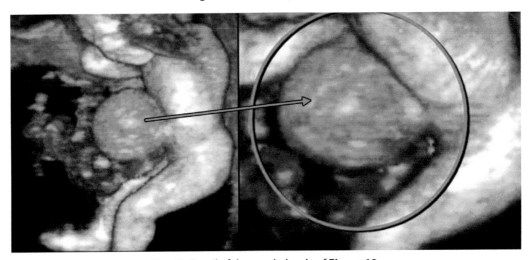

Fig. 20: Detail of the omphalocele of **Figure 19**.

the thin covering membrane is a very useful landmark for differential diagnosis.

The whole defect and its contents can be easily observed floating in the amniotic fluid (but coated by its membrane), as a malformation that comes out from the anterior abdominal wall, systematically accompanied by polyhydramnios, even when the defect is small.

Due to the fact that ascites or anasarca is also frequently accompanying signs, the herniated organs can be easily depicted.

The diagnosis can be established in the first trimester of pregnancy, but it is much easier, and is recommend waiting until week 12 to avoid confusion with a physiological herniation.

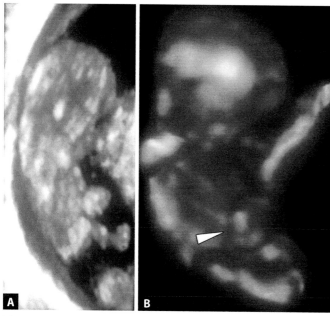

Figs. 21A and B: Physiological (A) and pathological first-trimester herniations. The normal ones disappear in week 11. The pathologic ones remained after week 11, are bigger than 7 mm, irregular, and sonoluscent (B).

The physiological herniation takes place between week 8 and the end of week 11. It is always round or oval, small, and homogeneous. At week 12, it has always disappeared. If it persists we must suspect on this defect, and proceed to other diagnostic techniques either in chorionic villi or amniotic fluid. An omphalocele can be suspected earlier than week 12, if the herniated sac is bigger than 7 mm, irregular, and/or nonhomogeneous **(Figs. 21A and B)**.

Differential diagnosis: It must be distinguished from gastroschisis, which is described below. Gastroschisis is a true disemboweling; intestinal loops float freely in the amniotic fluid without any coating membrane, through a small gap that is always localized on the right side of the umbilical cord, which is correctly inserted.

When an abnormal abdominal protrusion is detected before week 14, the differential diagnosis should include: omphalocele, gastroschisis, and prune belly syndrome, also known as Eagle-Barrett syndrome.

Gastroschisis normally appears later, because before week 16 the gap is very small and the abdominal wall muscles and peristaltic movements have not yet appeared (they are visible after week 12 and 14, respectively). In the second and third trimester, the external mass, consisting of bowel loops freely floating in amniotic fluid, is always located at the right side of the umbilicus and the opening is small, usually <1 cm, unless there is an exstrophy or another combined defect.

Prune belly syndrome is characterized by overdistension of the bladder, kidneys, ureters, or intestinal loops. All this leads to distension of the abdominal wall associated to some deficiencies in the muscles of the abdominal wall. It can also appear with some other nonobstructive kidney malformations, although these are the most frequent causes **(Fig. 22)**.

■ GASTROSCHISIS

Gastroschisis results from a partial failure of the midline abdominal closure **(Fig. 23)**.

The gut loops float freely in the amniotic fluid through a small gap located next to the umbilicus, practically is always located in its right side. However, the umbilical cord as well as its insertion in the abdominal wall is always totally preserved **(Figs. 24 to 26)**.

Through the opening the gut loops, and less frequently the liver or the stomach, come out. The most important difference with an omphalocele is the absence of a surrounding membrane and the small size of the exit gap.

Due to the contact of the amniotic fluid, the gut loops usually show thicker walls. This is because of the precipitation of fibrous and protein materials around the loops, a phenomenon that makes the intestinal torsions and obstructions to be very frequent. This means that, if a quick and proper surgical therapy is performed, the prognosis would be favorable; if it does not occur, and the majority of diagnosis in routine ultrasound is done, and the time that the loops are floating in the fluid is unknown, complications and intrauterine death are common.

Etiology

Even though the causing mechanism is unknown, it is accepted that the defect is the result of the lack of blood supply caused by a failure or a very early obstruction in the umbilical right artery (that is why the gap is always located in this side).

Also it has been proposed that early vascular failure would be located in the conduct's circulation. Any of them would produce a disruption in the blood supply of the structures irrigated by these arteries.

The aorta, initially, gives place to two omphalomesenteric arteries. In normal conditions, the right artery persists and the left one degenerates, becoming part of the mesenteric superior artery that replaces the vitelline vesicule. A vascular interruption of the blood supply will result on an ischemia in the right paraumbilical zone. If the proximal portion of this artery is also damaged, the resulting ischemia would produce a jejunal atresia, a commonly associated finding.

Finally, a new hypothesis has been proposed, the involution of the right umbilical vein.

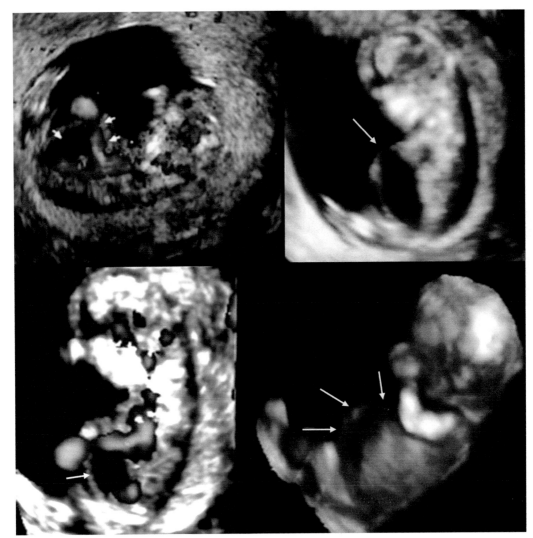

Fig. 22: 2D and 3D Doppler of a typical *prune belly* syndrome in first trimester.

Incidence

There are 0.3–2 cases in every 10,000 newborns. It is considered a sporadic malformation, although there have been family related cases, which suggest a dominant autosomal inheritance of variable expression.

Although its incidence is not different to that of omphalocele, less cases have been described in the first and second trimester because the gap is very small (at this stage <2–3 mm), and visceral herniation appears when the fetus is capable to increase its intra-abdominal pressure (i.e., with breathing movements) when abdominal muscles are contracted or when the peristaltic movements appear after the 14th week.

Diagnosis

Diagnosis is made by the identification of a cauliflower-shaped mass that contains uniform cystic areas in the anterior abdominal wall **(Figs. 23 to 26)**, or, sometimes, a solid cystic mass. Doppler imaging shows that these cystic bodies are not vessels.

The final diagnosis on the 14th week or later is more likely if 2D and 3D are combined, because it is possible to obtain better quality images using the orthogonal planes **(Figs. 24 to 26)**. It is not necessary to wait for further more explorations since the moment when breathing movements and peristalsis appear, which can be observed using 2D and 4D.

In advanced pregnancies, extra-abdominal mass movement and the loops can be observed by fetal movements as well as by shaking the transducers, or simply by observing the loops ballottement.

Differential Diagnosis

This malformation can be easily distinguished from omphalocele because of:

- Its position on the right side of the fetal abdomen.
- The presence of loops or intestines floating freely.
- The presence of a normal abdominal cord insertion side.
- The absence of a surrounding membrane.
- The absence of flow in the loops.
- Spontaneous or induced loop movements.

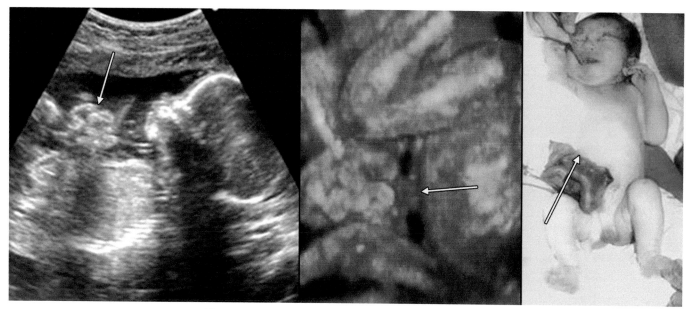

Fig. 23: Another case of gastroschisis in the third trimester.

With 2D as well as with 3D, segments of the gut loops can be seen and followed during a large trajectory.

The defect is nearly always accompanied by an increase in maternal serum alpha-fetoprotein (MS-AFP) and amniotic fluid alpha-fetoprotein (AF-AFP).

Finally, usually there are neither clinic nor ultrasound findings, because they are incidental diagnosis.

Chromosomal Disorders and Other Malformations

The existence of evidence suggests that gastroschisis is not related with chromosomal anomalies. However, 25% of the cases are gastrointestinal-related problems such as adhesion, stenosis, obstruction, atresia, and loop malrotation.

Additionally, restriction of the fetal growth and polyhydramnion are commonly associated. These are consequences of the vascular etiology defect already mentioned or the contact of the viscera with the amniotic fluid.

Although it is considered a sporadic malformation, familial cases have been described, suggesting an autosomal dominant inheritance of variable expression.

Recently, associated cardiac pathology findings have been described in 15% of the cases, much less than the 45% affected by omphalocele.

■ PENTALOGY OF CANTRELL

Cantrell, Haller, and Ravitch described the pentalogy of Cantrell for the first time in 1958. It is a constituted defect of:

- The lower portion of the sternum
- Defect of the midline supraumbilical abdominal wall closure

- Anterior diaphragm deficiency
- Diaphragmatic pericardium defect
- Intracardiac defects.

It is a very rare congenital anomaly, with <1 case in every 100,000 live births, affecting in the proportion of 2:1 for male/female gender, respectively. The females affected usually present more severe symptoms.

The embryologic origin of the sternum and abdominal wall defects relates to a defect in the migration of these mesodermal primordial structures. As for the defects in the pericardium and diaphragm, there is partial or complete failure of the epimyocardium development, structure that forms the cardiac wall composed of the myocardium and visceral pericardium.

The etiology of this anomaly is not totally clear. Family related cases were described suggesting a probable recessive inheritance connected to X-chromosome. It also described its association with viral infection, mother abuse of beta-aminopropionitríte, and chlorine inhalation. As for the chromosomal pathologies, there have been reported associations with trisomy 21, 18, and 13 chromosomes.

Other anomalies may be associated to the pentalogy of Cantrell determining variants of this entity such as: omphalocele, gastroschisis, caudal regression syndrome, anal atresia. Exencephaly, body—stalk síndrome, among others.

It is classified in two ways:
1. Thoracic form (classical)
2. Thoracoabdominal

The classical form presents the following findings: sternum defect, lack of the parietal pericardium, encephalic orientation of the cardiac apex, and small thoracic cavity. The thoracoabdominal form presents partial lack or gap of the sternum lower part, and there is usually a diaphragmatic

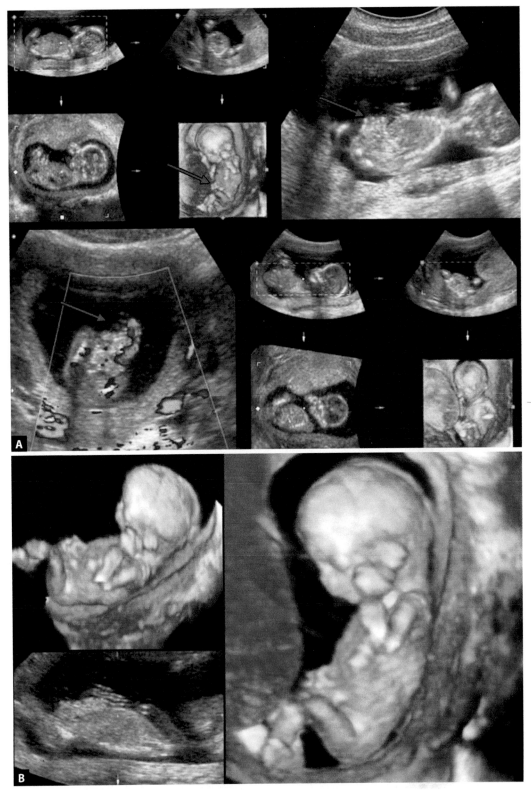

Figs. 24A and B: Gastroschisis in week 18.

defect of the parietal pericardium; normally omphalocele can be observed.

The prenatal ultrasound diagnosis is extremely important in the detection of structural malformations and in the planning of postnatal surgical correction, when possible. The diagnosis is usually performed at the beginning of the second trimester when the classical alterations are showed, however, there are described cases diagnosed in the first and third trimesters.

This happens in early stages and its consequence is the exteriors outcome of the heart, known as ectopia cordis. This finding is essential for its classification.

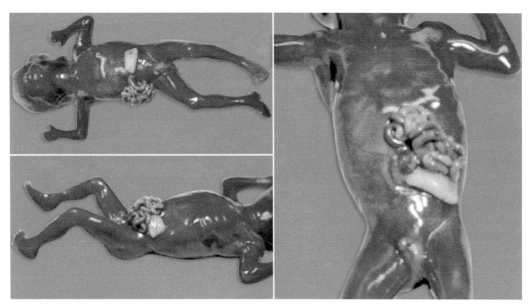

Fig. 25: Gastroschisis in week 18. Detail of the fetus.

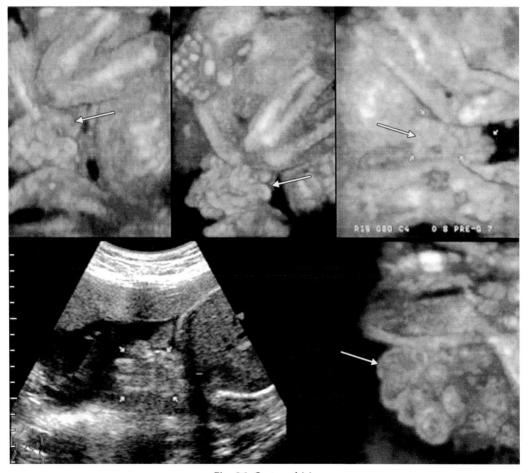

Fig. 26: Gastroschisis.

For diagnosis, it is essential that the heart lies outside the thoracic cavity, whether or not is associated with epigastric omphalocele and the existence or not of a herniation of the organs.

The heart can be seen beating outside the thorax, and at times floating freely in the amniotic fluid **(Figs. 27A and B)**.

The combined use of 2D and 3D is essential for the detection of cases associated with omphalocele, where it is extremely important to see the herniation of the organs with 2D and other superficial malformations using 3D, like in the cleft lip case; frequently it is accompanied by oligohydramnion, which difficult the diagnosis. It should

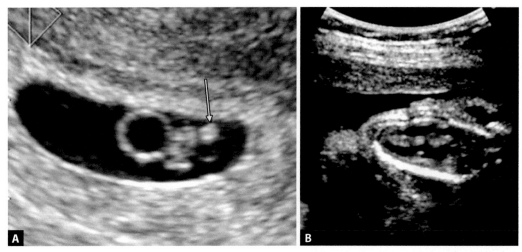

Figs. 27A and B: Ectopia cordis. (A) A 9th-week pregnancy abdominal ultrasound; (B) A second-trimester ultrasound.

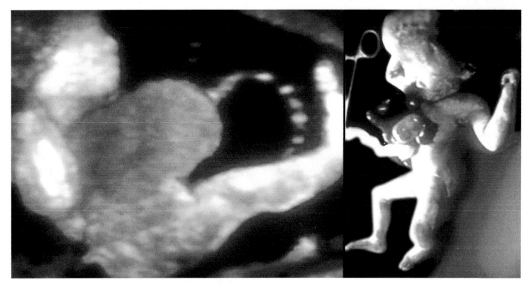

Fig. 28: Cantrell pentalogy.

be kept in mind the difficulty in the observation of cardiac defects due to the altered position of the heart.

In most cases associating epigastric omphalocele results in great diagnosis help. If this is related to the abdominal wall defect, the wall usually is very large **(Fig. 28)**, due to a joint failure of the cephalic and lateral folds.

Pentalogy as well as other cranial wall defects are commonly associated with chromosomal anomalies, especially of pair 18 (or Edwards Syndrome).

Prognosis is usually dismal due to the associated malformations.

■ BLADDER AND CLOACAL EXSTROPHY

If the defect affects the inferior fold, bladder or bladder and cloacal exstrophy is produced. The incidence is 1 case in every 30,000–40,000 newborns, and three times greater in males. Cloacal exstrophy is even rarer, 1 case every 200,000 newborns.

If it is a small defect, only epispadias may result with no further or minimal consequences. Large defects result in bladder exstrophy or bladder and cloacal exstrophy. The urinary tract and the cloaca remain open, and in direct contact with the amniotic fluid **(Figs. 27 and 28)**.

This mesoderm defect, which usually happens by day 29 of development, provokes three different anomalies:
1. *Cloaca septum failure:* The urethra, ileum, and the hindgut remain open.
2. *Rupture of the cloaca membrane:* It is the result of exstrophy of pubic branches and omphalocele.
3. *Medullar canal hernia:* Abnormal vertebrae appear in the lumbar-sacrum region.

When there is bladder exstrophy, its posterior wall can be seen because of the wide separation of the pubic branches. The navel lies low, the penis is short, and the testicles are not descended. In females, the clitoris is forked and the anus remains imperforated or stenotic. The typical cloacal exstrophy consists of evisceration of the gut loops in the ileo-caudal region, imperforated anus, duplicated bladder exstrophy, each with its own urethra, omphalocele, vertebral anomalies, and anomalous external genitalia **(Figs. 29 and 30)**.

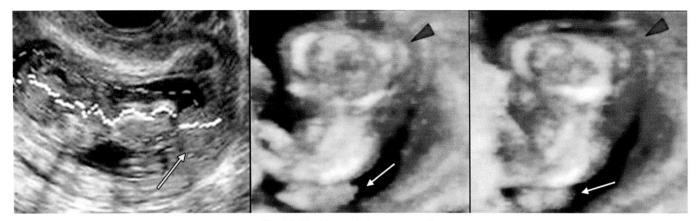

Fig. 29: Bladder and sigma exstrophy.

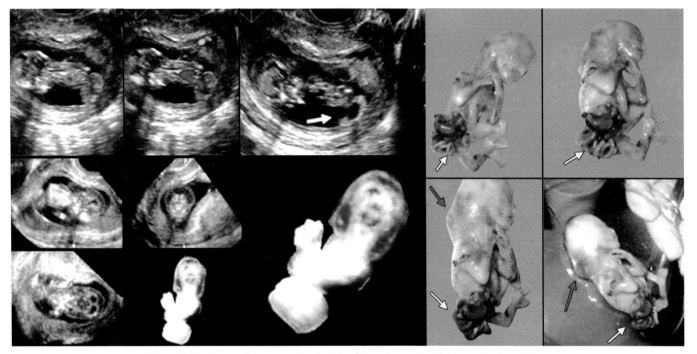

Fig. 30: Bladder and sigma exstrophy. The fetus shows also the typical evisceration.

The prognosis is even worse in cases of superior and inferior fold defects, in comparison with other defects of the abdominal wall.

Even though, 30% of the abdominal wall defects in the second and third trimester are superior and inferior folds, only 15% of them are diagnosed due to the high mortality associated.

BODY STALK COMPLEX

It is a lethal anomaly, due to the failure of fusion of the four-fold abdominal wall, and the developmental absence of the navel and umbilical cord, with an incidence of 1 in every 14,000 live births, which probably is the highest, because of early intrauterine deaths (in the first 12 weeks).

The abdominal wall with herniated organs is fused to the placenta, reason why they have been sometimes confused with gastroschisis. This is associated with numerous malformations (neural tube defects, gastrointestinal and genitourinary system, pericardium, heart, liver, and lungs).

MECONIUM PERITONITIS

Meconium peritonitis is a chemical aseptic peritonitis produced by a perforation of the digestive track during prenatal or postnatal life, consequence of an ischemic obstructive process. There are three types:

1. *Fibro-adhesive peritonitis*, characterized by an intense adhesive peritoneal reaction without intestinal peristalsis.
2. *Cystic peritonitis*, which shows a localized cystic cavity formed by adherent contiguous gut loops.
3. *Generalized peritonitis*, which shows no calcifications or adhesions. The generalized form is seen when the intestinal perforation occurs prior to delivery.

The incidence is 1 in every 35,000 live births. Most of them are diagnosed in the postnatal period, during an evaluation of

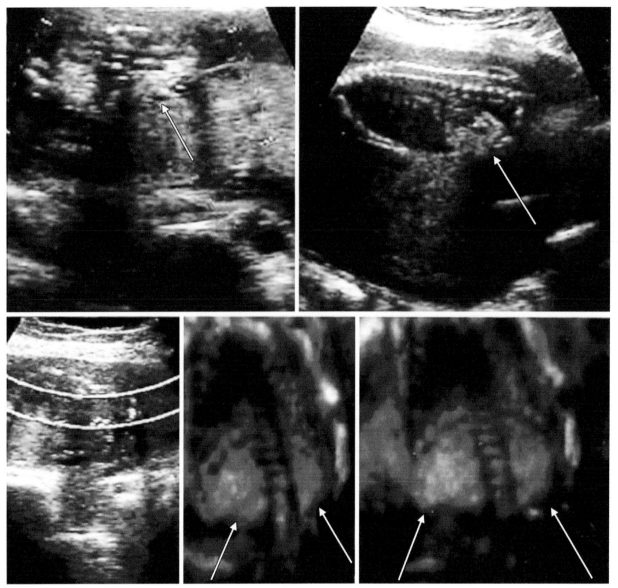

Fig. 31: Diffuse meconium peritonitis.

the neonatal vomiting, accompanied by acidosis, abdominal distension, and radiological images of diffuse abdominal calcification.

It is commonly associated with cystic fibrosis and 65% comes along with intestinal processes such as stenosis, idiopathic obstruction, atresia, or ischemia. Less frequently could be seen along with intestinal volvulus, intestinal invaginations or herniations, intestinal duplication, appendicitis, Meckel's diverticulum, accidental fetal puncture during the amniocentesis, or cases of imperforated anus. This can be associated with infections due to cytomegalovirus, with trisomies, but the etiologic factor only is found in 50% of the cases.

Ultrasound findings suggesting meconium peritonitis are: a simple echogenic mass or multiple intra-abdominal masses that are not well delimited, which its refringency is greater than the rest of the gut loops, nonhomogeneous,

shown acoustic shadows, especially if it is associated with polyhydramnion and ascites.

During an ultrasound examination diffused and small calcifications (at times very large) can be found, forming rings strongly alike to inferior acoustic shadows and anechoic central region **(Fig. 31)**.

Infrequently small peripheral abdominal echoes are found corresponding to other calcification areas. These are consequences of the existence of meconium in the abdominal cavity, where it tends to cause fibrosis and eventually, calcification.

Meconium that escapes from the peritoneal cavity causes a fibro-adhesive process that obliterates the peritoneal space and produces calcification in perforated areas or in areas where meconium has spread. This perforation generally occurs at the site where intestinal stenosis or loops obstruction (65% of the cases) is found **(Figs. 31 and 32)**.

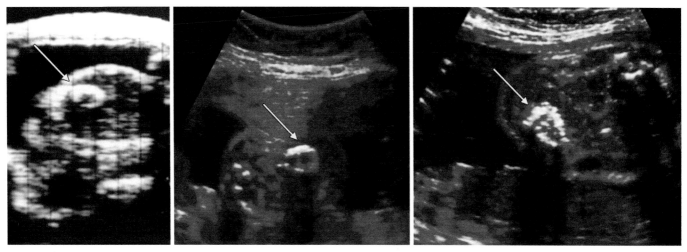

Fig. 32: Calcified meconium peritonitis.

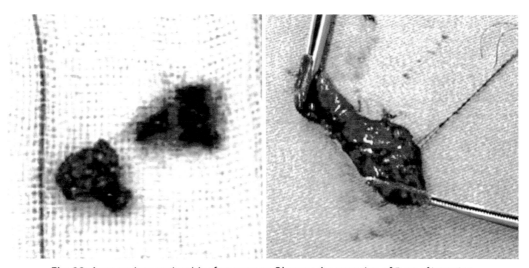

Fig. 33: A meconium peritonitis after surgery. Observe the resection of 5 cm of intestine.

On ultrasonographic examination, the following might be found:

- The walls of the intestinal loops are generally hyperchogenic with double contours, high density content, and active peristalsis.
- There is a greater abdominal circumference.
- Polyhydramnion is not always present. However, when observed, it is associated with intestinal obstruction.
- Ascites and anasarca.
- The other abdominal organs (liver, spleen, kidneys), as well as the uninvolved segments of intestine, the genitourinary tract, and the placenta, are usually normal.

As a general rule, peritonitis appears after week 20, although is known that peristalsis and presence of meconium start to appear in week 14.

The free-flowing meconium in the cavity can be encapsulated and/or calcified, forming pseudocysts. The diagnosis should be considered meconium peritonitis, if the fetal bowel is dilated, or whenever an area of fetal intra-abdominal hyperchogenecity is detected. The existent

possibility of a perforation increases if a small rim of ascites is observed.

Intestinal perforation can be clinically overlooked at birth, and manifest itself by the presence of meconium hydrocele. The meconium passes to the scrotum through the vaginalis testis process that communicates freely with the peritoneal cavity through the canal of testicular descent. When prenatal diagnosis is made and immediate postnatal surgery is performed, prognosis is usually favorable **(Fig. 33)**.

The differential diagnosis of hypoechogenic bowel must be performed with conditions that produce ascites and intra- or extrahepatic calcifications. Extrahepatic calcifications have been described in cases of hydrocolpos, urinary ascites, and neonatal biliary ascites. Intrahepatic classifications are observed in cases of infections caused by toxoplasma, cytomegalovirus, or calcified hemangiomas.

The differential diagnosis should also include **(Fig. 34)**:

- Intra-amniotic hemorrhage
- Precocious ascites
- Fetal hypoxia

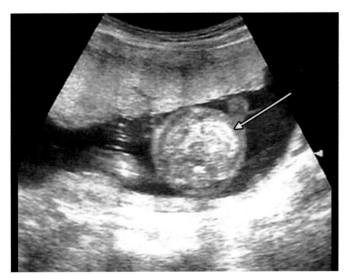

Fig. 34: Hyper-shrunken intestines. This image suggests a meconium peritonitis, cystic fibrosis, Down syndrome, or severe infection that affects the fetal intestines.

- Chromosomal anomalies
- Cystic fibrosis.

When meconial ileum and bowel hyperechogenicity are present in early stages (weeks 16–18), 75% of the cases are associated to cystic fibrosis.

Prevalence of cystic fibrosis in fetuses with prenatal diagnosis of intestinal obstruction is up to 10%, and this develops a meconium peritonitis in 7.7–44% of the cases.

In cases where an association of meconium peritonitis with chromosomal anomalies is suspected, chorionic villus sampling, amniocentesis, or cordocentesis is always indicated, regardless of the gestational stage. The amniotic fluid must be examined to determine the concentration that is always diminished of intestinal microvilli enzymes such as alkaline phosphatase, glutamyl transpeptidase, aminopeptidase, maltase, and sucrose.

It is recommended to use magnetic resonance imaging (MRI) in these cases to eliminate any doubt and to complete the diagnosis. The perinatal prognosis is ominous; the mortality is 50%, all of them during the postnatal stage.

■ HIRSCHSPRUNG DISEASE

The congenital absence of parasympathetic nervous glands and the sympathetic intramural plexus in a segment of the colon characterizes the disease. Its incidence is 1 in every 10,000 live births, and four times more frequent in females.

It is produced by an emigration defect of the glanglionary cells, from the neural crest.

Usually it affects the sigmoid and rectum, that lack of peristaltic movements, resulting in hyperperistalism, intestinal dilation, and hypertrophy in the proximity of the defect, but almost always after birth.

Anal atresia, meconium plaques, Hirschsprung disease, and other colon and rectal malformations are characterized

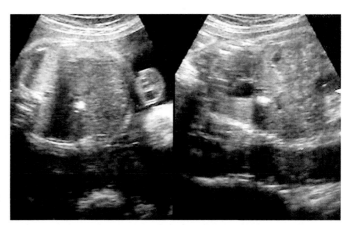

Fig. 35: Gallbladder stone.

by a hyperechogenic colon or dilated colon. A dilated intestinal segment in form of a V or a U in the minor pelvic area makes most likely the diagnosis of anorectal atresia. When dilatation of a segment of the colon is detected, it should always be kept in mind that Hirschsprung disease could be present.

There are very few intrauterine descriptions, but any abdominal distension must be informed to the pediatrician.

■ DISORDERS OF LIVER, SPLEEN, AND BILIARY TREE

Disorders of Liver

Hepatic Cysts

These are rare and result from obstruction of the hepatic-biliary system. Are typically found in the right lobe. They usually appear as unilocular and have been reported in a prenatal stage.

Gallbladder Anomalies

Gallstones may cause the appearance of fetal intra-abdominal calcification. They have been described before birth **(Fig. 35)**.

Hepatosplenomegaly

Isolated hepatomegaly is rare, but occurs in a variety of conditions. The etiology includes immune and nonimmune hydrops, hemolytic anemia, congenital infection, and metabolic disorders.

Tumors may also cause hepatic enlargement.

Hepatic hemangioma is a benign tumor, although it is associated with a high mortality rate (81%) secondary to congestive heart failure due to arterial venous shunting. The sonographic appearances are usually of a hypoechogenic structure within the liver, but hyperechogenicity or a mixed appearance is seen on occasions.

A hepatoblastoma may be suspected if calcified areas are seen, and in these cases maternal serum alpha-fetoprotein levels are elevated (in 90% of cases).

Other causes of hepatic calcification include intrauterine infections. Cystic liver changes are found in 30% of cases of adult polycystic kidney disease, and care should be taken to inspect the fetal kidneys.

Nonbowel Cystic Masses

Abdominal cystic masses are frequent findings at ultrasound examination.

The most common are:
- Renal tract anomalies
- Ovaries
- Mesenteric, omental, and retroperitoneal cysts
- Uterus.

Although the correct diagnosis may not be possible by ultrasound examination, the position of the cyst, its relation with other structures, and the normality of the other organs usually suggest the most likely diagnosis.

■ REFERENCES

1. Bonilla-Musoles F, Machado L, Osborne N. 3D of the new millenium. Madrid: Aloka; 2000.
2. Bonilla-Musoles F, Machado LE (Eds). 3D-4D Ultrasound in Obstetrics. Madrid: Panamericana; 2005. pp. 289-304.
3. D'addario, De Salvia V. Fetal malformations: the central nervous and gastrointestinal systems. In: Kurjak A (Ed). Textbook of Perinatal Medicine. London: Parthenon Publishers; 1998. pp. 299-324.
4. Thorpe-Beeston JG, Nicolaides KH. The fetal abdomen. In: Chervenak F, Isaacson GC, Campbell S (Eds). Ultrasound in Obstetrics and Gynecology. Boston: Little, Brown & Company; 1993. pp. 953-65.

Index

Page numbers followed by *b* refer to box, *f* refer to figure, and *t* refer to table.